The Nurse Communicates...

The Nurse Communicates...

April Sieh, RN, MSN

Assistant Professor
Nursing Division
Delta College
University Center, Michigan

Louise K. Brentin, RN, MSN

Associate Professor
Nursing Division
Delta College
University Center, Michigan

W.B. SAUNDERS COMPANY
A Division of Harcourt Brace & Company
Philadelphia   London   Toronto   Montreal   Sydney   Tokyo

W.B. SAUNDERS COMPANY
A Division of Harcourt Brace & Company

The Curtis Center
Independence Square West
Philadelphia, Pennsylvania 19106

Library of Congress Cataloging-in-Publication Data

The nurse communicates . . . / April Sieh, Louise K. Brentin.

p.   cm.

Includes bibliographical references.

ISBN 0–7216–4173–3

1. Communication in nursing.   2. Nurse and patient.   3. Nurse and
   physician.   I. Brentin, Louise K.   II. Title.
   [DNLM: 1. Nursing process.   2. Communication—nurses' instruction.
   WY 100 S571n 1997]

RT23. S565 1997

DNLM/DLC   96–30276

THE NURSE COMMUNICATES . . .   ISBN 0–7216–4173–3

Printed in the United States of America.

Last digit is the print number: 9   8   7   6   5   4   3   2   1

To my son Andy,
and to the memory of my husband,
Michael Slabchuck.

AMS

To Bob, Stephanie, Suzanne, and Lindsay
—my greatest blessings.

LKB

Preface

The impetus to write *The Nurse Communicates*... came out of our teaching experiences with students. Students very often find it difficult to apply communication theory in clinical situations, and textbook discussions related to communication primarily focus on conceptual content rather than on practical application. This often leads to student frustration and decreased student effort toward development of nurse–client communication skills. It is our intent to provide a resource that both stimulates the students' interest in the development of these skills, but also helps them see the importance of these skills in working effectively with clients, families, and the health care team.

The Nurse Communicates... has been designed to provide a sound introduction to the nature of communication and to augment basic nursing fundamentals textbooks. It assists the student to move from initial communication concepts to their application with clients and their families. The text addresses communication issues across the life span and in a wide variety of circumstances and practice settings. It also covers effective communication with colleagues and other health care team members. Note that each chapter title completes the sentence started by the book's title, *The Nurse Communicates*....

Thorough, concise, and contemporary in its focus, *The Nurse Communicates*... covers many clinical aspects of communication that are often not found in current textbooks. Case scenarios that illustrate key points, along with examples of communication techniques utilized in a clinical context, aid student learning. Application of concepts is reinforced through Practical Applications at the end of each chapter.

Effective communication skills are mandatory if timely, positive outcomes are to be reached with clients. However, these skills are often the most difficult to learn. *The Nurse Communicates*... facilitates development of these skills in a straightforward, clinically oriented manner that brings communication concepts to life.

In our role as educators, we believe it is important to provide effective tools for students to use in the development of their skills. It is in this spirit that *The Nurse Communicates*... has been written.

APRIL SIEH, RN, MSN
LOUISE K. BRENTIN, RN, MSN

Acknowledgments

We give thanks to all of the people who made this book a reality—our students, colleagues, families, friends, and the staff of the W.B. Saunders Company.

The spark for this book came from the nursing students at Delta College. We feel grateful for all of the things that we have learned from our students.

Our colleagues provided great help by reading chapters and providing suggestions for improvement. We know that this book is better because of the guidance that they gave.

Our families lived with a lot during the writing of this book. Piles of paper on the dining room table, hours spent in front of the computer (which meant that our children couldn't do their homework or play computer games), and quick meals were the order of the day for the four years during which we wrote this book. Even so, we didn't hear complaints. Our families knew how much the book meant to us. We thank you for your loving support.

On a long project such as this one, it's easy to get bogged down and discouraged. Our friends helped by providing the encouragement we needed to hear.

The staff at Saunders has been wonderful to us. Without their help and suggestions this book would be just a wistful dream.

We thank all of you.

APRIL SIEH, RN, MSN
LOUISE K. BRENTIN, RN, MSN

Reviewers

Contents

xiii

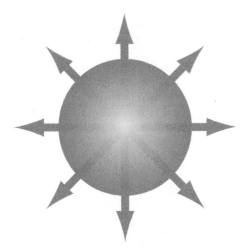

With People: General Principles in Communication

In this chapter, we will discuss:

- How people communicate in general
- Role/relationship patterns that can affect communication
- Environmental factors that can affect communication
- Guidelines for assessing communication effectiveness
- An interpersonal communication skills inventory

How Do People Communicate? What's The Process?

The majority of people communicate with at least one other person in some way every day. It would seem that, with all the exchange of information, thoughts, feelings, and ideas, we all would have a good, accurate understanding of each other's thoughts, feelings, ideas, and behavior. But somehow, this is often not the case. Just because we say or write something, or behave in a certain way for a reason, does not guarantee the person receiving the message, if it is received at all, understands its intended meaning. The process of communicating is often much more complex than it appears.

For communication to occur, there must be a sender and receiver of messages. The role each person plays in the exchange determines if the communication is a one-way or two-way interaction. A one-way interaction occurs when the sender of the message is in control, and flow of information goes from the sender to the receiver and little, if any, response is expected in return. Although this type of communication is efficient and quick, it is very limiting if feedback from the receiver is desired. In contrast, two-way interaction involves a dynamic exchange of message sent, message received and interpreted, and response(s) given. By its nature, two-way communication requires more time, energy, an openness to questions and clarification, and active listening (Bradley and Edinberg, 1982). The fact that a message sent is not always the message received supports the use of two-way communication in the majority of our interactions with others, whether they are family members, friends, fellow workers, clients, or other persons with whom we carry on conversation throughout the day. It allows responses (feedback) to messages we send and provides us the opportunity to clarify, or at least attempt to clarify, any miscommunication that occurs. It also demands awareness of word usage, jargon, and nonverbal cues that are all part of messages we send.

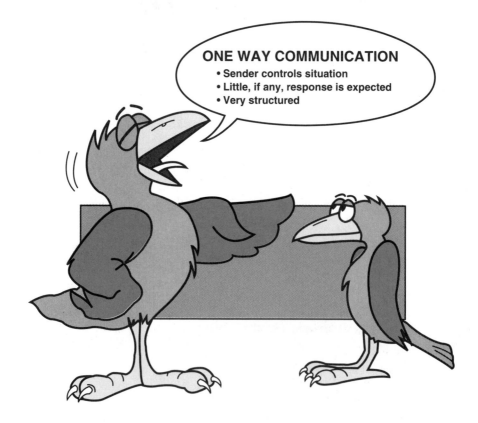

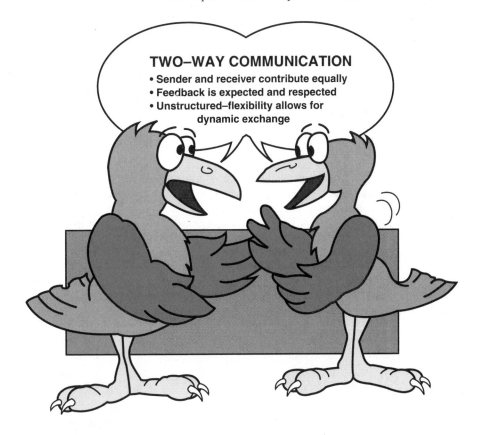

Consider This Scenario

Karen felt rushed getting to the unit staff meeting. She arrived just as the meeting was about to start. As she entered the room, she scanned the room quickly for a seat and then walked to the closest one available. She did not notice the handouts, which explained the terms of the proposal that was to be discussed, that were on the table just inside the door.

As the meeting progressed, she quickly realized she needed to listen closely to the discussion, take notes, and try to understand the proposal. She would pick up the handout on her way out. She remained very focused throughout the meeting and didn't pay attention to friendly comments going on around her.

After the meeting, as the group was beginning to leave, she smiled at a coworker beside her, who then stepped back and commented loudly and sharply, "I can't believe you can smile now, when all throughout the meeting you acted so cold and distant. You wouldn't even look or talk to us."

This really took Karen by surprise and she was very embarrassed. She reached over and touched the coworker's arm and jokingly said, "Some days I can only do one thing at a time, and this was one of them! I am sorry I gave the impression I was purposely ignoring you."

"Well, you usually are friendly at meetings, and we thought that the new job you have now was changing you, making you feel you don't need to associate with us anymore. . . ."

This scenario demonstrates several key factors that play large roles in communication:

- Verbal messages
- Nonverbal messages
- Use of humor
- Context in which message was sent and received

Verbal Messages

Word selection, including professional jargon, impacts the message sent and one's ability to receive and respond to it. Use of unfamiliar terminology without explanation inhibits the ability of the receiver to understand or respond to what is said in a timely manner. The listener can get lost in trying to understand the words used, rather than focusing on what the message is and its intent. Overuse of buzz words or jargon can give the impression that one is immature or too eager to impress others and can undermine one's credibility (Klinkenberg, 1992). Because Karen did not have access to the handout that explained the terms of the proposal being discussed, she had to expend much effort to understand and follow the discussion. It put her on the defensive when trying to figure out what was being said. As a result, the situation became a one-way type of communication, with Karen as the receiver.

Nonverbal Messages

Nonverbal communication "speaks" very loudly and, if not consistent with what is said verbally in a given set of circumstances, can cause much confusion. At times, it can completely override the sender's intended message. Comprehensive study of inconsistent messages found that nonverbal cues and behaviors were, most of the time, much more powerful than verbal cues in determining the meaning of the interaction (Mehrabian, 1981). Nonverbal cues include:

- Voice: tone, rate, organization, and volume of speech
- Use of silence
- Eye contact
- Physical appearance
- Use of touch

Each one has an impact on how the message sent is interpreted. People are usually very observant of, or at least subconsciously affected by, such behaviors, and care must be taken to keep verbal and nonverbal communication consistent with the intended message. In the scenario, Karen's focused listening prevented her from tuning in to peripheral conversation, as was expected of her by fellow workers. This resulted in what was perceived by her coworkers to be offensive, snobbish behavior.

VOICE   Tone, rate, and volume can convey emotion and degree of interest in what is verbally being said and may also reflect the confidence of the speaker. When speaking, we are often not aware of these nonverbal cues unless they are pointed out. Tone refers to the inflection used when speaking and often reflects emotion or mood. Tone is often emphasized by changes in voice volume. In the scenario, the coworker commented "loudly" and "sharply," which conveyed to Karen that her coworker was upset. If a person mumbles or is very soft spoken, it is hard to be interested in what is said because it is hard to follow and, because it portrays a lack of clarity, it may reflect a lack of confidence. Lower pitched tones and deep resonance of voice suggest authority and believability. If the rate of speech is fast, it can signal a con job, embarrassment, or awkwardness, whereas a moderately slow rate can convey conviction, thoughtfulness, interest, or sincerity (Fast, 1991). A normal rate of speech can vary, depending on individual style, geographic location, and ethnic background. For example, people in the Northeastern United States often speak quickly, whereas people in the South often speak more slowly. Those of Hispanic background tend to speak more rapidly than those of Caucasian background.

USE OF SILENCE   Silence is a very powerful nonverbal behavior. Karen's silence was not an intentional behavior, but it demonstrated how lack of interaction when it is expected can create discomfort or be misinterpreted. Just as Karen needed time to think about what was being said, others may also need time to think and sort out ideas during a conversation. Purposeful use of silence can convey respect, understanding, or support and is often used with therapeutic touch. Long periods of misunderstood silence, however, may cause feelings of uneasiness. As you develop skill in the use of silence, be aware of facial expressions and other behaviors that can indicate uneasiness (fidgeting, darting eye contact, nervousness) or comfort (relaxed, thoughtful, intermittent and direct eye contact) with the situation, and be aware of your own comfort level.

EYE CONTACT   How one uses eye contact conveys a message. Fond, long gazes convey intimacy. Long stares convey intimidation. Eye darts (eye contact for less than 2 seconds) convey being frightened or very uneasy. Looking just over heads or at only one to two people can convey lack of connectedness with a group. Averted gaze or no eye contact can convey uncertainty, lack of interest, or lack of involvement in the situation. (This is what happened with Karen, even though it was unintentional.) Making eye contact for 2 to 6 seconds when interacting helps you involve the other person in what is said without being threatening or intimate (Decker, 1985). It is important to note that eye contact patterns can have different meanings in various cultures. In contrast to eye contact being viewed as important to credibility in the general American culture, in some Native American, Hispanic, Japanese, Chinese, and Indian cultures it is considered a sign of disrespect or invasion of personal privacy (Snowdon, 1986). Being sensitive to your own eye contact patterns and the patterns of those with whom you communicate will help you to be more perceptive of what is occurring in the communication process.

PHYSICAL APPEARANCE   Studies have shown that words account for only 7% of the impact of our message, vocal quality for 38%, and the way we look and act for 55% and more in some other cultures (Mehrabian, 1981). Physical appearance, including dress, grooming, posture, gestures, and ease of movement, conveys attitudes about oneself and about others with whom one is interacting. The image one projects is a sum effect of all nonverbal activities as perceived and interpreted by the observer.

> Your appearance is an indication not only of your self-respect, but also of the respect you have for the person with whom you are dealing. If you can't make the effort to appear at your best, you imply that the person you're dealing with is not worth the effort. The resulting assumption will be that the quality of work or service to be

expected from you will probably be no greater than the quality of your appearance. . . . (Klinkenberg, 1992).

This excerpt has particular impact when applied to the highly scrutinized area of health care, where customers may often heavily weigh the appearance and mannerisms of the health care worker in their evaluation of the quality and appropriateness of care they received. There is no consensus in the literature on use of gestures, and often gestures are determined by culture. However, one common theme does prevail: gestures should be used to emphasize important or major points. Facial expressions should reinforce the message being conveyed. Random gesturing for no apparent reason may detract from what is said. Rely on choice of vocabulary to enhance clarity of expression.

When interacting with another person, conscious awareness of your stance, gestures, movements, word choice, and voice can assist you in establishing rapport with that person and impact the outcome of the interaction. Open posture is a relaxed stance with arms and legs uncrossed as you face the other person(s). Closed posture is a formal, more distant stance with arms and legs tightly crossed. You can mirror or reflect back to the other person certain aspects of their behaviors by using the same behavior(s) in a similar, though not exact, fashion. When this is done, the person often responds in a positive manner to the similarities between you, often feeling very comfortable and at ease (Brooks, 1991).

In Karen's situation, it was not *what* she said, but what was *not* said, and her behavior that caused miscommunication. Her being hurried, getting a seat at the last minute, realizing the need to listen closely, being "silent," and failing to make eye contact with fellow workers changed her usual social behavior pattern, which without any explanation left her unexpected nonverbal behavior open for misinterpretation.

In response to her coworker's loud, uncomplimentary comment and her withdrawing stance, Karen used a nonverbal approach that can be very helpful: touch. Karen reinforced her sincerity in her response by reaching out and touching her coworker on the arm. Therapeutic touch, in a communication sense, is using touch appropriately to convey concern, caring, empathy, support, or comfort. A touch on the hand, arm, or shoulder or sometimes a hug can be used to convey such messages. However, care must be taken to respect the client's personal space or comfort zone. As with eye contact, in some cultures use of physical contact when routinely interacting with others may not be viewed as appropriate behavior. This is true in China, Japan, Taiwan, Australia, Britain, and France (Snowdon, 1986). Touch should be used when it can benefit the interaction; because touch can be seen as aggressive, threatening, or indicative of sexual overtones, it must be used thoughtfully and purposefully. If there is hesitancy on the receiver's part to include others in his or her personal space (i.e., the person moves away or tenses up when others get too close), then it is best to demonstrate concern in other ways. The same is true for you. If you are uncomfortable or hesitant, it will most likely not be an effective approach. Karen reached out and gently entered the person's space in a limited, yet sincere, gesture that supported what she said verbally. It provided connectedness, something her fellow worker thought they had perhaps lost.

Use of Humor

Humor can be very effective in relieving tension and dealing with anxiety or stress. It has the remarkable capacity to help us control how we see what is going on, and in doing so it allows us the opportunity to choose how to view and react to what happens to us (Metcalf, 1994). It can assist us in facing our fears, embarrassments, and concerns that may be very difficult to address initially in a direct manner (Buxman, 1991). However, it must be used carefully. Humor that makes fun of a person or a person's ways is neither funny nor appropriate. To use humor effectively, you must know the person involved fairly well to anticipate what his or her response would be to humorous remarks and when to use it. At times, you can take your cues from the person and their significant others and their use of jest. Do they use humor or jest in dealing with daily activities and events, or are they more serious and reserved? Use humor with caution when dealing with persons of different backgrounds, because word meanings and appropriate use of humor can vary greatly from one culture to another. Karen, through her remark, defused the situation by poking fun at her own limitations and taking responsibility for her own behavior.

Context in Which Message Is Sent or Received

Karen's focus on hearing and understanding what was being said was misinterpreted by others for two reasons: it was not her usual way of interacting with fellow workers, and the fellow workers were interpreting or judging her behavior in light of her new position, a context not even considered by Karen at the time. As senders of messages to those we know, we must be aware of our own behaviors and how consistent they are with our usual patterns. To those we do not know well, do our behaviors clearly reinforce what is being expressed, or are there nonverbal behaviors that detract from what we are trying to communicate? It is also important to be aware of others' nonverbal behaviors during interactions with them, to help us identify signs of miscommunication or the need for clarification. For example, when a person who communicates in a very casual, conversational manner interacts with someone who is very formal, the casualness may be viewed as being very unpolished, and what is said may be viewed as lacking authority and importance. The formal person most likely will show a lack of interest in what is being said. In the casual person's eyes, the formal person could be seen as snobbish. However, if a person acts aloof, preoccupied, or disinterested in what is being said, consider that comfort, emotional needs, or a more urgent situation may be taking priority over your interaction.

Role Relationship Patterns That Affect Communication

Within any organizational group, be it a family, an educational organization, a large corporation, or possibly a social gathering, each person plays a certain role(s). Each role has attached to it certain expected behaviors, which determine how persons are to perform and how persons in the various roles relate to each other.

These behaviors may be explicitly written out, or they may be traditionally and culturally implied based on long-standing customs. Often, expectations are a mixture of both. The manner in which communication is carried out is directly related to the expected behaviors and the perception and understanding of them. An accurate understanding of role relationship patterns within a group is extremely valuable when deciding what, when, how, where, and to whom to communicate at any given time.

Consider This Scenario

Kathleen Watkins, 42, was completing the first week on her new job in the nursing division as an instructor.

John Peroni, a student (who was older than Ms. Watkins) in her clinical group, walked into Ms. Watkins' office and looked around. "It looks pretty nice in here. Well, what's it feel like to give orders to us 'older men,' Kathleen? Good, eh?" he asked.

Ms. Watkins replied, "I'm getting to know the ropes fairly quickly, Mr. Peroni. As we discussed in this morning's meeting, it's my philosophy, as well as the nursing division's, that we work as a team, and everyone is accountable for meeting the course outcomes. Age isn't an issue."

She noticed Mr. Peroni's behavior did not seem to be consistent with the reserved and considerate behavior observed earlier in the general meeting. She then asked him to have a seat as she pulled up a chair beside her desk. As he sat down, she asked him in a serious, concerned manner, "Does it bother you that your instructor is a woman who happens to be younger than you are?"

"It's just going to take some getting used to, I guess. Growing up, my Mom was always at home, cooking, making homemade pastas and breads, taking care of all of us. It was a big event when my wife continued to work after we got married. I just never imagined that I would be taught and evaluated by a woman younger than me," Mr. Peroni replied.

This scenario addresses several role relationship patterns that impact on communication:

- Social/cultural
- Superior/subordinate
- Male/female
- Personal/professional

Social/Cultural Patterns

The United States is a country rich in ethnic and gender role diversity and will continue to be even more so as we enter the 21st century.

> Not only will ethnicity and gender issues continue to need resolution but also cultural and language issues will become increasingly complex. . . . Employees themselves must recognize the part they play in creating a diverse work force. They must make personal commitments to work on changing their own discriminatory and stereotyping attitudes and behavior . . . (Fernandez, 1991).

The degree of diversity and how it is expressed or not expressed within a setting can have major effects on communication patterns that occur. The degree of comfort a person experiences when in a group of persons with varied backgrounds depends a lot on prejudices learned when growing up and the number of opportunities one has had in getting to know and interact with others from different backgrounds. A lack of understanding for languages, customs, dress, religions, lifestyles, and mannerisms different from our own serves as good breeding ground for stereotyping, prejudices, intolerance, and even fear. A common response is to avoid interacting with those who are different. This inhibits communication, and the lack of understanding escalates. Research has demonstrated that a large percentage of the American population is very bothered when others speak in a language they do not understand and that there is much greater acceptance of French, British, and German accents than of Spanish and Asian accents (Fernandez, 1991).

In the scenario, Mr. Peroni was having some difficulty knowing how to relate to the new, younger female instructor. Not having any previous experience with women in a senior position created discomfort for him and led to behavior not characteristic of him. Think how much more upsetting and confusing it would have been for someone whose wife did not work because "the woman's place is in the home" and "men are the ones who are always in charge!" Personal belief patterns and attitudes run deep in the soul, and when they make themselves evident in a situation in which other people are dramatically different, they can take us by surprise. Exploring new territories can be unsettling, but taking time to listen, clarifying what the other person is saying verbally and nonverbally, and exploring differences can increase tolerance and comfort levels. This will support ongoing communication efforts and positive role relationship patterns. In a multicultural work setting, diverse cultural communication patterns must be discussed and cultural sensitivity strategies undertaken to avoid unnecessary misunderstandings between staff members as well as between staff members and clients. See Chapter 4 for a more detailed discussion of cultural issues.

Superior/Subordinate Patterns

This type of relationship pattern implies that one party has power over the other. This power can be in the form of expertise, knowledge, position, or status. Examples of such patterns can be seen in family (parent/child or elder/younger sibling), teacher/student, supervisor/employee, and royalty/commoner situations. These relationships can be either mutually supportive or antagonistic or dynamic along the continuum of these two extremes. How the relationship boundaries are established varies. Title or position most often provides structure to such role relationships, which are reinforced positively or negatively through use of nonverbal and verbal cues discussed previously. Also, work cultures vary in different parts of the country, tending to be more formal on the East Coast, less formal in mid-America, and fairly informal in the South and West. Usually, the more formal the work environment, the more definitive the boundaries are between roles.

The person who has or is perceived to have the most power is most often viewed as the controller of the situation. However, the distribution of power in relationships influences the way in which individuals choose to communicate with each other. It also influences their interpretations of the communication that takes place. If the messages being sent are not clear, then clarification is needed.

In the scenario above, Ms. Watkins reinforced the professional status between herself and Mr. Peroni by addressing him as "Mr. Peroni" in response to her being addressed as "Kathleen": a gentle, very clear approach to establishing the formality of their instructor/student relationship. Restatement of her philosophy, consistent with the division's, reinforced what is expected of all students and clarified the age issue. She also acted on a hunch based on the change she noted in Mr. Peroni's behavior and sought to clarify with him what was driving his behavior. It is important to clarify what is really being communicated, when necessary, rather than run the risk of misinterpreting a message. For Ms. Watkins, it was important to understand clearly what Mr. Peroni was saying to ensure she addressed his true concerns.

In work situations, take cues from your instructor and professional nurses in the clinical agencies. There are certain expectations regarding dress, manner of addressing others, and workplace behavior. These are usually reflected in the instructor's and professional nurses' behaviors. This does not mean all department members should act and look the same. It means if the dress code specifies professional uniform, do not come to work in blue jeans and tight-fitting shirt or blouse. When working, your appearance nonverbally reflects the organization, and thus should reflect consistently the set standards of the organization. If you are addressed formally as Mr., Ms., or Mrs., then always address staff members in the same manner or until invited to use a first name. Even when on a first-name basis, do not assume that you are on a personal friendship basis (Klinkenberg, 1992). A solid relationship is grounded in work well done and goal achievement. Even when it is appropriate to use first names with supervisors in the office or private setting, formal titles should be used when in the clinical or public setting.

The same respect and courtesies apply to support staff members. Clear communication of requests, awareness of workloads, negotiating deadlines when necessary, remembering please and thank you, private review of performance concerns, and open acknowledgment of work well done will help build rapport and loyalty. This is invaluable, especially when knowledge of how to work through the system is needed. In this world of technology, the members of the support staff are key players, often experts, in information management and should be acknowledged for their roles and contributions.

Male/Female Role Patterns

Male and female communication patterns are often closely related with cultural, familial, and lifestyle patterns learned over a lifetime. There are dangers in categorizing how men and women communicate differently, but to not do so would avoid bringing differences to the discussion table.

> Pretending that men and women are the same hurts women, because the way they are treated is based on norms for men. It also hurts men who, with good intentions, speak to women as they would to men, and are nonplussed when their words don't work as they expected, or even spark resentment and anger (Tannen, 1990).

Several differences have been identified.

One difference relates to head movements. Women tend to nod or respond verbally as another person talks, to indicate they are listening. It does not mean they are agreeing. Men tend to nod only when they agree with what the other person is saying (Heim, 1992). Needless to say, men may often think women are agreeing with them, when in fact they are not, and women can easily interpret men's behavior as not attentive because they are not nodding. Other head movements can also be misread. A woman, tilting the head to one side or assuming a chin down with eyes gazing upward stance, while talking, signals a subordinate status posture. Men have the habit of holding their heads erect when speaking.

A second difference relates to conversation patterns. Men tend to interrupt when they believe it is necessary and do not apologize. Women usually wait for a pause by the speaker and often apologize (Klinkenberg, 1992). Again, both types of behaviors can be misinterpreted. These communication patterns can be presented in a different way. Men often see life as a contest, conversations being negotiations if a hierarchical social order is sensed, to maintain the upper hand and independence. Women often negotiate for closeness, confirmation, and support and seek to reach a consensus and avoid conflict (Tannen, 1990). As a result, when women express ideas more tentatively and men more assertively, the ideas expressed by the men are often valued more highly.

A third difference addresses smiling. Smiling is generally thought to be an expression of happiness and congeniality. It can put people at ease and encourage interaction. However, many women also unknowingly smile when they feel vulnerable or to cover up feeling unhappy. For example, a woman may unknowingly smile when she is criticized, which conveys weakness or powerlessness. This can create confusion, and true feelings are not identified accurately by the receiver. This can leave the woman feeling exasperated and not heard. In contrast, men will most often show no reaction when criticized or feeling vulnerable, and thus they convey a position of strength or control in the situation (Heim, 1992).

Fourth, a person's posture can also reveal one's emotional response in a situation. When threatened, one tends to recoil or pull oneself into a protective position—shoulders rounded, chest pulled inward, and head receding into shoulders, a posture called "getting small" (Heim, 1992). In contrast, when one feels powerful, shoulders are up and back, head is held high, and overall one tends to spread out, or "get big." When one is most often very confident and feels in control, this type of posturing becomes habit; the reverse can also be true. It is very

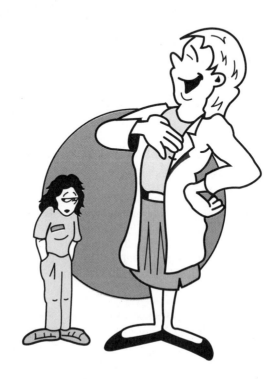

important to be aware of your posture and do a posture check, especially when you are not feeling "powerful." When standing, assume an erect posture, feet parallel at a comfortable distance; when sitting, again maintain an erect posture, arms relaxed at sides and resting on the arms of the chair—avoid getting small. Such posturing tends to come more naturally for men. Posture awareness can be especially helpful for women when confidence and strength need to be projected.

The point to be made here is that no one must be made to conform to only one way of conversing, but each person needs to be aware of how differently men and women communicate and how differently what or how something is said can be interpreted. Also, some women may have assertive behaviors most often seen in men, and some men may have more affiliative characteristics more often seen in women. Appreciation of differences allows for flexibility in expectations and prevents hastily drawn conclusions about social interactions. In the scenario, Ms. Watkins sensed she was not clear on the meaning of Mr. Peroni's comments and behavior, and she sought to clarify what was bothering him. She facilitated the discussion by deemphasizing the differences in role status: she offered him a seat beside, not across, her desk.

Personal/Professional Role Patterns

Personal relationships are built on a mutual "give and take" between persons, with each party giving and receiving fairly equally. However, in the professional arena, the focus is primarily on client outcomes. One's performance in a health care organization is generally evaluated on the basis of work done with clients and others. Effective client care is dependent on one's ability to work with others up and down the organizational structure to achieve positive client outcomes in an efficient and cost-effective way. This team approach requires commitment of team members to work and support each other, using each other's expertise to achieve the desired outcomes (Katzenbach & Smith, 1993). This makes very evident that your ability to communicate with others in a professional and positive way is a highly valued attribute.

DO   Listen to what is said, with eyes and ears. Seek feedback to verify that sent messages are interpreted correctly. Treat others professionally: (a) know and use proper etiquette; (b) respect others' spaces, work style, and expertise; and (c) acknowledge contributions made by others.

DO NOT   Use profanity or terms of endearment. In general discussion, do not (a) whine, (b) complain about another's performance or "quirks," and (c) talk about personal problems or affairs. If you are in a physical or emotional state that could result in negative nonverbal behaviors (i.e., anger, distress, preoccupation, etc.) toward others and their misinterpretation, arrange work coverage (this is a must if work cannot be done appropriately). When this is not possible, then you need to explain briefly to those with whom you work that extenuating circumstances may impact your usual manner of behavior that day so they understand (Lipkin, 1992). If your situation is overwhelming, professional assistance may be needed to cope with personal problems effectively. Seeking out support services is recommended. As a coworker in this situation, offer support and listen. Ask how you can be of assistance. If a work situation is the cause of a problem, address this in private with the appropriate person(s).

Environmental Factors That Can Affect Communication

Communication never occurs in a vacuum. The surroundings in which it occurs can impact the manner and the degree to which a person chooses to communicate. The environment sends many nonverbal cues that are then interpreted. These interpretations then contribute to a person's behavior, consciously or unconsciously.

Consider This Scenario

Mrs. Torres arrived at the clinic for the first time. It was dark and rainy outside. What a day to have to be out! As she went through the front door, she realized it was a much larger, busier place than she had anticipated. The lobby area seats appeared stiff and uncomfortable but were almost all occupied. Some people looked very ill or tired. The lighting was not very bright, the skylights reflected the dark skies, and the lobby was chilly. There were no direction signs, so she worked her way to the large information desk. As she waited her turn, she noticed how involved the staff people were in their work. It was like they were unaware of all the activity going on around them. The person at the information desk was answering the phone and answering questions. She looked tired and never smiled. When Mrs. Torres reached the counter, she asked for directions in slightly broken English.

The receptionist frowned and said, "Could you please repeat that? I have no idea what you just said."

Mrs. Torres was very embarrassed, but repeated her request. When the directions were given to her, she did not understand, but she elected not to ask anything more and just said, "Thank you." Feeling angry and overwhelmed, she walked down one of the hallways, looking at each sign she saw.

A few minutes later, a volunteer came by, and noting the lost look and frustration on Mrs. Torres' face, asked if she needed assistance.

Mrs. Torres, in her frustration, tried to explain her situation in a mixture of English and Spanish.

The volunteer listened, but all that was understood was something about blood pressure and appointment. So the volunteer asked, "Are you here to have your blood pressure checked?" because the hypertension clinic appointments were scheduled for today.

"Yes, yes!" Mrs. Torres' eyes lit up. The volunteer smiled and said, "I'll take you to the right clinic area."

Mrs. Torres relaxed a bit, and as they walked, she told the volunteer how much she appreciated the help. "It's so hard for me to come to a new place. I get so nervous and then I tend to talk in Spanish, and then no one understands me."

The volunteer asked if this was her first time here. When Mrs. Torres said yes, the volunteer told her that this was always their busiest day and could understand how all the people and activity could be upsetting. When they got to the clinic area, the volunteer introduced Mrs. Torres to the secretary, who then explained they were expecting her and showed her how to sign in.

As Mrs. Torres sat down, she noticed how cluttered the waiting room was: the chairs were close together, some were stained a little, and magazines were lying around. There were several large stacks of charts on a table behind the secretary, and equipment was

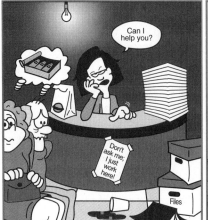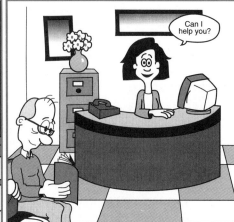

pushed up against the wall. This was so different from the doctor's office, and she wondered if she had made the right decision in coming here. Soon her name was called.

The secretary introduced her to the nurse, who smiled and led her into the office. The office was clean, neat, and quiet. "It's so good to know someone by name here," Mrs. Torres said. "I hope next time I will remember where to go."

"Let's take care of that right now," the nurse replied. "Here is a map of the clinic and parking lot. I'll highlight the way to get here and then we'll go over it together. I'll write my name and phone number on the bottom, too, so you can call me if you have any questions."

Mrs. Torres felt relieved and said, "I can feel my blood pressure coming down already and we haven't even gotten to it yet. Maybe this will work out OK."

This situation illustrates two major aspects of environment that can impact one's communication.

- Physical characteristics
- General atmosphere

Physical Characteristics

The physical characteristics and layout of a setting can nonverbally communicate information. For example, the type and arrangement of furnishings, floor plan, lighting, degree of privacy, neatness, organization, and cleanliness can all contribute to one's perceptions about the degree of formality and management of the setting. These perceptions then impact how comfortable one feels in the setting, which in turn affects how willing or able one is to communicate effectively. Men and women view their environment differently. In assessing an office, women place more emphasis on how functional it is: lighting, bookcases, enough seating, comfortable and supportive desk chair, and pleasing decor. Men tend to look at how an office communicates position within the organization, such as square footage, location, window size, and quality of materials used in furnishing the office. Therefore, both functional and status aspects of the work environment are important, and one must be astute to the role each aspect plays (Heim, 1992).

The clinic's appearance contributed negatively to Mrs. Torres' perception of the setting. Its size, lack of user-friendly signs, chilly temperature, low lighting, and lobby appearance all projected an unwelcoming environment. The rainy, dark weather outside reinforced the dreariness. Even the appearance of some of the persons in the lobby chairs contributed to the negative physical atmosphere. The large information desk, staffed by a person with aloof, inconsiderate behaviors, seemed to loom as a hurdle to be faced rather than being a place where information could easily be obtained. The lack of familiarity with the environment and an unsuccessful attempt to gain direction made the situation more frustrating than it had to be, and the frustration then contributed in her decreased ability to express herself. When upset, she tended to speak more in her native language, which made understanding her difficult. In the waiting area, the stains on the chairs, the magazine clutter, the equipment lining the walls, and the chart stacks reflected to Mrs. Torres that possibly the clinic was not well managed, and this caused concern. The interior of the nurse's office, however, helped alleviate some of this concern.

General Atmosphere

The degree of formality and the sensed pace within a setting can impact communication in several ways. A very formal atmosphere, highly structured in nature, has the capacity to alienate persons unfamiliar with the setting. This capacity may be real or perceived as real. Nonverbal behaviors seen in this type of setting may be described as stiff or aloof, with little, if any, small talk or facial expression. Openness to questions or offering of assistance may not be seen. Such behaviors can lead to limited and possibly inaccurate, exchange between persons involved. Lack of familiarity with the environment, coupled with being unsure of the correct meaning of the nonverbal behaviors, led Mrs. Torres to react with nervousness. This then severely hampered her ability to communicate her needs clearly. The lack of sensitivity by the receptionist only led to more frustration, and Mrs. Torres decided to withdraw from the interaction altogether by just saying "thank you."

In contrast, more casual, informal interactions may include some social small talk to assist persons to become more at ease. Accompanying nonverbal behaviors, such as eye contact or a smile, are more "other" directed. Information or assistance is often offered when it is needed, rather than waiting for it to be requested. The volunteer demonstrated a sensitivity to Mrs. Torres' frustration and sought to help her. The volunteer also served as a link between Mrs. Torres and the secretary, who then continued to be helpful and reassuring by letting Mrs. Torres know she was expected and assisted her with signing in. The nurse demonstrated an ability to listen to Mrs. Torres' needs and addressed them before focusing on the purpose of the appointment. The positive interaction with these persons helped to offset the negative perceptions Mrs. Torres had from her earlier interaction. Degrees of formality in a situation can vary depending on the styles of those involved in the interaction; however, an overall atmosphere usually prevails based on the perceived dominant styles.

The pace of a setting, defined as the number of persons and events occurring at the same time in a setting, is another factor that may impact one's desire and possibly one's ability to communicate. If there are many persons hurriedly and actively involved in tasks that seem urgent and important, as Mrs. Torres noticed, then one may be hesitant to interfere or may do so in a very limited manner. Also, one may not know or be able to identify with whom to communicate.

It is important to understand that one's perception of the situation, whether accurate or not, can determine whether attempts to communicate will be made, and, if they are made, how one will choose to start the process. First impressions are tremendously important in all communication.

Guidelines for Assessing Communication Effectiveness

How does one evaluate the effectiveness of communication? Key questions can help in this process:

1. Did each person actively participate in the discussion?
2. Were the nonverbal behaviors consistent with what was being said? Consider tone, volume, and rate of speech; posture and body positioning; gestures used; eye contact; and word selection.
3. What was the context in which the message was sent and received: was it the same for both?
4. Were there any cultural factors reflected in the manner in which the persons expressed themselves? Were these factors understood and appreciated by all involved?
5. Were any role relationship patterns affecting the communication? If so, in what way?
6. Were there any environmental factors affecting the communication? If so, in what way?

If each person came away from the conversation feeling as though he or she was heard and respected, and the purpose of the interaction was achieved, then the interaction was an overall positive one. This does not mean everyone had to agree with each other. It means that each person felt able to voice concerns, viewpoints, and feelings and be heard by the others. The following are active listening behaviors (Arnold & Boggs, 1989).

1. Clarification of points is sought when necessary.

    Example

    Client: "I really sleep a lot during the day."

    Nurse: "What do you mean by 'a lot'?"

    Client: "My little girl is just not acting like herself."

    Nurse: "Not acting like herself . . . what do you mean?"

2. The listener restates what he or she perceives the other has said so any misunderstanding of a key point can be corrected.

    Example

    Student: "This is making me so nervous. I wish I had experience in giving injections."

    Instructor: "You are nervous because this is the first time you will give an injection to a client?"

3. Paraphrasing is used to clarify major concerns or themes that verbally have been expressed.

Example

Student: "There are just so many plusses about this job, but a few things keep coming up in my mind about it."

Instructor: "You are excited about your new job, but you have some concerns."

4. Reflection by the listener of the feeling tone(s) noted when the other was speaking can help validate the accuracy of feelings perceived, and this also provides the speaker the opportunity to explore the relationship between what was said and the feelings that were expressed.

Example

"You seem very angry since you received a C on the exam."

"You seem uneasy about doing your client assessment."

5. "Encouragers" are used to stimulate further communication.

Example

"Go on."

"That's interesting."

6. Open-ended questions are used to stimulate answers that provide information.

Example

"What factors do you feel contributed to your situation now?"

"What health problems have you had during the past 10 years?"

7. Silence is used selectively to allow the speaker to collect thoughts when speaking and then go on, or it can be used to show respect when one is expressing or sorting emotional feelings that arise out of the interaction.

Example

"It is just so hard to accept such a loss (speaker pauses, no interruption by listener); I know I can get through this, but I'm not sure where the energy will come from."

8. Respect for another's personal space and mannerisms is demonstrated.

Example

Allow approximately 1 1/2 to 2 feet between you and the other person when interaction is initiated. Never mimic or ridicule a person's mannerisms; focus on what the person is trying to convey.

A Personal Communication Skills Inventory

When evaluating your own communication skills, it is important to do three exercises. First, take time to consider your cultural background, learned patterns of gender and cultural behavior, knowledge of others' cultural patterns, openness to and level of comfort with others different than yourself, beliefs and attitudes,

Table 1–1 INTERPERSONAL COMMUNICATION SKILLS WORKSHEET

Skill	Good	Fair	Poor	Rating	Comment
Thought organization; clarity of ideas, feelings	Well organized; clear	Fairly well organized; somewhat clear	Disorganized; lacks clarity		
Effectiveness; able to get intended message across in positive manner	Message clear to receiver; approach supports two-way interaction	Message fairly clear to receiver; neutral manner	Unable to get message across; manner does not support two-way interaction		
Use of					
Gestures	Appropriate use; contribute to what is said	Neither add to nor detract from what is said	Inappropriate; detract from what is said		
Posture/positioning	Upright, open posture	Neutral effect on what is said	Negative stance; closed		
Eye contact	Intermittent, 2–3 seconds/ contact	Slightly prolonged or less frequent	Staring; lack of contact		
Personal space	Approximately 1½ feet	Person backs off or comes closer	Insensitive intrusion of other's space		
Tone	Appropriate inflection; moderate pitch	Some inflection; pitch varies	Overuse or lack of inflection		
Volume	Appropriate for situation; heard without difficulty	Slightly too loud or too soft	Inappropriately loud or too soft to be heard		
Rate	Moderate; easy to follow	Somewhat hard to follow; too fast or too slow	Hard to follow; too fast or too slow		
Language/word usage	Familiar word choice; sophistication matches that of receiver; proper grammar	Some use of jargon; occasional misuse of grammar	Poor grammar, overuse of jargon; slang, profanity		

level of self-confidence when interacting with others, and personality and style of interacting. Second, consider how these factors affect your ability to interact effectively in a variety of communication scenarios that occur every day. Identify factors that support effective interaction and those that do not. Third, use this information to enhance future interactions. Getting to know yourself can help you appreciate the complexity of other individuals, and it can generate a sensitivity to the multitude of factors that can come into play when persons interact with each other. Table 1–1 would facilitate this process.

PRACTICAL APPLICATIONS

1. With a partner, identify the boundaries of your personal spaces. How did you know when your space was invaded? Are your spaces about the same or are they different?

2. Reflect on a situation when you were misunderstood. What in the situation and in the communication seemed to have contributed to the misunderstanding? Share your experience with the group.

3. Describe a personal incident in which humor was used effectively to defuse the situation and an incident when it was used inappropriately. What made the difference?

4. Give clear instructions to the other members of the group on how to do a procedure, such as changing a flat tire or cooking a special recipe. Use the Interpersonal Communication Skills Worksheet (Table 2–1) to give each person feedback on their short presentation (approximately 5–7 minutes).

5. Give two examples of the following types of responses:
   a. Clarification
   b. Reflection
   c. Encouragement
   d. Open-ended questions
   e. Restatement

REFERENCES

Arnold, E., & Boggs, K. (1989). *Interpersonal relationships: Professional communication skills for nurses* (pp. 228–239, 258–259). Philadelphia: W. B. Saunders.

Bradley, J., & Edinberg, M. (1982). *Communication in the nursing context* (pp. 10–11). New York: Appleton-Century-Crofts.

Brooks, M. (1991). *The power of business rapport* (pp. 83–91). New York: Harper Collins.

Buxman, K. (1991, December). Make room for laughter. *American Journal of Nursing,* 46.

Decker, B. (1985). *Speak to win* [Audiotape]. Chicago: Nightingale-Conant.

Fast, J. (1991). *Subtext: Making body language work in the workplace* (pp. 42, 44). New York: Viking Penguin.

Fernandez, J. (1991). *Managing a diverse work force: Regaining the competitive edge* (pp. 6, 43, 261). Lexington, MA: Lexington Books.

Heim, P. (1992). *Hardball for women: Winning at the game of business* (pp. 159–163, 173–175). Los Angeles: Lowell House.

Katzenbach, J., & Smith, D. (1993). *The wisdom of teams: Creating the high performance organization* (pp. 49–56). Boston: Harvard Business School Press.

Klinkenberg, H. (1992). *At ease professionally: An etiquette guide for the business arena* (pp. 9, 22, 67, 223). Chicago: Bonus Books.

Lipkin, G. (1992). *Effective approaches to patient behavior* (4th ed., pp. 12–13). New York: Springer Publishing.

Mehrabian, A. (1981). *Silent messages: Implicit communication of emotions and attitudes* (2nd ed., p. 77). Belmont, CA: Wadsworth Publishing.

Metcalf, C. W. (1994). *Nurturing your sense of joy: Cultivating your personal assets* [Audiotape]. Chicago: Nightingale-Conant.

Snowdon, S. (1986). *The global edge: How your company can win in the international marketplace* (pp. 31, 63, 90, 105, 147, 161, 171, 184). New York: Simon & Schuster.

Tannen, D. (1990). *You just don't understand: Women and men in conversation* (pp. 16, 17, 24, 25). New York: Ballantine.

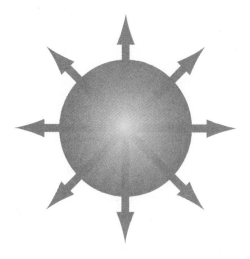

2

In Learning Environments

In this chapter, we will examine:

- Communication problems that can arise in the nursing education setting
- Communication tools within the learning environment
- Primary contacts in nursing education
- Qualities of a nursing student that can affect communication
- Communication issues that arise during clinical activities
- Communication roles: staff nurse as resource

Nursing school can be a very exhilarating, yet taxing, endeavor. Most nursing students report that nursing education is totally different from any of their prerequisite classes. Nursing education is unique.

Many nursing students relate that there is so much to learn and so little time in which to learn it. As a student, you will have to decide what is important to know and then learn it. To help you organize the material, there are mechanisms such as objectives for learning built into the learning environment. Faculty members, nurses in the clinical environment, and your peers will guide you on your way.

In any organization such as nursing school, part of the educational experience involves simply knowing how to use the system and information correctly. To maximize your nursing education, you'll need to know how to get answers to your questions, handle problems, and pass on information. To do this, you will need to be able to communicate effectively. In fact, your ability to communicate with faculty members, clinical nursing staff members, and your peers will affect your success in the nursing profession.

Another objective for nursing students is to discover what information they need to know. One of the most common questions a new nursing student asks is "How do I find out what I need to know?" This is an important question because there is a tremendous amount of information to learn in a limited amount of time. To help students narrow their data search, nursing schools have developed many forms of nursing communication, such as the course syllabus, student handbooks, and handouts (Table 2–1). However, many students do not take the time to read these vital communication tools! Companies that publish nursing textbooks have also developed methods to help you zero in on the important material.

Nursing education is largely composed of two areas: didactic learning (or theory) and application of that learning (the clinical practicum or simply "clinical"). In both areas, student nurses have to learn methods to communicate effectively. Although this may not sound difficult, it can be hard for a student to learn how nurses communicate because much of nursing communication is learned on the job.

While in nursing school, you must be able to understand what is expected of you. You need to be able to communicate on an effective level with the nursing instructor, peer group, health care staff, and clients. Problems can arise when students are unsure of what is expected of them and are unable to make their needs known.

Many students report that they find communication in the clinical arena to be

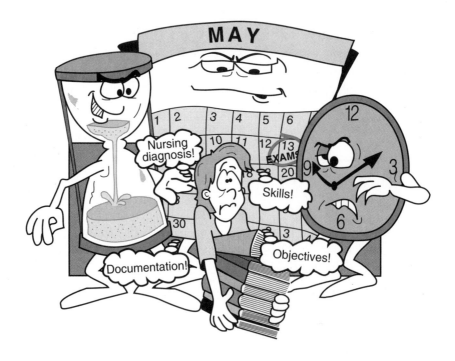

Table 2–1 COMMUNICATION TOOLS WITHIN THE LEARNING ENVIRONMENT

Method	What Is It?	When Do You Use It?	How Do You Use It?
Syllabus	This is a description of the course. Frequently, the course is broken down into units or modules. Each unit or module would have learning objectives.	This should be used every time you study. Compare your reading against it.	Pay attention to the learning objectives. They will tell you what is important to know.
Student handbook	A guide to policies of the nursing program, i.e., dress code, attendance policy, and chain of command.	Read it at the beginning of each semester.	Use it as a reference source.
Handouts	Written materials or charts that supplement other materials.	Use as a reference when you study.	Use as a reference.
Lecture	One person verbally provides information to a group of learners.	Used to provide a large amount of information in a small amount of time.	Pay attention! Read the objectives for the class before the session. Can you tape record the lecture and listen to it again? (Ask permission first.)
Small group discussions	Usually a topic is assigned to the group to research and present back to the total group.	Used to help you become more actively involved in your own learning.	Have each group member do a portion of the assignment. Make sure that you do your part!
Audiovisual materials	Supplemental materials are especially useful for the visual learner.	Typically assigned to supplement the lecture and reading content.	When viewing these materials, take notes. Pay extra attention to those that demonstrate skills to be used in clinical.
Textbooks	Books are chosen to provide information about health care problems and appropriate nursing interventions.	Read the assigned text materials *before* the lecture. Read the book slowly and carefully.	Read the preface and the chapter on how to use the book. Does the book have chapter objectives or chapter summaries? If so, read them!
Ancillary guides (care plan books, study guides, laboratory test books)	These books supplement the information in your required textbooks.	Use them when writing care plans and studying.	These reference books can be wonderful for writing care plans! They also can be very helpful for clinical.

difficult. There are several factors that can contribute to this difficulty, such as short clinical rotations, the severity of the client's illness, and the anxiety level of the student.

Lack of communication skills becomes very evident to a student when the clinical situation focuses on emotional care rather than physical care issues. Many nursing students are comfortable with interaction skills that relate to physical problems, such as "Are you comfortable?" But they are less likely to spend time with a person in emotional distress; students frequently say, "I don't know what to say to them" (Davis & Kurtz, 1991).

Who Are Your Primary Contacts in Nursing Education?

You will spend a great deal of time in nursing school with three groups of people: nursing faculty, nursing staff members, and your peers. Let's look at who these people are and what they do.

Nursing Faculty

Although the specific organization of each nursing school is slightly different, their general structures are similar. The school of nursing is headed by a division chair or coordinator who is responsible for the day-to-day operation of the program.

Many nursing programs use full-time and part-time faculty members. Full-time faculty members usually perform theory and clinical activities. Part-time faculty members are hired to fill in as needed and may teach either theory or clinical. Faculty members usually teach within their areas of specialization. Another nursing faculty position may be that of teaching in the simulation or nursing computer lab.

Nursing Staff Members

The nursing staff of a typical hospital nursing unit is composed of a variety of professional and support staff members. The *nurse manager* is responsible for the 24-hour management of the nursing unit. Nurse managers used to have the title of "head nurse," but the name was changed to reflect more accurately their management responsibilities, which include budgeting for the unit, ensuring appropriate client care, and hiring and evaluating staff members.

The *charge nurse* or *assistant head nurse* is in charge of the unit for a specific time frame. The charge nurse is typically found at the nursing station, overseeing the daily unit operations.

The *registered nurse* (RN) is responsible for the delivery of the client's care. This does not change even when a nursing student is assigned to the client. The nurse shares responsibility for the client's care with the student and faculty member. So you can see that it is really important to keep the lines of communication open among the nursing staff, faculty members, and students.

You might hear the term "staff nurse" or "professional nurse" used to refer to the RN staff. You may also hear the term "room nurse" used. This is another way of saying "the nurse assigned to the client's room." Keep in mind though that this nurse could be an RN or a licensed practical nurse (LPN).

Primary nursing is a method of delivering client care. In the strictest definition, the primary nurse is responsible for the client 24 hours a day, from admission to discharge. However, many care delivery systems use modifications of the primary care system. In some, the primary nurse is responsible for the planning of the client's care but doesn't have 24-hour responsibility for the client. The primary nurse is assigned to the client each day until the client is discharged.

Licensed practical nurses or *vocational nurses* provide bedside nursing care. In many institutions, they can give medications and perform many direct client care activities. The LPN's responsibilities vary from one institution to the next. The institutional policy manual will describe the role of the LPN.

Many institutions use unlicensed personnel such as *nursing assistants* or *aides* to help the nursing staff in providing care. Many institutions are using creative names, like "care associates" or "care technicians," for their bedside care providers. No matter what the name is, they provide care under the supervision of the nursing staff. Remember that the supervising nurse, whether an RN or an LPN, is ultimately accountable for safe client care.

Some institutions are training their nonlicensed staff to be able to perform several functions. For example, the unit aide might also know how to be a housekeeping aide. Cross-training in this fashion allows more flexibility in staffing patterns. The person the unit aide reports to depends on the job function the aide is performing.

Unit secretaries or *ward clerks* are responsible for maintaining the flow of oral and written communication at the nursing station. They spend much of their time transcribing client orders from the client chart and answering the telephone. Unit secretaries and ward clerks have a wealth of information available: If you have a question about anything to do with institutional rules (but not nursing procedures), ask them! The unit secretary or ward clerk reports to the nurse manager.

Peers

You will spend a great deal of time with your peers—maybe even more time than with your family. Your peer group can be a great resource to you as a support system. After all, they know what you are going through. Another great thing about a positive peer group is group studying. Many study groups are made up of friends or acquaintances made in the classroom.

You'll meet all kinds of people in nursing school. It's probably natural to compare yourself with others in your nursing program, but it is important to remember that each person is unique, with personal strong points and weaknesses, just as you are unique. Some students learn information quickly, and others need more time to catch on. Some students have difficulty getting good grades but have an excellent bedside manner. Others may get great grades but don't seem to enjoy working with people. Some students are very down-to-earth, and others seem to lack common sense. Some nursing students arrive directly from high school, whereas others have many years of life experiences behind them. Some students enter nursing school with experience in the health care field, whereas others have never held a paying job.

Are there any aspects of peer groups that can be viewed in a negative manner? Yes! Let's think about gossip and the rumor mill. In many nursing programs, rumors seem to occur with regularity. This seems to happen especially around test time, the end of the semester, and other stressful occasions. Perhaps the very nature of a difficult curriculum combined with the time limitations contributes to this.

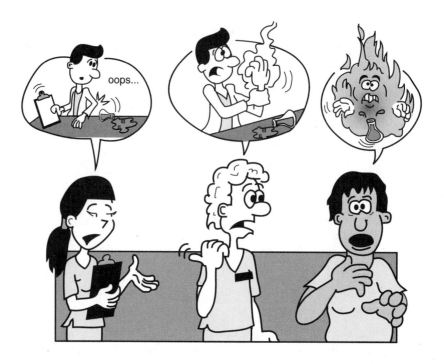

Be careful when listening to gossip. Rumors can have very serious consequences. If you hear a rumor and accept it as truth, you may base actions on incorrect data, which happens often. If you tell people incorrect conclusions, you will be contributing to the body of incorrect information. You also could be harming someone personally or professionally. There might even be a basis for legal action against the person(s) spreading the incorrect information.

If you hear a rumor, before you accept it as fact, do some research. Go to the source of the gossip and ask for verification of the information. If you find out that an incorrect rumor is floating about, try to squelch it.

What Nursing Student Qualities Can Affect Communication?

Because communication is so much more than simply the words we say, student nurses need to think about how other factors can influence a listener. The way you look, your mannerisms, your verbal presentation (including grammar), and your level of interest can all play a part in how you are perceived.

The client's perception of a student's abilities can be affected by the way the student looks. A nursing student's appearance should reflect that required of the nursing profession. Although no one is suggesting that students wear expensive clothes or conform to a certain height or weight, it is important to be neat and clean. You must look as if you are a professional.

Another aspect of appropriate communication is attitude. Good students are able to express their needs in an appropriate manner, without becoming angry or defensive. Throughout a nursing career, there will be times that do not go according to plan. Then, even more than during other times, a nurse will have to be able to communicate in an appropriate manner.

Nursing students need to be interested in learning and able to think in an inquiring manner. When they don't know something, they need to ask. You might hear a student use the phrase "I don't know about that, but I will find out about it."

Another aspect to consider is that of poise and self-confidence. Clients rely on care providers to know what they are doing. This includes students, too! To reassure clients, care providers must project the attitude that they know what they are doing. It can be really hard for students to be confident of their own abilities, much less project confidence to clients. Students continually encounter new things and sometimes have limited opportunity to practice their skills, which can create anxiety. Some tips to improve your self-confidence include:

- Practice your clinical skills until you know them very thoroughly.
- Before you perform a procedure, talk yourself through the steps. (Don't do this within the client's hearing, though!)
- Observe other students and staff nurses as much as possible.

Confidence and self-poise are skills that you will need to work on all the way through nursing school and even after graduation. Most students gain confidence after they gain experience in the health care field.

Consider This Scenario

Today is the first day of your nursing clinical experience this semester. Your instructor has given you your assignment: providing care for an elderly man, Mr. Lawrence, who has developed pneumonia after an abdominal operation. You've been oriented to the nursing unit and can find important things such as the medication room and the bathroom. You know that your instructor will be available but he has 10 students to help. You worry, "What if I need something when he's not available?"

As you arrive on the unit to do your client assessment, one of the first things you notice is the noise level around the nurse's station. Although there seem to be 20 or 30 people in the nurse's station, you know there really aren't that many; it's just that they're moving so fast. You know that you will have many questions but believe you will be hesitant to ask them because everyone looks so busy.

You have met Mr. Lawrence; reviewed his health history, physical assessment, and laboratory values; and read the progress notes in the chart. You also reviewed the established care plan. You have read about his condition and you know about his medicines and treatments. Based on this information, you have sketched out your plan of care but you wonder how much you can do yourself and how much assistance you will need.

After analyzing your client's needs, these are the interventions the client may require:

- Vital signs
- Physical assessment
- Medications: oral, topical, IV push, IV piggyback
- Assisted bed bath
- Linen change
- Positioning in bed
- Monitoring oxygen therapy
- Incentive spirometer
- Charting
- Reporting on and off
- Capillary blood glucose

- Abdominal dressing change
- Monitoring IV therapy
- Ambulate three times a day

You consider these activities, thinking about your experience and level of education. You remember that your instructor told you that he wanted to be present for IV bag changes.

To keep things straight, you decide to break the above list into things you can do yourself, things you need help with, and things you cannot do in clinical. Here is how the list looks now:

Clinical Interventions Needed by Mr. Lawrence		
Can Do By Myself	**Need Help With**	**Cannot Do**
Vital signs	Physical assessment	IV push
Bed bath	Oral medications	
Linen change	Topical medications	
Positioning in bed	IV piggybacks	
Monitoring oxygen therapy	Charting	
Incentive spirometer	Abdominal dressing change	
Reporting on and off		
Capillary blood glucose		
Monitoring IV therapy		
Ambulate		

Now that you know what you can and cannot do for the client, you can communicate this to the nurse who is also assigned to the client.

Review the Situation

This scenario illustrated the types of concerns that a nursing student might have during the first days in a clinical setting.

- Do you know what types of nursing interventions you can do independently in the clinical setting?
- What types of procedures do you need help with?
- How much help do you need?
- What can't you do for the client?

As a new nursing student, you are concerned that if you ask questions you may be perceived as not knowing what you should. But if you don't ask questions, you might do a poor job of providing care for your client. You know that you really want to be a good nurse and you must provide safe care. But who will guide you? You know that you will have many questions during the day. Who can you ask for help?

Finding Out What You Can and Cannot Do in Clinical

As a nursing student, you know that you are liable for your actions regarding client care. There is a common misperception that nursing students practice nursing under the umbrella of the instructor's nursing license and therefore are not liable for their own actions. This is not true; allowances are made for nursing students in the state Nurse Practice Acts. Student nurses would be held to the same standards as practicing nurses for content materials already covered. So you can see that nursing students must assess their skills and abilities and seek help when they are unsure of nursing procedures. They must ask for help when needed (Lessner, 1990).

But how much help do you need? You can't really answer this question until you know what types of nursing interventions your client will require. After you receive your clinical assignment and understand the care needed by your client, think about your ability to perform these interventions. Look at the following table. List your client's required nursing interventions according to your ability to perform them.

What Can You Do Without Help?

At this point in your nursing career, what types of nursing interventions can you do without any help? Consider your educational level in your nursing program, past experiences, and demonstrated skill competence. What is your comfort level with the procedures the client may need? What does your instructor want you to do independently?

For example, if the client needs IM injections, have you been cleared to do this independently or do you need assistance or supervision? As a rule, it is better to ask for help if you are the slightest bit unsure than to *not* ask for help when you need it.

What Do You Need Help With and What Type of Assistance or Supervision Is Needed?

If you need help when providing nursing care, what type of help is needed? Do you need help with physical care, such as turning a client? If so, you could have your instructor, another student, an aide, LPN, or RN help you. Or perhaps you need help with a skilled activity such as IV therapy and want someone to help you hang an IV bag. Depending on your level of experience, your instructor may need to observe you perform skilled activities such as this or this may be delegated to one of the staff nurses. Ask your instructor which person should help you with specific clinical skills.

A problem can arise when you recognize that you need help, ask for help, and yet don't get anyone to help you. This could occur for several reasons: you may not have made your needs known, or the others simply may be too busy to help you. Think about why others aren't helping you. If you didn't make yourself clear about the help that you need, then ask again, stating your need more distinctly. If you really need help and don't get it, notify your instructor.

Clinical Interventions Needed		
Can Do By Myself	**Need Help With**	**Cannot Do**

Perhaps you may need help from your instructor, who is currently busy. Many students do not want to bother their instructors when they are busy. But you must tell your instructor what you need to allow the instructor time to rearrange priorities and be able to help you. Another possibility is that the instructor might ask a staff nurse to help you.

What Can You *Not* Do for the Client?

Does the client need nursing care that you cannot provide at this point in your nursing career? A beginning nursing student may be assigned to provide basic care for a client who has cancer, but the instructor may want the student to do only the physical assessment, bed bath, and linen change. The room nurse is responsible for the other aspects of client care, such as administering the client's chemotherapeutic drugs. This information must be communicated at the beginning of the shift so the room nurse can plan time to deliver the care needed.

If there are care aspects that you cannot perform, who is responsible for getting them done? Is the room nurse going to do them, or perhaps your nursing instructor? In any case, it is important to be sure that someone is aware that he or she is responsible for the care aspects that you cannot deliver. This should be discussed as early as possible so that time can be allotted for the intervention.

There will be occasions in which you aren't comfortable performing activities even though you are supposed to know how to do them. This could occur because you didn't practice your psychomotor skills thoroughly or because you simply forget how to do something. Whatever the cause, if you aren't comfortable doing an intervention, don't go on until you have assistance. It is your responsibility to review the policy and procedure manuals and review the procedure with your instructor. If necessary, arrangements can be made to have the intervention completed by another person.

Communication Issues That Arise During the Clinical Experience

The clinical practice setting can be very interesting and yet frightening to the typical nursing student. For the student to achieve optimal learning and for the client to receive optimal nursing care, it is important for the student nurse and staff nurse to be able to communicate effectively. When the staff nurse is giving you information, be sure that you understand what is being said. Staff nurses can use so much nursing jargon that it may seem as though they aren't speaking English. If you don't understand something, ask for a definition.

The Scenario Continues

You see on the assignment sheet that Meribeth Hollally, RN, is assigned to provide care for Mr. Lawrence today. After she gives you report, you tell her your plans for Mr. Lawrence. "I'm going to do his physical assessment and write it out when he is having breakfast. I'll help him with his bath around 10:00 and we'll ambulate after he rests. I see that he needs to ambulate three times today. So we will do it again after lunch. I have made a list of nursing interventions he needs and figured out who will do them. Let's look at it. I'll need some help when I do his physical assessment. I am not sure of my findings when I'm listening to breath sounds. My instructor will be present when I do his oral, topical, and IV

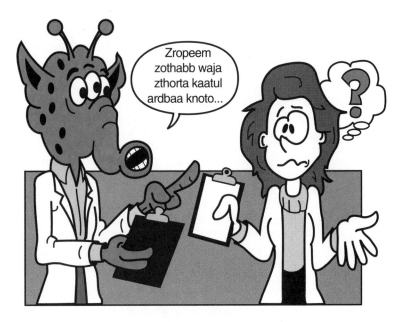

piggyback medications. He will also help me with Mr. Lawrence's abdominal dressing. I notice that Mr. Lawrence needs to have IV Lasix at 9 a.m. I can't give IV push medications this semester, so you'll have to give that."

Ms. Hollally asks you what Mr. Lawrence's primary nursing diagnosis is. You tell her that you plan to work on his ineffective airway clearance. She agrees that this is his primary problem. You also tell her that your personal goal for the day is to hang an IV bag with minimal supervision. You will be on the nursing unit from 7 a.m. until 2 p.m. Ms. Hollally is going to lunch at 11 a.m. so you plan to go to lunch at noon.

Review the Situation

Many events occur during the course of the clinical experience. It is important to know when and where you need to talk to the clinical staff members.

- What should you do at the beginning of the day?
- Where should you talk to the nursing staff members?
- After report, then what?
- How long will you be on the unit?
- What are your goals and your client's goals?
- What do you need to know?

At the Beginning of the Day

As soon as you arrive on the unit at the beginning of a clinical day, find the nurse(s) assigned to your client. If the care management system is a team approach, you may be working with RNs, LPNs, and aides who make up the team. Find out what aspects of client care each team member would be responsible for if you were not here to provide care. This information will be helpful in knowing who you might go to for help. Also, note their break and lunch times. This can help you plan your break and lunch time. In the scenario, the student planned her lunch time to alternate with that of the room nurse.

Typically, the next action is to obtain report from the client's nurse. You may be obtaining report from the nurse on the previous shift or the nurse on the current shift. See Chapter 10 for help on how to obtain report.

Students sometimes believe that they do not obtain enough information during report to enable them to provide safe client care. The report may not have included enough detail to help the student formulate a plan of care for the client. There could be several reasons for this. The nurse could have been extremely busy or perhaps could have thought that the student already knew the client. If you don't think that you receive enough detail during report, ask the staff nurse for more information. This would be a great time to practice assertiveness skills. The most important thing to remember during clinical is this: If you don't know something, you must ask someone. The point of asking questions is to obtain enough information to be able to deliver safe, appropriate nursing care.

To help you understand what a typical nurse's day is like, see Table 2–2.

Table 2–2   SAMPLE STAFF NURSE SCHEDULE FOR DAY SHIFT (7:00–3:30)

Time	Activity
7:00–7:10	Count narcotics.
7:10–7:15	Look at assignment sheet.
7:15–7:30	Get report from off-going nurse.
7:30–7:45	Make a quick check of the clients.
7:45–8:00	Discuss clients with LPNs, nurse aides. Decide who will do what.
8:00–8:25	Prepare client for surgery.
8:25–9:00	Do 3 client A.M. assessments.
9:00–9:15	Give 8:00 medications.
9:15–10:00	On phone to make arrangements for client to be transferred to rehabilitation unit (5 calls). Skip break.
10:00–11:00	Make rounds with physicians and nurse practitioner.
11:00–12:00	Get first client back from surgery. Do his postop assessment. Before set up his PCA pump notice that the client is allergic to the medication ordered for the PCA pump. Have to call the surgeon for an alternate medication. Another client's IV infiltrates, so you restart the IV.
12:00–12:30	Go to lunch. Another RN is covering for your clients. The LPN working with you will go to lunch after you get back.
12:30–1:30	Finish paperwork for the client being transferred to the rehab unit.
1:30–2:00	Get second client back from surgery. Do his postop assessment and find everything is okay.
2:00–2:30	Although you have been interacting with the LPNs and nurse aides throughout the day, you collect information for report from the LPN and nurse aide.
2:30–2:50	Check all client charts to ensure completion of orders, check charting for accuracy, check medication sheets to ensure all medications given, check all IVs to ensure patency, and measure IV level.
2:50–3:00	Count narcotics with on-coming nurse.
3:00	Ready to give report. Second shift not ready yet.
3:15	Give report.
3:30	Go home!!

Where Should You Talk to the Nursing Staff Members?

It is always best to communicate in a quiet place such as a conference room. But it can also be very useful to have the nurse give you shift report in the client's room. This way, the nurse can *show you* as well as *tell you* about the client's condition. You can also easily ask questions if you aren't sure of what the nurse is telling you (remember that the client is listening also).

After Report, Then What?

After you have received report, you will need to discuss the following items with the nurse with whom you are working:

- Time you will be on the unit
- Client goals
- Student personal goals
- Client routines
- Nursing interventions—who will do them

How Long Will You Be on the Unit?

How long will you be on the nursing unit? Do you have to leave the unit for a conference with your instructor or to attend an inservice? Will you be having a break, lunch, or both? It works well to take your break and meal at different times than the nurse assigned to your client. This way, there is consistent staff coverage for the client. Always tell the room nurse when you are leaving the unit, where you are going, and when you expect to return.

What Are Your Goals for the Day?

What do you want to accomplish today? You should have a goal each clinical day. It can be personal, professional, or a combination of the two. In the scenario, a personal goal of hanging an IV bag with minimal assistance was identified. To achieve your goals, you need to look for experiences that fit both within your goals and the parameters for your clinical experiences. Do you want to start an IV, do a complete physical assessment, learn how to do discharge teaching, or perhaps just be calm and composed while giving an IM injection? Because the staff nurse is more aware than you are of other experiences that may be happening on the unit, it is helpful to discuss your goal(s) with the nursing staff each day because they can also watch for these experiences.

What Are Your Client's Goals for the Day?

Because nursing care is client centered, you need to consider how your nursing care will affect the client's condition. What should your client be able to accomplish during your clinical day? Although all accomplishments may not be evident within one clinical day, the majority of clients do show some improvement. Be sure to discuss client goals with the nurse caring for the client and with the client. The nurse usually knows the client better and has more data than you may have as a student nurse.

What Do You Need to Know?

It is very important for a student nurse to know the nursing care interventions required by the client. Although some of this information will come from the chart and care plan, much of the information will come from the nursing staff, because the staff can describe how the interventions are actually done. Discuss your planned interventions with the nurse on a daily basis.

It is also important to learn the routines for the unit. What are routines? They can be described as nursing interventions that are done so often they have become routine. On many nursing units, they are the unwritten rules for client care. Remember, though, that these routines can vary considerably from unit to unit.

Another type of routine nursing intervention is called a clinical pathway. A clinical pathway is a series of specific nursing interventions to be followed for a specific medical diagnosis. For example, in a clinical pathway for a client who had an abdominal hysterectomy, nursing interventions are described for each day of the client's stay.

Examples of unit routines or clinical pathways could be:

- When can the client ambulate after surgery?
- Should the client take a shower or a bath?
- When is the surgical dressing removed?
- When can diet, activity, and pain medication be progressed?

There are several cautions to consider in regard to routines or clinical pathways. The first caution is that it's very easy to miscommunicate when a staff member tells you to "just do the routine." As a student, you may not even know the routine. To prevent errors caused by miscommunication, ask the staff member, "What is the routine here?" After the routine is explained, *restate it*. You could say, "Now, you are telling me that most second day C-section clients can take a shower? Is this correct?"

Another concern is whether routines should even exist. Client care should be individualized, not routine. You should never do an activity simply because "most clients do it this way." It must be appropriate for your client. As a student, you may find that routines are among the most frustrating areas of your clinical experience, simply because of your lack of knowledge of them and when to use or not use them.

It would be very good to go over your plans for the clinical day with the room nurse as well as your instructor. This might be seen as having a contract with the room nurse. Be as specific as possible. This is an especially good idea during your first semester in nursing school.

During the Clinical Day

As you begin your clinical day, you will see that there are many issues that must be expressed both to and about your client. It is very important to know with whom to communicate and about what information. You might find that communication with your client or health care staff members is difficult for a variety of reasons. As discussed in the client chapter (Chapter 3), specific approaches are used to overcome communication barriers caused by culture, feelings of loss, and distress. If you believe that these barriers impact upon your ability to communicate with your client, refer to these chapters (Chapters 4, 6, and 9). It will also be helpful for you to read the chapters on communicating with nurses and physicians (Chapters 10 and 11).

The Scenario Continues

> After you help Mr. Lawrence with his bath, you notice that he is tired, so you decide to have him rest for a while. A few minutes later, you come into his room and notice that he is now extremely short of breath. You do a quick assessment and note that his lungs are more congested than earlier in the day. Ms. Hollally walks by the room and you ask her to come to see Mr. Lawrence. You tell her that he was tired but not short of breath after the bath, so you let him rest. Ms. Hollally suggests that you elevate the head of Mr. Lawrence's bed. You do so and his breathing gets easier. Ms. Hollally tells you to discuss Mr. Lawrence's breathing problems with the nurse practitioner when she makes rounds.
>
> You see your nursing instructor a little while later and tell him about Mr. Lawrence's breathing problems.

Review the Situation

Because the client's condition can change rapidly, it is vital to keep the staff members informed of the client's condition.

- Keep the staff or room nurse informed
- Keep your instructor informed

Keep the Staff or Room Nurse Informed

If the client's condition alters, tell the staff nurse as soon as the changes occur. By keeping the staff nurse informed, you will have a resource person to guide you with planning care around these changes. Some examples of client condition changes could be:

- An alteration in vital signs
- Changes in physical or mental condition
- Equipment that isn't working properly
- Refusals by the client to do planned interventions such as a.m. care, ambulation, or dressing changes
- Lack of response to an intervention, such as intolerable pain despite the use of pain medication

Remember that this is a partial list and that there are many other client condition changes. If you have any questions about whether the nurse is aware of the client's condition, ask the nurse about it. In the scenario, the client had a change in physical condition and the student appropriately notified the nurse.

Keep Your Instructor Informed

Just as you need to keep the staff nurse informed of the client's condition, you need to keep your instructor aware of what is going on. Your instructor has a legal obligation to ensure that you are delivering safe, appropriate nursing care, which may require alterations caused by changes in client condition (Lessner, 1990). Your instructor will be able to lend assistance in altering your nursing interventions to reflect the changes in the client's condition. If you are unsure whether your nursing instructor is aware of alterations in the client's condition, it would be better to bring this to your instructor's attention, rather than risk not keeping your instructor informed.

At the End of the Clinical Day

Before you leave the nursing unit, you need to report off to the staff nurse. Provide the following information:

- Current client physical assessment
- Description of progress or lack of progress toward the goal
- Interventions or medications that still need to be completed before the end of the shift
- Significant events that occurred during the clinical day and the interventions required
- Requests of the client

Some problems regarding reporting off can arise. There are times when the nurse is too busy to listen to your report at the time you want to report off. Another difficulty can be the number of students a staff nurse is working with. Usually, the greater the number of students, the more the confusion. Another issue is that you may be giving report to a nurse who is covering for your nurse, who is at lunch or break. All these factors can contribute to poor communication. To lessen this problem, write your report on paper, review it with the staff nurse, and give the nurse the written report. Include the above information. List your name and your instructor's name because there may be questions later after you have left the unit.

Communication Roles

Staff Nurse as Resource to the Nursing Student

Members of the nursing staff can be a tremendous resource because they have an understanding of institutional policy and have the technical skill that every nursing student wants to have. Staff nurses can also be a great source of moral support and act as consultants to the students with whom they work.

Before you can really understand how to communicate with staff nurses, you need to know what their role is in regard to nursing students. The relationship between nursing staff and student nurses has changed over the years. Today, nursing students and staff nurses work cooperatively, rather than in a subordinate/superior fashion as in the past. With these relationship changes comes occasional confusion and even resistance to change. Not all nursing staff members understand how to work effectively with students, but the vast majority do.

Are staff members always happy to have nursing students on the unit? Although the majority of nurses are delighted to have nursing students on the unit, not all nurses work well with nursing students. Some nursing staff members are uncomfortable in the role of educator. Students report that staff members are occasionally rude or even hostile to them. Table 2–3 provides hints on how to manage difficult people. If you believe a staff member is being difficult, you must still act in an appropriate, professional manner. Discuss the staff member's behavior with your nursing instructor.

Table 2–3 WORKING WITH DIFFICULT PEOPLE

Because of the interaction of many interpersonal factors, some people can be difficult to communicate with. Before you label someone as "difficult," think about what other things are occurring on the nursing unit. If your nurse is swamped with work, you might interpret this as being uncommunicative instead of rushed for time. Remember, though, as a nursing student, you will not be with these people for very long times, so you need to learn how to communicate the best you can during this relatively short period. Here are some suggestions to help you communicate with difficult people.

Type of Problem	What Does It Look Like?	Interventions
Uncommunicative people	You talk to them and they answer briefly. They do not search you out to talk.	Keep attempting to talk to them. Use a quiet, yet direct, manner. Don't get angry because they will not talk to you. If you need information and you cannot get it from them, either talk to another staff member or your instructor.
Can't-make-a-decision people	When you present problems to them, they either give you multiple solutions or no solutions at all!	If they are providing multiple options, you could say, "Let's go over each choice to pick out the best one." If they aren't providing any options, you may need to suggest some. (Check with your instructor, though!)
Don't-appear-to-like-nursing-students people	When you talk to them, they answer you curtly or perhaps make fun of you.	Don't take this personally. They may be having a "bad hair day." Chalk it up as a learning experience. (Remember this when you have graduated and nursing students are on your unit.)
Forceful people	These people do not allow any choice other than their own.	To decide on the right course of action, you need to think about why they are acting this way. Do they have experience with this type of situation that you lack? Talk to them about other options you would like to use. You may need to include your nursing instructor in on the discussion.
Territorial	These nurses believe that the clients are "theirs" and don't want to give up control of "their" clients.	Many nurses worry about the responsibility of their job and thus have great difficulty delegating any responsibility to others. To work with this type of person, keep them informed of every detail of the client's care. This might help them to "share their territory."

Because staff nurses have multiple responsibilities, they may not always be immediately available to the student nurse. Students need to realize that events may be occurring on the unit that they are not aware of. So if the staff member appears hurried or states that he or she can't talk to you, be assertive and say, "When will be a good time to discuss this?" The staff member should be able to tell the student when he or she *will* be available to provide assistance.

Nursing staff members will frequently offer suggestions to you about client care. What do you do when these suggestions conflict with what you have been taught or with information given to you by your nursing instructor? This can really be a difficult situation. First, decide if this situation really reflects two opposing views. There is an old adage about "there's more than one way to skin a cat," meaning that there are frequently several ways to do something. Could it be that the staff nurse's method and your instructor's method are both correct, just different? It's sometimes very hard for a student to decide if this is so. Discuss this with your instructor and work out a solution.

Clinical Faculty Interactions With Staff Members

The nursing instructor is responsible for the supervision of the nursing students and the appropriateness of care delivered by the students. The clinical faculty members must work closely with staff members to keep communication lines open. They also serve as resource persons and troubleshoot student-related issues.

Before nursing students begin clinical rotation, the nursing faculty members have been collaborating with the nursing staff members to give students the best clinical experience possible. The nursing instructor will tell the staff members about the students' educational levels and abilities and what skills they are specifically looking for. This may be done verbally or written on student assignment sheets. See Figure 2–1 for an example of a student assignment sheet.

The faculty member usually makes the assignments, looking for clients who will provide good learning experiences for the students. The nursing instructor will discuss the clients with the nursing staff members to determine if they will be appropriate for students.

Because nursing staff members spend so much time with students, they can

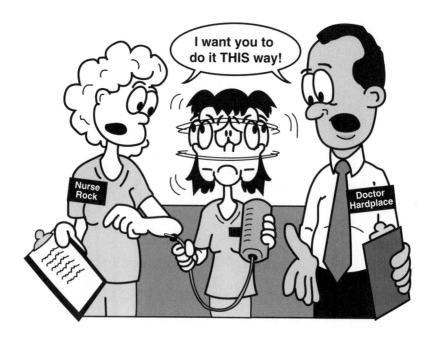

StLukes

STUDENT ASSIGNMENTS

CLINICAL UNIT __3 m__
DATE(S) __10-2, 10-3__
HOURS ON UNIT __7ª - 3ᵖ__
PRE/POSTCONFERENCE (TIME & LOC.)

AFFILIATING COLLEGE __Delta College__ INSTRUCTOR __April Sieh__ PAGER NO. __9125__
NURSING PROGRAM/COURSE/STUDENT LEVEL __RN program, Med-Surg;__
CLINICAL FOCUS/OBJECTIVES FOR THE WEEK __Cardiac__

EXPERIENCES/SKILLS NEEDED TODAY/THIS WEEK __telemetry, NG insertion__

SPECIAL NOTES _____

STUDENT RESPONSIBILITIES:

☒ HYGIENE (AM/PM CARE) ☒ VITAL SIGNS (P, R, T, BP)
☒ AMBULATION
☒ TOTAL PATIENT ASSESSMENTS ☐ DISCHARGES
__ ADMISSION ASSESSMENTS
☒ TUBE FEEDING
   X NG TUBE INSERTION
☒ MEDICATION ADMINISTRATION
   X ORAL   X EYE/EAR DROPS
   X SQ   no EPIDURAL
   X IVPB
   no IVP
☒ IV THERAPY
   X MONITORING   no BLOOD PRODUCTS
   X BAG/TUBING CHANGES X TPN
   X DISCONTINUATION
   no INSERTION

☒ FOLEY CATHETER
   X CARE
   X INSERTION
☒ DRESSINGS
   X MINOR   X SUTURE/STAPLE REMOVAL
   X MAJOR   X WOUND DRAINAGE DEVICES
☒ CHEST TUBE CARE
☒ TRACHEOSTOMY CARE
☒ OSTOMY CARE
☒ ONE TOUCH BG MONITORING
   (WITH SUPERVISION OF CERTIFIED OPERATOR)
☒ ENEMAS
☒ EKG TELEMETRY MONITORING
no HEMODYNAMIC MONITORING
no NURSE/PATIENT MGMT-LEADERSHIP FOCUS

OTHER _____

	STUDENT NAME	PATIENT NAME	ROOM NO.	BREAK TIME	MEAL TIME
1.	Nick Gushen	Tom Thornton	311 A	10:15	12:00
2.	Stephanie Miller	Jenny Cloud	317 B	10:15	12:00
3.	Connor Gushen	Maggie Smith	321 B	10:15	12:00
4.	Lillian Chylek	Charles Hough	309 A	10:30	12:45
5.	Mary Pintree	Caitlyn Larry	317 A	10:30	12:45
6.	LeeAnn Myers	Jill Chrysler	308	10:30	12:45
7.	Kyoto Lee	Harry Morcome	309 B	9:00	11:15
8.	Betty Kron	Cheryl Lakeheath	319 A	9:00	11:15
9.	Lucille Lennon	Albert Wright	317 C	9:00	11:15
10.	Betty Siehly	Tom Leonard	310	9:00	11:15

8/92

Figure 2–1. Example of a student assignment form. (Courtesy of St. Luke's Hospital, Saginaw, Michigan.)

provide input about students' clinical performance. The staff members often provide very insightful comments about student behaviors, provide excellent suggestions for improvement of student performance, and identify examples of good student performance.

Faculty-Student Interactions

What are some of the communication problems between faculty members and students? One of the most common communication problems is that students do not keep the instructor informed of their needs. This could occur because students may not yet know their own needs or because they do not want to give the impression that they do not know something. In any case, instructors cannot help students if they do not know what the students' needs are.

Sometimes students believe that they cannot understand or relate well to their instructor. Students need to remember that they do not have to like their instructors on a personal level. They simply need to work with them on a professional basis. After analyzing one's feelings, a student should ask the instructor for an appointment and have a frank discussion about the issue. The conversation should focus on "I feel," rather than "you should."

Another issue for students is that they may believe that each instructor has different expectations. This comment is most often made regarding client care plans. The student may believe that each instructor writes and grades care plans differently than the other instructors. Whether or not this is true, it is always a good idea to ask instructors about their expectations. If the concern is in regard to care plans, you could ask for examples of good and bad care plans. Or, you could write a sample care plan and ask for a critique.

Although students may view differences with faculty members in a negative fashion, working through these differences will help the students adapt to the varying expectations of the clinical agencies that may ultimately hire them.

Testing Considerations

Although the ultimate goal of most nursing students is to become nurses who can provide safe, appropriate, and compassionate client care, they have to make it through nursing school first. One of the real challenges in nursing education is relating information correctly on tests. In fact, many students see tests as roadblocks instead of measurement tools. If you find that you have poor test grades or simply have test grades that you would like improved, there are activities you can do.

The first is to determine what type of help you need. Are you studying the correct information or using the appropriate amount of study time? Can you read your lecture notes? Compare your lecture notes against those taken by an "A" student—are they the same? If not, what did the other student write that you did not? Do you understand the material? Do you get too anxious before the test? Are you unable to narrow the answer choices down to the correct answer? Many schools have testing or learning centers to help you determine your test-taking problem and formulate appropriate interventions.

The testing format in nursing education is often different from many other college disciplines. Testing is aimed at applying knowledge to situations, rather than just remembering facts. This type of testing format is needed because student nurses must be able to prove that they can apply their health care knowledge to client care, not simply memorize facts. However, this type of testing is typically perceived as more subjective than fact-recall questions, and disputes can arise about the accuracy of a test answer.

Although the intent of any testing format is to test in a fair and impartial manner, sometimes questions are perceived by students to be written ambiguously. As a nursing student you might encounter a test question that in your opinion has two correct answers, or maybe even no correct answers.

After the test it's very common for students to want to discuss the test and answers with the instructor. Although there are a variety of ways for students to contest a test question, the most common method is for students to crowd around the instructor after the test and try to convince the instructor to see the question in the way the student did. When mobbed by 30 students, the instructor may be overwhelmed and not really able to hear or understand your issue.

If you want the instructor to really hear what you are trying to say, it is important to do it correctly. Here is a better method to contest test answers: write the question on paper and include a paragraph supporting your choice of the answer. If you include any supporting documentation, such as a photocopy of a textbook page or lecture notes, use a highlighter pen to show the supporting text. Sign the paper and give it to the instructor. Ask when you can expect a response to your query (Dessner & McCoy, 1991). Another method is to make an appointment with the instructor to discuss the issue. Remember to bring all your supporting documentation. However, don't assume the instructor will change a question or an answer simply because you have challenged it.

Some nursing programs have specific guidelines to follow when challenging

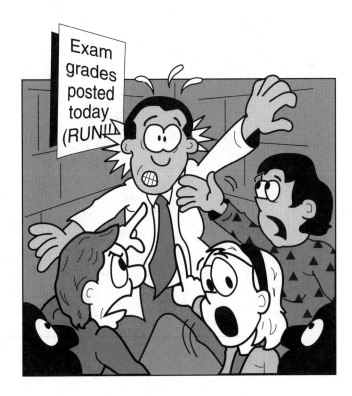

a test question answer. If your nursing program has guidelines, these must be followed.

When Should You Talk to Faculty Members?

You have to decide on the immediacy of the conversation, depending on the situation. For example, many clinical problems must be resolved quickly, and so you must talk to your instructor about the issue as soon as possible. For problems with grades and didactic content, you could probably make an appointment. However, if you are having problems with understanding content or are getting poor grades, you should try to talk to your instructor as soon as possible. To obtain test grades or get papers back, make an appointment. As stated earlier, don't rush or overwhelm your instructor after a test.

PRACTICAL APPLICATIONS

To conclude this chapter, let's look at two versions of a scenario. When you read it, keep in mind that it is not only what is said, but how you react to what is said that can make a big difference.

The **WRONG** Way

It is early in the clinical day and you have just arrived on the nursing unit. Because it is your second day there, you have some understanding of the unit's routines and layout. You wonder if you will be working with the same nurse as yesterday, but by the staff assignment sheet you see that you will be working with a different nurse, Chantrelle Puck, RN. You ask the unit clerk to point you in Ms. Puck's direction. You are directed to the conference room and see her sitting at the table.

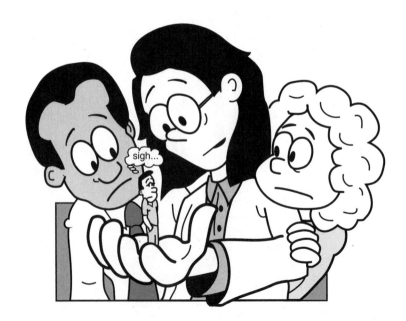

You say to her, "Hello, I'm going to be taking care of Mr. Turnbull. Can you give me report?" "Fine, but who are you?" she replies. "Oh, I'm Cindy Meyers, a first-year student at Learnmore College," you say. Ms. Puck begins to give you report. "Mr. Turnbull is a second-day open choley. They had problems last night with the N/G tube. He has normal saline going at 125." You interrupt her by saying, "He has normal saline going through his N/G tube?" Ms. Puck starts to laugh, "Boy, I don't know what they teach you at that nursing school, but his normal saline is the IV solution." Your face starts to turn red and you are really embarrassed.

Ms. Puck continues. "He has 500 up in the *normal saline*. Do you need to know anything more?" "No," you mumble, and walk away.

You go the restroom for a few minutes to compose yourself. As you go to your client's room to assess him, you see your instructor. You ponder whether to tell him what happened in report. You decide not to tell him, because he might think that you were dumb. Your instructor asks "What is your plan of action for today?" You tell him your planned goals and interventions, and he agrees with them. As he walks away, he says, "I'm going to check on the other students and I'll be back in about 15 minutes. Page me if you need me before that."

As you finish your assessment, it occurs to you that Mr. Turnbull is breathing much harder than yesterday. You recheck him and find the same thing. When you look over his nursing notes for the last day, you don't find any mention of difficult breathing. You consider asking Ms. Puck to come and see him, but after the way she treated you in report, you don't want to ask her anything. Your instructor said he'd be back in 15 minutes, so you decide to ask him about Mr. Turnbull's breathing then. As you begin to do his bath you think, "Maybe this breathing problem isn't anything. After all, nobody else noticed it."

After his bath, you notice that his breathing is really getting worse. Just when you decide you are going to go get help, he stops breathing. A code blue is called.

After the code blue, Mr. Turnbull goes to intensive care.

Afterward, you have a long talk with your instructor about Ms. Puck's making fun of you, your lack of confidence in your abilities, and your failure to keep Ms. Puck or your instructor informed of the client's status.

This clinical day surely wasn't what you expected.

Now Let's Re-Run the Conversation Using the Ideas From This Chapter the **CORRECT** Way

It is early in the clinical day and you have just arrived on the nursing unit. Because it is your second day there, you have a basic understanding of the unit's routines and layout. You wonder if you will be working with the same nurse as yesterday, but by the staff assignment sheet you see that you will be working with a different nurse, Chantrelle Puck, RN. You ask the unit clerk to point you in Ms. Puck's direction. You're directed to the conference room and see her sitting at the table. You say to her, "Hello, I'm Cindy Meyers, a first-year student at Learnmore College. I'm going to be taking care of Mr. Turnbull. Can you give me report?" Before Ms. Puck begins to give you report, she asks, "Have you taken care of him before?" You reply "Yes, I took care of him yesterday." "OK, then, I'll give you a brief report. Mr. Turnbull is a second-day open choley. They had problems last night with the N/G tube. He has normal saline going at 125." You interrupt her by saying "He has normal saline going through his N/G tube?" Ms. Puck starts to laugh, "Boy, I don't know what they teach you at that nursing school, but his normal saline is the IV solution." Your face starts to turn red and you are really embarrassed.

Ms. Puck continues. "He has 500 up in the *normal saline*. Do you need to know anything more?" "No," you mumble, and walk away.

You go the restroom for a few minutes to compose yourself. As you start toward your client's room to assess him, you see your instructor. You ponder whether to tell him what happened in report. You decide to tell him because you don't know whether it's better to confront Ms. Puck about embarrassing you or to just chalk it up to being a student. He suggests that you tell Ms. Puck of your embarrassment. He then asks, "What is your plan of action for today?" You tell him your planned goals and interventions, and he agrees with them. As he walks away, he says, "I'm going to check on the other students and I'll be back in about 15 minutes. Page me if you need me before that."

As you finish your assessment, it occurs to you that Mr. Turnbull is breathing much harder than yesterday. You recheck him and find the same thing. When you look over his nursing notes for the last day, you don't find any mention of difficult breathing. You go find Ms. Puck to come and see him. You plan to talk to her of your embarrassment, but you know that this isn't the correct time or place. After you and Ms. Puck enter Mr. Turnbull's room, you notice that his breathing is really getting worse. Just as Ms. Puck starts to assess him, he stops breathing. A code blue is called.

After the code blue, Mr. Turnbull goes to intensive care.

Later that day, you see Ms. Puck sitting alone in the conference room. You go up to her and say, "Ms. Puck, I'd like to talk to you about something you said in report today. When you were giving report, I interrupted you by asking if the normal saline was in his N/G. I know that I shouldn't have interrupted you, but I felt really embarrassed when you said that it was his IV solution." "Oh, I'm sorry," said Ms. Puck, "It was just so funny how you said it. It reminded me of nursing school. I didn't mean to embarrass you."

This clinical day surely wasn't what you expected, but as you leave, it occurs to you that you performed exactly as you should. You look forward to another exciting clinical day tomorrow.

REFERENCES

Browning, E., & Campbell, M. (1987). Evaluating student's communication skills: Tape recording. *Nurse Educator, 12*(1), 28–29.

Davis, D., & Kurtz, P. (1991). Assessing interaction patterns of students. *Nurse Educator, 16*(5), 9–11.

Dessner, S., & McCoy, C. (1991). A workable solution to test review. *Nurse Educator, 16*(6), 12–13.

Haggerty, L. (1987). An analysis of senior nursing students' immediate responses to distressed patients. *Journal of Advanced Nursing, 12*(4), 451–461.

Lessner, M. (1990). Avoiding student-faculty litigation. *Nurse Educator, 15*(6), 29–32.

Voignier, R., & Freeman, L. (1992, July-August). Helping staff help students. *Journal of Nursing Staff Development*, 165–169.

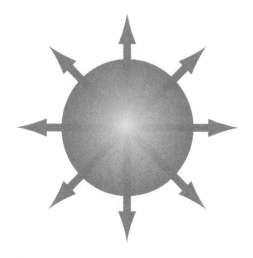

3

With Clients

In this chapter, we will discuss:

- Therapeutic communication
- Specific issues related to communication with clients
- Environmental factors affecting client communication in the institutional setting and in the home care setting

Therapeutic Communication

Therapeutic communication is purposeful communication defined as "any communication designed to increase the self-worth of the client or alleviate psychological distress; [it] implies unconditional positive regard for the client from the nurse and is done in a caring, concerned, and empathic manner" (Bradley & Edinberg, 1982). This requires an awareness of the client's "feeling" environment and the ability to respond to needs through the use of verbal and nonverbal communication skills, including therapeutic touch and active listening.

These skills are developed over time with practice. Because they require self-awareness, a nurse must be able to understand and value himself or herself as a person. Self-esteem and self-confidence are necessary to appreciate the value of one's presence for clients. The underpinnings of the helping role of the nurse are those words and actions that enhance the client's sense of person, meaning, and dignity. Effectiveness is often judged by what is done for the client, but it is often the being with and listening to the client that is most significant (Benner, 1984). For the nurse to know the client, the nurse must be with and listen to the client (Tanner et al, 1993). Beck (1993) reviewed four studies in which nurses identified the most important caring behaviors; the most important are identified as follows.

- Listening to the client; touching the client when comfort is needed
- Allowing expression of feelings
- Getting to know the client as an individual
- Calling the client by name; talking to the client
- Realizing the client knows himself or herself best; including the client in care planning and management
- Being perceptive of the client's needs; planning and acting accordingly
- Teaching clients how to care for themselves
- Providing information so the client can make informed decisions
- Valuing honesty, respect, patience, and responsibility
- Giving good physical care
- Putting the client first

This list should help to decrease the fear of saying the "wrong thing" to clients and increase the focus on offering a helping relationship with clients and families. These relationships can assist clients to new ways of understanding and coping with problems and can help them see their problems as approachable and manageable (Benner, 1984). The nurse's ability to build such relationships is dependent on the nurse's sensitivity toward the client/family situation. This includes awareness of role relationship patterns; environmental factors; professional language and jargon usage; knowledge of personal attitudes, assumptions, and beliefs; and how each impacts client/family and nurse communication.

Consider This Scenario

Mr. Rose is going to surgery at 8 a.m. The night nurse awakens him at 6 a.m. to ensure he has enough time to get ready. She reminds him not to eat or drink anything, and tells him to shower and then put on the surgical gown. As she lays the towels and gown in the bathroom, she goes on to say that after his a.m. care is done, she will get his IV going and help him put on TEDs. Mr. Rose says very little as he gets up.

As the nurse leaves she tells him, "I will be back shortly. If you need assistance before then, put on your call light."

Mr. Rose takes his shower, but he cannot understand why he has to be up so early. When he puts on the gown, he feels like his identity and dignity have been taken away. As he sits down at the bedside, he thinks about what is going to happen next. "I know the nurse last night went over what would happen today, but it's all a blur now. What IV line was she talking about—I don't even have a line to get going! Who is this 'Ted'? Boy, I really feel uneasy about all this stuff."

When the nurse comes back into the room, she notices Mr. Rose is very quiet and not making eye contact. Even though she has only known him for a few days, this seems so unlike him. He is an executive at a local company and always has lots of questions and has enjoyed being involved in his care. She says, "Mr. Rose, you seem unusually quiet this morning," and then pauses.

Mr. Rose hesitates a moment and then says, "You know, every morning I get up and get dressed, review my appointment schedule for the day over a cup of coffee, check my phone mail messages, and then plan out my day. But today, here I am wearing this silly gown, and in spite of what you all told me earlier, I have no idea what is going to happen

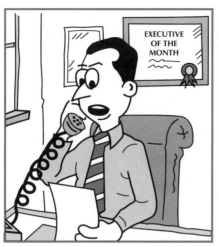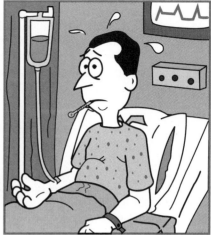

next. I don't even have an 'IV' line, let alone know how you'll get it going, and I have no idea who 'Ted' is. I guess it is just that I don't feel in control here and I'm not used to that."

The nurse brings Mr. Rose his bathrobe, and sits down. "I can see how this routine is really different. Let me go over a few things so you will know what will be happening and when. I'll give you a crash course in hospital English so you can understand much of what the staff are saying." She takes a pad of paper and her pen out of her pocket. "Here's a paper and pen in case you want to make notes. It's handy to jot down questions as they come up and then we can go over them." As she looks at her watch, she said, "There should be time between 7 and 7:30 a.m. for you to check your phone messages if you like. It may help you feel more connected to your usual routine. So, let's get started and clear up this IV issue. . . ."

This scenario addresses several key factors that come into play when communicating with clients:

- Alterations on role relationship patterns that can occur
- Use of professional jargon
- Use of assumptions based on belief patterns

Alterations in Role Relationship Patterns

When persons enter the health care system, they take on the role of client or patient, a role much different than the one they are used to. Role status and relationships are often supported or reinforced by external behavior patterns, personal space, and dress. When these reinforcers are taken away, a person's sense of control over the situation can be greatly affected. Needless to say, this can be very unnerving. Consider what happens when one enters an acute care setting. It is advisable to bring in only the necessities. Expensive personal items and jewelry should be left at home. Often, even one's pajamas are replaced with a hospital gown, short and open down the back. The client rooms all look pretty much the same and are usually small, with a shared bathroom and little space for familiar items. There are no "power" desks or status clothes, familiar faces, or comfortable work and family routines that carry a person through the day.

When the nurse noted a change in Mr. Rose's behavior, she provided him the opportunity to share his thoughts by commenting on his unusually quiet behavior and by giving him time to respond, which he did. She cued in on his concerns—losing his usual routine and role, feeling out of control, getting lost in jargon—and proceeded to address them, verbally and nonverbally. Handing him his own bathrobe acknowledged his concern about the gown; sitting down conveyed that his concerns were important and valid, and she was willing to address them with him. Letting him know when he could check on his phone messages conveyed she understood the importance of his morning routine. These behaviors set the stage for the positive verbal assistance she provided him. She helped to reinforce who he was as an individual and assisted him in learning more about his care routines.

Use of Professional Jargon

In many situations, groups develop their own language, which serves as a shorthand method of speaking. However, this type of speech can also serve as an exclusionary method to keep others from knowing what the group is talking about. As such, it could be used or perceived to demonstrate that one person has power and status over another (Bourhis, 1989). The health care profession has its own jargon, and it is common for groups within the health care field to use different terminology based on the areas of practice. This language is full of abbreviations and medical terminology, most of which is not understood by the general population.

Often we nurses take time to explain things to our clients, and we believe we have done a good job because there were few, if any, questions and the client seemed to nod at appropriate intervals as we spoke. It is only later that we find out through observing the client's behavior that the client had not understood. We become so familiar with a whole vocabulary of clinical terms that we do not realize we speak a different language. A recent study looked at physicians' perceptions of how well they communicate with clients versus the clients' perceptions of the same. The results indicated that even when the physicians thought they had communicated well, making efforts to avoid unfamiliar terminology, they still had often been unclear and had used terms with which clients were not familiar (Bourhis, 1989).

This study has implications for nurses. Nurses frequently have the responsibility to coordinate client care and must assist clients in becoming familiar with health care terminology. Using pictures, educational materials, and audiovisual and computer programs; engaging in group and one-on-one discussions; and providing hands-on practice are all viable ways of sharing information. Whichever mode is used, it should complement client needs.

Client educational level, the amount of information to be provided, general word choices, and sentence length should be considered when sharing information. Words with multiple syllables and long, complex sentence structure could make listening a hard task. This is particularly true when the client is ill, tired, stressed (physically, emotionally, or mentally), in pain, or medicated.

It is helpful to have clients write down their questions and then encourage or assist them in talking with members of the health care team. Writing questions down as they occur provides clients with a reference to use when their physicians and health team members make their rounds. Clients often forget what they wanted to ask, and this approach eliminates that frustration. Try to be with the client during visits by other team members. This provides the opportunity to assist the client in asking questions, to clarify what has been said, and to collaboratively clarify goals and approaches to care problems and concerns. Answers to questions could also be written down for client/family reference.

It is very important to seek feedback from clients to evaluate how well they understand information given. Corrections can then be made if miscommunication occurred. This helps ensure that clients are truly well informed. Clients often fear appearing uninformed or silly if they ask too many questions. One way of avoiding this would be to say:

> "I have given you some new information and I want to be sure I have covered it clearly. Explain it back to me—that way I can see if I have missed anything."

or

> "Now that we have gone over how to do the procedure, I want you to do it for me. That way I can see if I have explained it well and if we need to review any information. It is important to me that you can do the procedure confidently."

This approach puts some of the responsibility for sharing the information on the nurse as well as on the client. The client has the responsibility to speak up if the information is not clear. Statements like the ones above provide the opportunity for the client to do so.

In the scenario, Mr. Rose had been given information, but he was not able to absorb it and then recall it when he needed it. This usually occurs when too much new information is given too fast or if there is too great a time lag between the time the information was given and when it is to be recalled. Too many activities or changes in routine can also distract from the information flow. All these factors could have contributed to Mr. Rose's predicament.

Not only do care providers use jargon, but our clients may do so as well. Many groups within our society use their own jargon or have detectable speech patterns. For many years, teenagers have made up their own language, which changes from time to time. For example, a teenager may say, "I've been reversing gears for days!" In this case, "reversing gears" means vomiting. Gang members have their own version of the English language, often referred to as street talk. For example, "She fell out yesterday" means she fainted. If a client uses terminology that is not understood, simply ask what it means. Some emergency departments have prepared lists of teenage and street slang definitions for staff reference. Because such terms or phrases vary from place to place, it is important to verify their meaning. Avoid making fun of these variances in speech patterns, and do not try to imitate this kind of talk; this would come across as ridiculous and demeaning.

Use of Assumptions Based on Belief Patterns

It is easy to assume that if clients are well educated, they understand what is happening around and to them, and if they do not, they will ask. This is particularly true if it is known that a client works in the health care field. Consider Mr. Rose, an executive. Who would have thought he would feel so out of control in the acute care setting? The assumption in reverse may also occur: a client who is or appears to be not well educated, may be perceived as not being well informed about his or her health status or not caring to know. This does not make sense, but it does occur and seems to stem from beliefs based on stereotypes.

Similar general assumptions are sometimes made about persons ascribing to certain religious faiths or belonging to certain ethnic groups. Assumptions and beliefs are formed by the information to which a person has been exposed and by the experiences one has had. These then form one's attitudes. The validity of these is directly related to the accuracy of the information and the breadth of the experiences as well as to the degree to which these mind sets seem to fit into one's overall scheme of things. Awareness of your attitudes and belief patterns and an openness to those of others helps you realize that each client is a unique human being. When this approach is taken, the individual needs will most often be identified and addressed. Attitudes are often communicated very clearly through nonverbal behaviors. Care must be taken to keep verbal and nonverbal messages to clients consistent. If they contradict each other, then confusion, insincerity, and lack of concern for the client will be communicated. See Chapter 4 for a more focused discussion on cultural diversity.

The sensitivity and comfort level felt when talking with a client about needs and concerns are very much impacted by your own life experiences. Life experiences and interpretations of them are a complex combination of learned attitudes, beliefs, and behaviors based on religious, cultural, and social mores. For example, if you come from a background where health and personal matters were considered private and not addressed with others, then you might be uncomfortable asking clients about these areas. Reaching a comfort level would take much practice, and finding a balance between personal background and behaviors necessary for practice would also be required. The same is true when learning to talk with other professionals, authority figures, and ancillary help. This is addressed further in Chapters 9 and 10.

Student nurses are quite amazed at the variety of clients for whom they provide care. Many clients fall outside cultural and social patterns with which the student is comfortable. A student might provide care for a client shot in a robbery attempt, for a client injured while under the influence of alcohol, or for a client who is simply annoying. Taking care of such clients can be very interesting, yet distressing. Are nurses obligated to provide care for clients they may not personally like or approve of? The answer is yes. As a nurse, one is obligated by the American Nurses' Association Code of Ethics, which states: "The nurse provides services with respect for human dignity and the uniqueness of the client unrestricted by considerations of social or economic status, personal attributes or the nature of health problems" (American Nurses' Association, 1985). Does this mean the nurse must personally like all clients or approve of their actions? No, it means the nurse must provide safe, appropriate, professional nursing care in a nonjudgmental fashion.

At times, you may have such strong feelings about a particular issue, such as abortion rights, and believe you cannot provide care for a client undergoing this procedure. In this type of situation, if you are absolutely unable to provide care to a client because of beliefs, you are obligated to arrange for the client to receive care from another care provider (Zerwekh & Claborn, 1994). Such conflict can be avoided. As a nurse, it is your responsibility to seek employment only in those settings in which activities are congruent with personal beliefs.

Specific Issues Related to Communication With Clients

Communicating with clients on a daily basis brings to life many issues that are not always evident. You will interact with a great variety of persons: clients, family members, other health care team members, and ancillary personnel involved in health care settings. The form of interaction may be verbal—in person, via telephone or other telecommunication devices, or over intercoms—or in writing and via computer entries. Your communication style must be modified appropriately depending on the format used, who will be the receiver of the information, and the type of information that is being shared. The human element demands that you consider many factors that can affect the ability of clients and families to receive and respond to information. The sensitivity of the information and confidentiality must be respected.

Consider This Scenario

Mr. Lopez, RN, is beginning his morning assessment rounds. He knocks on the door, waits 2 to 3 seconds, and then enters the room of Mr. Wiggins, who was admitted the previous evening. Mr. Wiggins is sitting on the side of the bed. Mr. Lopez introduces himself, "Good morning, Mr. Wiggins, I am Mr. Lopez. I am a registered nurse and will be working with you, supervising your care today." He extends his hand and offers Mr. Wiggins a firm handshake as he makes eye contact and smiles gently. "How was your night here?" he asks, and then waits for a response.

Mr. Wiggins responds, "It took a while, but once I fell asleep, I stayed asleep. It felt awkward to be away from home. Being in the hospital is a new experience for me. I was surprised by the number of people who work here. When I came in, I must have talked to three or four different staff people, then there were the lab and x-ray techs, I guess you call them."

Mr. Lopez agreed that there are many types of employees, and encouraged Mr. Wiggins to let him know if he had any questions about his care or related procedures. He pulled the curtain and proceeded to do his nursing assessment, explaining its purpose to Mr. Wiggins as he went along. He finished with an explanation of the morning care routines and the x-ray Mr. Wiggins was to have later in the morning.

A short while later, as he passed out medications, Mr. Lopez met Mrs. Wiggins, who appeared very upset, in the hallway. In talking with her in a quiet sitting area, he found out Mr. Wiggins had been feeling ill for the past several weeks and had been unable to work. This had put much strain on their finances, and the hospital expenses were very worrisome. (This was information Mr. Wiggins had not relayed.) Mrs. Wiggins stated that although neither of them knew much about seeking assistance, even though it was embarrassing, she felt they needed to talk with someone.

Mr. Lopez asked, "Would you like me to contact the social services representative to arrange a meeting for you and Mr. Wiggins to discuss your concerns?"

Mrs. Wiggins readily agreed with this, and they both went in to talk with Mr. Wiggins before a call was made. Mr. Lopez provided privacy and, realizing how embarrassing the situation was for the couple, spoke in a soft tone as he reviewed what Mrs. Wiggins had discussed with him outside the room.

Mr. Wiggins said, "It's so hard for me to admit we are having money problems. It's never happened before. I can't seem to get better enough to go back to work, and that scares me, too. What if I can't go back to work soon? This whole thing has me so upset inside. I guess it would be a good idea to talk with someone who may be able to help us through this. Just talking about it now helped take a little pressure off. Thanks, Mr. Lopez."

This scenario illustrates specific issues that are addressed as one communicates with clients:

- How to address the client
- Types of information communicated
- Confidentiality
- Psychosocial factors that affect the ability of client and family to communicate

How to Address the Client

In American society today, there often tends to be a certain informality in the way we dress, behave, and interact with others. This contributes to a more relaxed atmosphere as we go about daily activities. However, as a professional, the initial interaction with a client should be more formal. When the client meets you for the first time, the way you, as the nurse, present yourself has a subtle but distinct impact on the client's perception of your professional or nonprofessional image and competence. Using a client's first name, especially without permission, connotes a social relationship, not a professional one (Campbell-Heider & Hart, 1993). Use of more formal language with clients can elicit feelings of self-esteem in the client, which is important as we foster active client participation in care activities.

After taking care of many clients, nurses become comfortable with physical assessment and care of clients, and it is easy to forget that these activities totally invade their clients' personal spaces. Because of the nature of the health care setting some degree of this is expected by clients, but personal space must be respected whenever possible. By establishing credibility and demonstrating respect for clients and their cultural beliefs related to touch and space, you can greatly reduce the level of stress related to frequent invasion of personal space before performing these care activities.

Introduce yourself using your name and title, and address clients using their proper title, i.e., Dr., Mr., Mrs., Ms., or Miss, and their last name. This gives the client the opportunity to tell you how she or he would like to be addressed. If he says, "Call me Bill," then you can do so, but take your cues from the client and your comfort level. If a client seems too casual, you can help control the situation through use of a more formal, business-like approach. Also, inform the client of your role and when you will be involved in care.

Example

"Good morning, Mr. Smith. I am Mrs. Jones. I am a student nurse from Learnmore College. Today I am here to meet you and gather information about your care so I will be prepared to take care of you tomorrow and Friday."

When you do not know the client's name, "sir" or "ma'am" in most instances indicates respect. However, it is best, whenever possible, to introduce yourself first and then seek to learn the client's name. Addressing adolescents as "Ms." or "Mr." suggests you view them as their own person and not as a child. Simply using adult reference may enhance their sense of self-care responsibility (Campbell-Heider & Hart, 1993). Do not use terms such as "honey child," "dear," "Granny," or "Grandpa" to refer to clients or visitors. These terms can be impersonal labels or reflect a close personal relationship, which in most instances is not true. Use of these terms is unprofessional.

A client may attempt to shift the focus of the interaction back onto you by asking personal questions such as "Are you married?" or "Why did you become a nurse?" Responses to such questions will vary. It is best to answer such a question in a brief manner, if it seems appropriate, and then to redirect the conversation back to the client.

Example

"Yes, I am married, Mrs. Smith. I noticed you are, too. Will your husband be able to visit you here in the hospital?"

"I enjoy working with people and nursing gives me the opportunity to do that. What I need to do now is check your blood pressure. How do you feel since you started on the new medication to help keep it down?"

Occasionally, a client may make offensive or sexually aggressive comments. You may feel uncomfortable or angry, which is normal. Appropriate responses should take into consideration (a) possible reasons for the client to act this way and (b) the need for the nurse to clarify or reinforce the necessity of maintaining a professional relationship. Illness may negatively impact a person's self-esteem and feelings of sexual adequacy and may cause inappropriate behavior. When this happens, respond in an honest, yet respectful and professional, way (Jarvis, 1992).

Example

"Mrs. Smith, your comments make me uncomfortable. It is important that our relationship be a professional one. Your comments seem so out of character for you. It seems as though something may be bothering you?"

"Mr. Wirtzik, please don't make those kinds of comments to me. You know our relationship is a professional one. Could it be your long stay in the hospital is causing you to make those comments?"

These types of responses would give the client an opportunity to appropriately explore the situation with you and reflect your professional concern for the client as well as establish limits on the behavior(s). If offensive behaviors persist, seek assistance from other health professionals who are skilled in dealing with such client behavior.

When Mr. Lopez entered the new client's room, he addressed Mr. Wiggins by name and immediately let him know who he was and that he would be working with him and overseeing his care that day. Note also the nonverbal behaviors Mr. Lopez used. Before entering he knocked and waited a few seconds, which showed respect for client privacy. The firm handshake, steady eye contact, and smile conveyed a confident, interested attitude on his part. These behaviors were validated as Mr. Lopez inquired about Mr. Wiggins' night and asked if he had questions about care or procedures. These nonverbal and verbal statements demonstrated respect and concern for Mr. Wiggins and set the tone for the assessment Mr. Lopez proceeded to do. The curtain was pulled to ensure privacy.

Closure of a nurse-client relationship is also important, especially if you have cared for the client over a period of time on a fairly consistent basis. What is said depends on the circumstances and the persons involved. If the client has made a remarkable recovery, it is usually a happy, fun moment. If a client remains quite ill or needs further recovery, it may be a time to share a few caring words of encouragement and concern. At times, a caring touch, such as a warm handshake, a touch on the arm or shoulder, or even a hug may be all that is needed.

Types of Information Communicated

The purpose of asking clients questions is to obtain information related to and necessary for client care. This can involve many questions concerning the client's health history as well as present health problems. When information is sought, it is important to identify yourself and your role, what information is needed, and how it will be used, just as Mr. Lopez did in the scenario. As noted above, nonverbal, professional behaviors, such as providing client privacy and being sensitive to client needs and concerns, reinforce the nurse's genuineness in dealing with the client. You may need to explain that nurses frequently pursue a different line of questioning than do physicians. Nurses ask clients more questions about how the clients are able to function in their daily lives with respect to their health status and needs, whereas physicians spend most of their time focusing on known or suspected pathology (Zungolo, 1994).

Seeking information for its own sake or because it is interesting is inappropriate. When the client is the victim or perhaps the perpetrator of an act of violence or trauma, you might be tempted to ask, simply for the sake of curiosity, how the situation occurred. But, unless you have a specific health care reason for this line of questioning, do not pursue it. There are times when it is appropriate to discuss events that led up to violence or trauma, particularly when there is evidence of repeated occurrences, and the information will be used clinically to address health and safety needs of the client.

When interacting with clients, nurses obtain, provide, and reinforce information, examples of which are shown in the box.

Before the 1960s, clients were discouraged from knowing details about their health status. Now clients are encouraged to know as much as possible about their condition and care. Who supplies the client with information? A general rule is that each professional answers questions that fall within his or her scope of practice. Nurses can provide client information related to nursing activities. For example, you can tell the client about findings on the nursing assessment, vital signs, medications, when and why treatments will be done, when the client's therapy appointments are scheduled, and available support services that may be helpful. When clients ask questions that fall within the realm of collaborative practice, consider

Examples of Information Communicated

Type of Interaction	Examples
Obtaining information	Doing assessments, asking questions, acting as client sounding-board, talking with family
Providing information	Teaching formally and informally, informing clients about day's activities, explaining jargon, answering questions, sharing knowledge of supportive resources
Reinforcing information	Verifying what was said, ordered, or previously taught

the type of information that is requested: is it related to a specific area of expertise? If so, it is best to communicate the client's request to the person with that expertise. Examples of such questions include: What were the results of my biopsy? Why did the doctor put me on this drug rather than the new one that is being advertised? The dietician told me how much fat and protein I need to eat at home and I can't remember now; how much do you think I should eat? If the question relates to general procedures and policies, then answer the question accordingly. If you do not know how to answer a client's question, be honest, "I am not sure how to answer your question, but I will find someone who can and will get back to you." Be sure you follow through.

There are so many disciplines involved in caring for clients and so much information to be relayed. A key to good communication with clients is good communication within the health care team. Each member contributes different knowledge and skills to client management, and understanding each other's approaches will facilitate communication with the client.

Mr. Lopez became aware of the family's financial concerns through his interaction with Mrs. Wiggins. Realizing this was not an issue he could address personally, he offered to arrange for them to meet with the social services representative and provided the opportunity for them to talk about their dilemma. This approach helped ease some of the tension the situation was creating for them.

Confidentiality

The issue of confidentiality comes into play when communicating with and about clients. Often, clients are concerned about confidentiality when they are asked to share personal information. They may ask questions such as, Who will see this information? Why do you need it? How will it be used? Think about how many persons interact with clients in an acute care setting within a 24-hour period. Most of these persons have access to the client's record. This was one of the first observations Mr. Wiggins made after entering the hospital. Clients often do not know or remember the names or professional status of persons they talk with, perhaps because of the proliferation of scrubs, use of lab coats by a variety of personnel, disappearance of the nurse's cap, hard-to-read name tags, and an increase in the number of students in the various settings. Clients have the right to expect that any information obtained by health care providers will be kept confidential and used only for health care purposes. Failure to keep information confidential can result in civil litigation (Annas, 1989).

Consider these questions regarding client confidentiality:

1. Do you NEED this information?

   Is this information needed for the care you are going to provide? If so, this information should be obtained. Otherwise, do not pursue it. The information needed varies depending on the situation.

2. Do you have a RIGHT to know this information?

   Does the information pertain to health care concerns? If someone begins to tell you gossip about a client and the information is not relevant to the care, tell the person sharing this information that it is unnecessary information and that you are not interested in hearing it.

3. WHERE are you discussing the information?

Are you discussing client information in a secure place? When you are having a conversation that has anything to do with hospital business, remember to think about your location. It must be held in a place where you cannot be overheard. When Mrs. Wiggins started to talk about her husband in the hallway, Mr. Lopez had her continue the conversation in a quiet sitting area to ensure privacy. Areas where client information is discussed, such as conference rooms or staff lounges, should have doors on them, which are kept closed when the room is in use. Voice volume should be moderated to prevent being heard outside the room. Many nursing stations have an open type of layout, which allows for easy transfer of information to anyone standing nearby. Be very cautious of what you are saying when you are in this type of area. Also, avoid any hospital or client discussion in public restrooms, hallways, elevators, or cafeterias. Even if you couch your discussion into generalities, such as "the man I'm taking care of" or "the woman on 7 North," it may be possible to figure out about whom you are talking, or others may incorrectly assume they know about whom you are talking. It is best to simply make it a habit not to discuss anything to do with the care setting in a public place.

4. With WHOM are you discussing it?

One of the most common errors made concerning confidentiality is discussing information with people who should not be hearing the information. You should discuss client information with (a) the client, (b) health care personnel directly involved in the client's care, and (c) persons suggested by the client to receive information.

When providing information to another health care provider, make sure you know who they are. This can be difficult when there are many people passing through a typical nursing unit. It is easy to assume that if individuals are wearing lab coats and stethoscopes around their necks then they are physicians or other health care providers. Remember, though, that appearances may be deceiving. Look for a name or hospital identification tag. However, be aware that many health care personnel, especially physicians, do not wear name tags and many do not wear lab coats. If you do not know who someone is, ask the person. You could say, "I have not had the pleasure of meeting you. I am Mike Jubicyzk, an RN student from Learnmore College. And you are . . .?"

Family members often want information about their loved one's condition. Before you discuss client information with the family, however, you must explore how much or how little information the client wants others to know.

Example

Nurse to client: "Family and friends often call or stop by the desk to ask nursing personnel about the client's status. What type of information concerning your condition, and with whom, do you want shared if someone should inquire?"

Client: "If my Mom and my sister, Sayonda, ask about me, it is OK to tell them anything about me."

This should also be documented. An example of a narrative note is:

1/23/96   Discussed type of information concerning condition that could be shared,
0900   and with whom; stated, "If my Mom (Mrs. Pam Meckle) and sister (Sayonda
           Meckle) ask about me, it is OK to tell them anything."—K. Blitz, RN

Without such a statement, be very cautious when giving out information, in person as well as over the telephone. In most settings, all that can be discussed without client permission is a general statement of the client's condition. For example, "The client is in fair condition." If a family member or friend calls inquiring about the client and no permission has been given to convey information to them, you could offer to transfer the call into the client's room, and the client could then relay any information she or he chooses to share. Because obtaining client information over the phone is convenient for friends and family, some institutions have developed specific telephone policies that should be followed.

Occasionally, a client may request that information shared with you be kept confidential. This may make you feel privileged that the client is confiding in you. However, if it is information that impacts on the client's care and needs to be shared with the health care team, you must tell the client you cannot comply with his wishes.

Example

Client: "I am so sick and I really don't want to be resuscitated, but my family won't hear of it. Please don't tell anyone, but if I die when you are here, don't bring me back."

Nurse: "You know, Mr. Sea, that is something I cannot do unless there is a formal Do Not Resuscitate order on your chart. I can, though, help you talk to your doctor and the nurse manager about this during their rounds today. It can be very difficult for family members to discuss this kind of decision. Would you like help in talking with your family about this?"

Such situations provide opportunities to help the client address the issue that is causing concern.

When collecting and recording client information for educational purposes, client names and addresses must be omitted from paperwork forms used. Problems can arise when client information is taken beyond the classroom or clinical agency. Because nursing brings new and different experiences, it is tempting to discuss these experiences with family and friends. You may be asked if you saw mutual acquaintances at the hospital. A good response to this is, "I was so busy today. I did not see them." If requests for information are consistently politely refused, the requests usually stop. It is very important that client information not be shared with *anyone* outside the care or learning environment. It is important that you know and follow the institutional policy and procedures related to confidentiality issues.

Psychosocial Factors That Affect the Ability of Client and Family to Communicate Their Needs

Effective communication takes energy and the ability to focus on the other person and what the other person is saying. There are times when clients are unable to do this or to do it well:

- When clients are very ill or in pain, their energy is usually focused on their physical stress.
- Emotional stress can cloud thought processes.
- Medications such as analgesics or sedatives can also alter their ability to take in, process, and respond to information in a coherent and appropriate manner.
- Nearly all hospitalized clients report an increase in stress levels, which contributes to varying degrees of anxiety. This may lead to inability to concentrate on other thoughts and activities going on around them. For some, such worry can almost become incapacitating as day-to-day responsibilities become harder to perform.
- Many hospitalized clients report difficulty obtaining adequate amounts of sleep. Sleep deprivation can lead to irritability, depression, disorientation, emotional lability, and physical exhaustion.
- Already present communication difficulties can be magnified when the client is in a new environment.

These factors cause concern if decisions regarding treatment need to be made by the client during these times. As nurses, we need to be able to assess for potential communication barriers. Consider:

COGNITIVE FUNCTION   Is the client alert and oriented? Does she or he have difficulty concentrating or following directions? What is his or her educational level? Does he or she speak and understand English? If not, what is the native language? Are there any auditory, visual, or neurological deficits that affect reception and processing of verbal and nonverbal communication cues?

AFFECTIVE BEHAVIOR   What is the general attitude? Has it changed? If so, in what way? Is the client calm and rested or angry and agitated? Upset? Does the client take an interest in what is happening around him or her and in the care routines?

SITUATIONAL CIRCUMSTANCES   Is the client in the midst of crisis? Severe fatigue or pain? Mr. Wiggins and his wife were very worried and embarrassed about the financial situation that resulted from Mr. Wiggins' prolonged illness. This added much additional stress to that of not knowing what was causing his illness. By addressing this stressor with the help of social services, more of his energy could then be directed toward getting better.

There are many situations in which family members are also overwhelmed. Lack of sleep, anxiety, and loss of familiar routines contribute to their decreased ability to communicate, similar to those stressors seen in the client. Stressors unique to the family can include coordination of child care and work schedules and home routines (laundry, meal preparation, shopping, and housekeeping) in addition to the need for time to be with the ill family member. This is magnified if it is the primary caregiver who is ill and young children are involved. Financial matters can be a major concern if the primary income earner is ill and has been depended on to take care of financial concerns or if both incomes were necessary to meet expenses. Single-parent families are particularly stressed when illness must be faced. Such stressors can be overwhelming, especially when illness is prolonged and if specific family roles had been very well defined and structured. This can lead to a variety of feelings that are expressed. Dealing with these feelings, especially ones perceived as negative, such as sadness or anger, can be quite difficult. Further discussion on how to talk with clients and families about their feelings can be found in Chapters 6 and 9.

There are many definitions of family today. Twenty years ago, a family was defined as persons related by blood or marriage. Even the legal system had its definition of family. Today, there are heterosexual and homosexual marriage relationships, divorced couples and single-parent family units, and common law arrangements. Although there is increasing acceptance of various definitions of family, it can be hard for some persons to accept alternative family relationships. In this book, "family" is defined as "caring significant others." A group of individuals who provide a support system for each other may say they are a family, and they are one, at least socially and emotionally. This support system is significant and must be recognized when providing care. However, such family units may not be recognized legally, and administrative guidance must be sought when clinical issues related to guardianship and next of kin occur.

In caring for clients, it is important to identify the family unit, who the caring others are in the situation, and who the spokesperson is overseeing the family unit. This may be one or several persons. When the client is unable to participate fully in his or her health care decisions, identify the family spokesperson. If the spokesperson is not a good communicator, has difficulty with the English language, or is having difficulty dealing with the situation, the nurse may have to diplomatically assist the spokesperson or identify others who can assist that person. Here are two examples of how this could be addressed:

Example

"Mrs. Link, you seem so overwhelmed and very tired. Who in your family could best assist you in keeping up with all you need to do? It would be very beneficial to have a relief person that could cover for you on a regular basis. This would allow you time to rest and take care of business, and still have continuity here at the hospital."

"Mr. Lopez, we need to communicate well so you understand what is happening to your wife. This is Mrs. Cortez, a medical interpreter who can translate for both of us."

Consider the family's comfort level. Does the family know how to visit? Have they ever visited a family member in the hospital before? Observe them as they enter the client's room. Do they move up close to the client or stand far away from the bed? Do they seem nervous or uneasy? How do they address the client? If family members seem uneasy or anxious, provide them with tips to make their visits more productive and enjoyable. Go in with them. Model for them how to talk to the client, whether the client is alert and oriented, disoriented, or comatose, and encourage them to do the same. Explain that familiar voices can be very soothing, even if the client cannot respond appropriately. The family may not know what to say when the client cannot communicate verbally. Tell them to talk as they normally would have before the illness. Suggest they talk about what is happening at home and what is happening with others in the family. Other activities include reading the newspaper or cards received. Explain what the bedside equipment is for and how they can safely touch the client. Many family members fear that if they touch or move anything, they will hurt the client. Provide as much privacy as possible.

Explore with the family members how involved they would like to be in the care of their loved one. Do they wish to do some of the care or do they prefer that

Clients at High Risk for Complex Psychosocial Needs
Elderly
Those living at home alone
Children abused, neglected, or with birth anomalies
Those transferred from another institution
Those heavily dependent on community resources
Multiple or recent readmissions
Clients with
Financial problems
Terminal illness
Out of country residency or poor command of English language
Care intensive disease, catastrophic illness, chronic illness
Multiple chronic illnesses
Newly diagnosed disease, or recent disabilities
Few or no visitors
Substance abuse problems
Suspected abuse (elderly, women)
Family problems
Psychiatric disorders
Poor living conditions

the staff do the care? Cultural customs or family roles may play a role in their decision. Fear of hurting the client or doing something wrong often may also contribute to the decision made. If the client was very ill at home for a period of time before admission, family members may be very fatigued and emotionally drained. Family member responses will vary and should be respected.

It is important to assess the client's and family's psychosocial status on an ongoing basis to identify client and family needs as they arise. Be sure to follow through with assisting them to learn about available support services and appropriate contact persons. Multidisciplinary team planning is a successful approach to providing this kind of assistance and is routinely done in most institutions and care agencies. A Red Flag List (box) has been developed to assist nursing staff identify clients at high risk for complex psychosocial needs and concerns that may need a more focused assessment (Rankin & Stallings, 1990).

Once identified, these clients and their families must be reassessed more frequently to identify needs early and intervene appropriately.

Environmental Factors Affecting Client Communication

Nurses face barriers to communication that originate from the type of practice environment they are in and its related performance expectations. It is helpful to acknowledge these factors and take steps to minimize the negative impact the environment can have on nurse-client communication. Environmental factors in an institutional setting vary greatly from those seen in the home setting. Each setting will be discussed separately.

Consider This Scenario *in an Institutional Environment*

Mrs. Tea was admitted last evening to a semiprivate room on a busy medical-surgical unit. She was very ill and was exhausted on admission. Her IV was started shortly after her arrival, multiple IV medications were being administered throughout the day and night, and an IV pump was being utilized. Staff members were very nice but always seemed to be in a hurry. She was in a bed nearest the door and bathroom. Whenever her roommate needed to use the bathroom, which she frequently needed to do, she had to pass right next to Mrs. Tea's bed. The roommate's spouse visited most of the day and evening. The frequent beeping of the alarm on the IV pump, the bathroom trips, and the light being left on were very irritating to her. As the night got later, Mrs. Tea just wanted to sleep. But the IV medication schedule required the nurse to be in the room frequently with the light on, and even though she was efficient and gentle, it still woke her.

"If I could just go home," she thought. By 3 a.m., she was in tears when the nurse came in with another dose of IV medication.

The nurse sat down. She took Mrs. Tea's hand and softly said, "What's wrong, Mrs. Tea?"

Mrs. Tea told her, "The lights, the pump noise, the busy hallway . . . there's no privacy or quiet . . . I'm so overwhelmed. . . . "

The nurse listened. She then said, "I am so glad you told me how you feel. I will see if there is another room with a bed available near the window that you could transfer into in the morning. That would give you a little more privacy and less interruptions. The IV schedule I can't change at present, but I will ask the doctor in the morning for a sleeping medication for use if you feel you need it tomorrow night. I have a few extra minutes, Mrs. Tea. Would you like a back rub to help you relax and possibly sleep for a few hours?" Mrs. Tea agreed to have a back rub. Afterward, the nurse closed the curtains around Mrs. Tea's bed as she left. When she checked back 30 minutes later, Mrs. Tea appeared to be sleeping. Those few extra minutes with Mrs. Tea were worth it.

This scenario presents several key environmental factors that affect clients in an institutional type setting:

- Limited privacy
- Noise or sensory overload
- Pace of unit activities

Limited Privacy

Most people want their own space. So, it is rather incongruous that when people often feel their worst, they receive a complete stranger for a roommate in a semiprivate room. Some problems seen with this type of arrangement are related to differences in roommates' needs and customs. One roommate may find lots of visitors and activity comforting when ill, whereas the other may prefer total quiet, privacy, and few visitors. Clients have very little, if any, control of their "new" environment. In Mrs. Tea's case, her being so close to the bathroom that her roommate needed to use frequently gave her very little private time in her new "space" within the hospital room. Nurses need to intervene when possible on clients' behalf to make their environment as comfortable as possible, as occurred in the scenario. If this is not possible, it is important to assist clients in meeting their needs in spite of the environment.

With the increasing public awareness of contagious diseases, many clients are concerned about "catching something" while hospitalized. They may perceive their roommate as a source of disease, especially if discussion about a disease is over-heard. If such feelings are suspected, the nurse could say, "You seem concerned about possibly coming down with another disease while you are here. You can lessen that possibility by not sharing care items and making sure the bathroom is clean before you use it. Tell us if it needs cleaning." After morning care, be sure bathrooms are checked and ensure the environment is kept neat and clean. When-ever possible, discuss client information in private. Use private conference rooms when available for client/family discussions related to illness and care.

Noise/Sensory Overload

Simply being in a hospital environment has an impact on many people. Some have a fear of hospitals and do not even want to enter one. The sights, sounds, equip-ment, and overall environment can cause considerable sensory overload. When a person is ill, such sensory stimulation can easily be overwhelming. For Mrs. Tea, the sense of being overwhelmed built up gradually. The frequent interruptions and the fatigue finally took their toll.

It is easier for nurses to block out some of the sensory bombardment because of the business of the unit and tasks to get done, but for clients who are primarily bedfast, there is no "getting away." When clients are overwhelmed, they may react by lashing out or withdrawing, or they may have difficulty thinking clearly. Mrs. Tea held in her feelings until fatigue won and she broke into tears. It is important to note and respond to such feelings of the client. This helps defuse them and provides the opportunity for the client to talk about them if she or he so chooses. The nurse responded immediately when she noticed Mrs. Tea was crying. Her sitting down and touching her hand conveyed concern and respect for Mrs. Tea's feelings, which was reinforced as she allowed Mrs. Tea to express them. She enhanced Mrs. Tea's ability to rest by giving her a back rub and providing privacy.

Modifying the environment whenever possible, such as pulling the curtains around the bed, helps to decrease or control sensory stimulation. In this scenario, it also provided the client with a sense of her own private space, something very important for Mrs. Tea. If hall noise is a problem, closing the door may help. Some institutions have quiet times throughout the day to provide a quiet rest time on busy units, usually in early afternoon and mid to late evening. Equipment alarm volume may be adjustable; check equipment instructions and agency policies re-garding this. Clients may not understand what equipment alarms mean, which contributes to client stress. When a piece of equipment with an alarm is used, make sure that the client or family members understand its purpose, what the alarms mean, and what should they do when an alarm activates.

Pace of Activities

Nurses sometimes believe that good communication takes time, a rare commodity on a busy unit. If nurses do not believe they have time to communicate with their clients, then they feel like something is missing, and they are right. Even though the nurse may be short on time, she or he must find ways to interact productively with their clients as they move through the day. A skilled nurse is able to meet most client/nurse communication needs as other tasks are carried out. The nurse caring for Mrs.

Tea seized the moment when Mrs. Tea started to cry, listened, helped her to relax, and explored relocation options with her. The effectiveness of this short, but important, time with Mrs. Tea was reflected in her ability to get some rest.

It is important to understand that the pace of a unit does not necessarily determine the extent to which client/staff communication is valued, but it can impact client and staff perceptions of the types of activities that are most important. These perceptions are then either reinforced or changed depending on their experiences on the unit. When clients perceive staff members as being very busy, they can be very hesitant to express their feelings or ask questions. However, if staff members are busy and yet still are sensitive to and respond to clients' expressed feelings, such as the nurse did with Mrs. Tea, clients will feel more at ease about discussing their concerns. The same situation can occur with staff members. If staff members tend to measure their productivity by the number and speed with which tasks are done, their care focus tends to be primarily getting things done, whereas if the focus is more client centered and flexible, based on client needs, they tend to be more client focused. Often, as student nurses rotate through a variety of clinical settings in a relatively short amount of time, they sense these differences in approaches to care and unit activities.

Consider This Scenario *in a Home Care Setting*

Ms. Catalbo was on her way to her initial home visit with Mr. Osaka and his family. Mr. Osaka had just come home from the hospital where he had been given care after an acute stroke. The referral the nurse had received from the hospital nurse indicated he was very independent in nature and was frustrated when he was unable to do his own care and when restrained for safety reasons. The residual effects of the stroke left him with complete left-sided paralysis. He returned to his daughter's home, where he had been living for the past several years.

On entering the home, Ms. Catalbo was greeted by Mr. Osaka's daughter, who seemed somewhat bewildered. "I am so glad to see you. The two days he's been home have been hard."

Ms. Catalbo introduced herself and said, "It can be very hard to care for someone who has just been brought home from the hospital." She noticed the house was very quiet and her client was not in the living room. "Is Mr. Osaka awake?"

His daughter said, "No, he just fell asleep. It seems so unkind to say this, but I really enjoy these quiet times. Just to have a cup of tea without interruption is so nice."

Ms. Catalbo noticed how tired she looked. "Why don't we just talk a bit before I see your father. Your input is very helpful to me in assessing how I can be of most assistance to you and him. Would that be all right?"

"Oh, yes. Come into the kitchen. Do call me Kay. Would you like some tea with me?" the daughter replied.

"That would taste good," Ms. Catalbo said as she followed her into the kitchen. As she sat down in the chair Kay offered her, she continued, "Tell me how Mr. Osaka has been and how you have managed since he came home from the hospital."

This scenario helps illustrate how home care is different from institutional care. Major differences are:

- Home care nurse as "guest"
- Flexibility is mandatory
- Nursing takes on more independent role

Home Care Nurse as "Guest"

"Control belongs to clients in the home, a fact that must always be kept in mind. The nurse may be the deliverer of care, but the setting is borrowed and every interaction is negotiated with respect to this. As a result, nursing's power base differs; this piece alone is often nursing's greatest adjustment" (Stulginsky, 1993a and 1993b). Just as each individual has personal space that must be respected, families, too, have their spaces that must be respected and entered into slowly and thoughtfully. There are times when the family space is closely guarded and the nurse may not be invited into it very far. Remember, clients are free to accept or reject the services the nurse has to offer.

The initial contact with the client and family can affect how well the relationship develops over time. The nurse needs to be very astute to the needs of those involved. The client's and family's perceptions of their needs take priority over how the nurse views them, at least initially, until the whole picture can be seen and evaluated by the nurse. This does not mean the nurse is all things to all clients, but it allows time to learn what their perspective is and to assess overall priorities and care problems. Only then can resources be aligned to meet the situation's demands. In the scenario, Ms. Catalbo was interested in seeing the client, but in meeting with the daughter first, it became clear to her that the daughter had some concerns related to caring for her father. With the client asleep and the daughter needing some quiet time, she switched her focus to the daughter. She took advantage of the opportunity for them to get to know each other and discuss the daughter's concerns.

By taking time with Kay, Ms. Catalbo also validated the importance of Kay's feelings. She acknowledged this when she stated it is hard to care for someone just home from the hospital and then took the time to learn about those "two days," thus reinforcing her concern for Kay as the caregiver. This concern lays the groundwork for a good client/family/nurse working relationship. It is out of growing rapport and trust and exchange of feelings and ideas that exploration of care options and willingness to try new approaches can occur (Stulginsky, 1993a and 1993b).

Flexibility is Mandatory

No two clients, nor homes, nor care expectations, nor routines are ever the same. In the hospital setting, there is a certain amount of control over the activities of the day. Each unit and shift has "routines" that are followed. In the home care setting, each visit brings different ground rules and routines based on the individual client situations. This requires an ability to shift gears very frequently and to be realistic about what can be accomplished (Stulginsky, 1993a and 1993b). Client and family priorities often take precedence, as indicated in the above scenario. Ms. Catalbo demonstrated flexibility while still maintaining clinical effectiveness. Many times, immediate needs of food and shelter come first and health care ranks down the list. The nurse may go to a home and find the client has no money to purchase his medications, is very ill, and cannot get into a clinic for 2 weeks. Their lives can be as complicated as their care. "What am I going to do now?" is a question that the client might ask the nurse (Carr, 1993), and one that the nurse may ask herself or himself. The ability to deal successfully with acute needs that often occur unexpectedly and still maintain a focus on the overall plan of care requires flexibility and resourcefulness on the nurse's part.

Nursing Takes On a More Independent Role

In an institutional setting, many resources are established within the system and can be tapped during care when supportive services are needed. In home care, supportive services are not readily accessible. Phone calls can be made when necessary, but on-site persons to assist the nurse are not a reality. Problem solving becomes more independent in nature. Ongoing accurate assessments are vital in problem identification and appropriate intervention. Knowledge of communication behaviors and cues and the ability to communicate well with clients, families, and supportive and health care team members are tools the nurse must use to maximize the accuracy of these assessments and thus the appropriateness of the interventions. See Chapter 13 for a more detailed discussion of home care issues.

In Conclusion: Importance of Client's Expectations

How successful nurses are in providing competent, coordinated, quality care depends greatly on the extent to which the *client's* expectations were met. "It's not enough to provide excellent quality medical and nursing care if the [client] doesn't perceive it as such. Our first task as nurses is to understand who our [clients] are and what they expect from us" (Messner, 1993). So much hinges on your ability to communicate well with clients, families, and colleagues. Here is a summary of what client satisfaction surveys reveal is important from the client's point of view (Messner, 1993):

1. Listen to clients: they tell us what they need.
2. Don't dismiss their concerns.
3. Treat clients like people, not like a disease.
4. Talk to clients, not at them. Make eye contact; let them know who you are.
5. Respect client privacy.
6. Explain delays in treatments, test results, and respond to their requests.
7. Assist the client in understanding what he or she needs to know or do, how to do it, and why, in a way that is meaningful.
8. Keep the client informed and involved in evaluating progress.
9. Remember: clients are individuals.
10. Let clients know you care and look out for them.

PRACTICAL APPLICATIONS

1. Choose a partner and decide who will be the client and who will be the nurse. In a simulated laboratory setting, the client puts on a gown and gets into a hospital bed. The nurse then interviews and does a basic physical assessment of the client. As the client, consider how it feels to be in attire and surroundings in the client role; what does it feel like giving personal information to the nurse? How did you feel during the physical assessment?

    As the nurse, how comfortable did you feel asking the client personal information questions? How did the client respond? How did client responses and comfort level affect your ongoing line of questioning? Did the client seem at ease or uncomfortable? What behaviors tell you so? Consider your questions: were they open? closed? What nonverbal behaviors did you display? How at ease did you feel doing the physical assessment activity? Why?

Switch roles.

2. Choose a partner to be the client. You are about to start an intravenous line in your client. Explain to him or her what you are about to do. Your partner is to listen and write down the clinical words or jargon you used in your explanation. Do you think a real client would have understood? Switch roles and explain a different procedure.

3. In a clinical setting, assume an observer role. First, stand near the nurse's station. For the next 15 minutes, record the number and types of personnel interactions with the unit secretary or the charge nurse at the desk. Note how many times the phone rings, the page/call system is used, and visitors ask questions. What kinds of verbal and nonverbal behaviors are exhibited by the secretary and nurse? What is the atmosphere at the desk area? How would you approach the people at the desk? Compare your experience with that of a fellow student who did the same activity on a different unit. How do you feel this activity will influence your behavior as you enter client care settings in the future?

REFERENCES

American Nurses Association. (1985). *Code for nurses with interpretive statements*. Kansas City.

Annas, G. (1989). *The rights of patients* (2nd ed.). Carbondale: Southern Illinois University Press.

Beck, C. (1993). Caring relationships between nursing students and their patients. *Nurse Educator, 18*(5), 28–29.

Benner, P. (1984). *From novice to expert: Power and excellence in clinical nursing practice*. Menlo Park: Addison-Wesley.

Bourhis, R., Roth, S., & MacQueen, G. (1989). Communication in the hospital setting: A survey of medical and everyday language use amongst patients, nurses, and doctors. *Social Science Medicine, 28*, 339–346.

Bradley, J., & Edinberg, M. (1982). *Communication in the nursing context* (p. 346). New York: Appleton-Century-Crofts.

Campbell-Heider, N., & Hart, C. (1993). Updating the nurse's bedside manner. *Image, 25*(2), 133–139.

Carr, P. (1993, November). Home care: "What am I going to do now?" *American Journal of Nursing, 93*(11), 24.

Jarvis, C. (1992). *Physical examination and health assessment* (p. 71). Philadelphia: W. B. Saunders.

Messner, R. (1993, August). What patients really want from their nurses. *American Journal of Nursing, 93*(8), 38.

Siegler, E., & Whitney, F. (Eds.). (1994). *Nurse-physician collaboration: Care of adults and elderly* (pp. 4–5). New York: Springer.

Stulginsky, M. (1993a, October). Nurses' home health experience, Part I: The practice setting. *Nursing and Health Care, 14*(10), 405–406.

Stulginsky, M. (1993b, November). Nurses' home health experience, Part II: The unique demands of home visits. *Nursing and Health Care, 14*(1), 477.

Tanner, C., Benner, P., Chesla, C., & Gordon, D. (1993, Winter). The phenomenology of knowing the patient. *Image: Journal of Nursing Scholarship, 25*(4), 273–280.

Zerwekh, J., & Claborn, J. C. (1994). *Nursing Today, Transition and Trends* (p. 299). Philadelphia: W. B. Saunders.

Zungolo, E. (1994). Interdisciplinary education in primary care: The challenge. *Nursing and Health Care, 15*(6), 288–292.

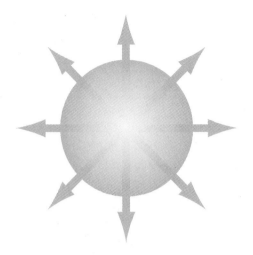

4

With Culturally Diverse People

In this chapter, we will discuss:

- What is culture?
- Why is transcultural understanding vital to nursing?
- What are cultural differences and similarities across the major cultural groups in the United States?
- What approaches should be taken when communicating with those of a different culture?

What Is Culture?

Culture is a learned and distinct dynamic way of viewing yourself, your life activities, and the world. Immediately after you are born and gradually through interacting with others close to you, distinct patterns of speech and language, attitudes, and social behaviors develop. These gradually become an integral part of you and are reflected in characteristics of your family and social group as a whole. Each of us is, then, a member of a general cultural group that displays a certain set of behaviors and values unique to that group. Certain factors, however, can affect our individual behaviors and perceptions, including:

- Region
- Family structure
- Occupation
- Gender
- Travel
- Socioeconomic level
- Political viewpoints
- Ethnicity
- Education
- Age
- Social activities
- Peers
- Geographical location of our homes

Sometimes sociologists study larger groups to identify group or subgroup patterns or behaviors that can determine public policies. Study results can also help establish group identities. When this is done, however, the risk of stereotyping persons and groups is high. We must not assume all persons within an identified specific group will think, act, and feel exactly the same way. All members of a group may have many other subgroup affiliations that impact their behaviors, beliefs, attitudes, and perceptions (Jarvis, 1992). Subcultural groups that have received much media attention include homosexuals, youth gangs, baby boomers, generation X'ers and homeless persons.

People tend to make assumptions about cultural groups or subgroups based on either experiences and information gained from various sources (articles, television, books, videos, stories, etc.), which may be biased, or lack of experiences with others different from themselves. Such assumptions are based on the belief that one's own perspective and cultural norms are correct. This assumption is called ethnocentrism. It can lead to cultural imposition, in which one's own cultural beliefs and ways, because they are thought to be right or the best, are forced upon others, without recognition or knowledge of the different culture (Leininger, 1978, 1991). Taken to an extreme, cultural imposition can lead to feelings of distrust and even fear of those who are different from oneself.

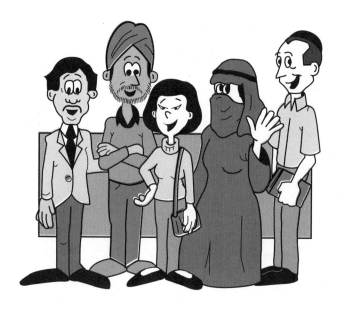

Table 4–1 QUESTIONS TO HELP YOU GET IN TOUCH WITH YOUR CULTURE

1. What family roles do you have? How were these roles established?
2. How do you carry out your gender role? What expectations are linked to your gender role? Why?
3. What are your religious beliefs? Customs? Are they the same as those of your parents? If not, how are they different? Why?
4. What holidays do you and your family celebrate? How are they celebrated? What traditions do you carry out?
5. How are elders addressed and cared for in your family?
6. What are your mealtimes like? Who prepares the food? What food is enjoyed? What kind of communication occurs during mealtime?
7. What kind of education have you experienced? Schools? Grade level? Travel?
8. What is your ethnic background? What activities or personal practices do you relate to it? Are your practices similar to those of your parents or relatives?
9. Do you live in an area where most people are of similar background and experiences?
10. Do you speak a language other than English? If so, how did you learn it?
11. How do you like to dress? Why?
12. What health practices have you learned through your family and relatives? Do you use them? Why?

Interestingly, often cultural assumptions are made without thinking, as reflected in this brief exchange:

"Mommy, why do we do things the way we do?"
"Well, because that's the way it is—it is the right way."

Two things make true communication impossible: (a) lack of understanding another's cultural ways and beliefs and (b) lack of seeing the importance of understanding another's cultural ways and beliefs.

The important first step toward increasing your cultural awareness and understanding of other cultures is to explore your own culture. Table 4–1 contains questions that will help you identify your own cultural beliefs and behavior patterns. Once you realize the many factors that have made you the person you are now, you can begin to appreciate how others from varying backgrounds may act and think differently than you do. Only then are you able to see your own prejudices.

Why Is Transcultural Understanding Vital to Nursing?

Consider this quote by a prominent leader in transcultural nursing:

By the year 2010, it is reasonable to predict that nurses and other health personnel will be interacting with clients, families, and other health consumers from virtually every place in the world. Many of these "cultural strangers" will necessitate new kinds of knowledge related to transcultural nursing. No longer will nurses be focusing primarily on heart, kidney, and medical disease pathologies, but with people whose lifeways, living conditions, stresses, and concerns are transculturally based. Nurses will be required to provide truly holistic care informed by knowledge of different world views and environmental conditions. Increasing numbers of travelers, immigrants, and cultural groups to the United States and to other countries in the world will make most nurses want to make accurate holistic care assessments, nursing care decisions, and to respond confidently with these cultural strangers (Leininger, 1994).

This is quite a challenge.

This demand for culture-sensitive care is already occurring in some areas and will continue to increase. Consider these trends:

- Racial minorities (African-Americans and Hispanic-Americans) are gradually becoming growing majorities in some cities in the United States.
- White males already comprise less than half the labor force.
- By the year 2005, three fifths of children will be from minority groups (Malone, 1993).

With these increasing demands for transcultural care skills, it is becoming evident that staff inabilities to deal with a wide mix of languages, cultures, and backgrounds are creating barriers to effective care (Hagland, Sabatino, & Sherer, 1993). More specifically, in nursing, these difficulties have led to an inability to develop therapeutic relationships with clients, which has led to major areas of frustration and stress (Murphy & Clark, 1993). There is also underrepresentation of minorities, i.e., black, Hispanic, Asian, Native American, and Alaskan Native, in the health professions, which limits first-hand professional expertise in cultural-based care (Bureau of the Census, 1990; Rosella, Regan-Dubinski, & Albrecht, 1994). Even when nurses of different cultural backgrounds work side by side, there has been limited sharing of cultural beliefs and practices (Burrows, 1983).

Gradually, concepts of cultural diversity are being introduced into nursing educational programs, and positive attempts are being made to identify a variety of approaches that are successful in increasing transcultural sensitivity and care (Bernal, 1993; Eliason & Macy, 1992; Rooda & Gay, 1993; Smith, Colling & Elander, 1993). As a member of the nursing profession, you will be faced with a challenge and an opportunity to redefine your world view and see clients and their lifeways from an entirely new and broadened perspective. To be open to this challenge you must be open to:

- New understandings of what health care is
- Where, when, how, why, and by whom health care is carried out
- Evaluation of care effectiveness across cultural boundaries
- The similarities and differences between cultures

Knowledge and insight gained from this holistic approach will help you provide care that maximizes the "assets or strengths of your client's culture that keep them well and prevent illness" (Leininger, 1991).

What Are Cultural Differences and Similarities Across the Major Cultural Groups in the United States?

Presently, the dominant cultural group in the United States consists of white, middle class Protestants, typically those whose ancestors came from northern Europe two or more generations ago. From this background has come the dominant values of individuality, material wealth, comfort, humanitarianism, physical beauty, democracy, newness, cleanliness, education, science, achievement, free enterprise, punctuality, rationality, independence, respectability, self-discipline, effort, and progress (Herberg, 1989). However, there are numerous subcultures within this overall culture, as well as other cultural groups increasing in the population, that provide the rich diversity of people, ways, and customs in the United States. With such diversity comes the challenges of understanding and appreciating the lifeways of these various and ever-changing groups without stereotyping them. This section presents a general overview of cultural practices and belief patterns that may be seen in major cultural groups in the United States. Such information is intended to provide a framework for appreciating the uniqueness of each group and the varying degrees of commonalities between them. Culture has great impact on a person's view of "appropriate" approaches to health, wellness, illness, and death. To be effective as a health care provider, you must become aware of and use cultural information as you interact with and provide care for clients of diverse backgrounds. It is a valuable base from which to work.

Table 4–2 addresses practices and beliefs (relating to health, approach to illness, family structure, communication, and perceptions of the health team and time) of the cultural groups often encountered in the United States. Not all members of the identified cultural group will necessarily practice or profess the beliefs indicated, or they may do so in a selective way. With clients of a different background, it is wise to explore the degree to which they and their family members participate in culture-specific practices and beliefs. This tells them their culture is recognized and valued, and it will help prevent misunderstanding.

What Approaches Should Be Taken When Communicating With Those of a Different Culture?

"Members of a profession whose concern is with the health of the whole person and who use themselves as a means of healing have a particular obligation to understand the world, both around and inside them" (Rogers, 1988). This statement focuses our discussion very well. To communicate with others who are different from ourselves requires our initiative to learn as much as possible about:

- Oneself and one's beliefs, values, concerns, support system, language, customs, and perceptions of a given situation
- Other persons and their beliefs, values, concerns, support system, language, customs, and perceptions of a given situation

It is in this learning process of understanding what you do, why you do it, and what you expect from an interaction with another that you learn to appreciate and value why others have their own way of behaving the way they do. These behaviors may be totally different, but the appreciation that there are reasons for a person's behaviors is invaluable insight. The information in Table 4–2 gives clues to what might be the reasons behind certain cultural behaviors. The information can facilitate interactions that are more sensitive and open to the needs, concerns, and behavior of clients. If, when reading through Table 4–2, you react to the information with impatience, disbelief, or dislike, then the opportunity to explore those reactions and consider possible reasons why they occurred is yours. It is in the examination of such reactions that true participation in cultural awareness occurs.

Table 4–2 CULTURAL COMPARISONS OF MAJOR ETHNIC GROUPS IN AMERICA

Group	Practices and Belief Patterns
African-American	*Health.*—Varied, with acute care focus for many; illness may be viewed as related to bad luck, chance, domestic problems, poverty, violence or unemployment; some lack understanding of or have misconceptions about biomedical approaches that limit their seeking medical attention. *Approaches to illness.*—Home care remedies often tried first before seeking medical care; biomedical; culture/folk practitioners, as above. Cost of private health care often prohibits preventative health care; may have beliefs or understandings about biomedical interventions (true or not) or past experiences with acute care systems that impact greatly on health care decision making. *Family structure, roles.*—Mixed, often matriarchal, single-parent family structure; grandmother may be decision maker and primary caretaker of children. Women often find support in each other. *Communication patterns.*—Touch: common with family, extended family members; language: black English speech dialects have much cultural value but can contribute to lack of understanding or misunderstanding when interaction occurs with those outside their cultural group. *Interaction with health team.*—Use of nonstandard English may make accurate history taking difficult for health care providers not familiar with dialect and may make client understanding of care instructions problematic; may not feel comfortable relating home care remedies tried before medical attention for fear of being misunderstood or criticized. *Time perception.*—Varies; some groups focus mainly on present, others more future and goal oriented.
Chinese	*Health.*—Health promotion important; attribute upset in body energy to cause of disease and health as state of spiritual and physical harmony with nature; may resist surgery because of belief they do not own their bodies, that soul will escape from body and be lost forever; may refuse blood to be drawn because of belief blood does not regenerate and is source of life; taking medications when feeling well may be alien cencept to some; mental illness stigmatized. *Approaches to illness.*—Holistic; traditional; includes moxibustion, acupuncture, herbal medicine. *Family structure, roles.*—Very strong sense of family and community; family unit more important than individual; elderly have high status, cared for by children; young defer to old in decision making; roles based on age, gender, generation; expanding roles and status of women. Father/son and mother/son relationships strong; eldest son responsible for all arrangements for deceased parent; both parents make decisions regarding children; children taught to be unselfish and function competitively within a group. *Communication pattern.*—Touch: not accustomed to being touched by strangers; nod or slight bow acknowledges introductions; eye contact: lateral gaze, avoidance of direct eye contact when listening is polite and respectful; direct contact may be used with elderly; personal space: increased, greater than arm's length; language: silence may mean speaker wants listener to think about what has been said before continuing; pain: strong negative feelings and emotions suppressed (considered sign of weakness); because it is considered improper to accept something first time it is offered, pain relief medications may need to be offered more than once. *Interaction with health team.*—Health care providers authority figures; may not express concern or seek information regarding treatments or care; polite and may express thoughts indirectly. *Time perception.*—Tend to have a patient, inexact, broad sense of time; plan for the future.
Eastern Indian	*Health.*—Acute sick care only; diseases believed to be caused by upset in body balance. *Approaches to illness.*—Biomedical, traditional; strong spiritual values; males often receive preferential treatment. *Family structure, roles.*—Unquestioned obedience to elders expected; women dependent in traditional families, some educated, and more involved in decisions; male children very desirable; children rarely praised to avoid evil eye; Sikh religion forbids shaving of body hair, turbans worn; older women have higher prestige. *Communication patterns.*—Touch: handshakes between men only; women may be greeted by men with palms together and slight bow; upper arms and shoulders never bared; eye contact: direct contact considered disrespectful, an invasion of privacy; pain: quiet acceptance of pain; pain relief medications accepted; language: head motions for "yes" and "no" opposite than those used in U.S.; avoid saying "no" directly. *Interaction with health team.*—Terminal illness may be shared by professionals with family but not client; nurses may not be able to influence health care decisions of clients and work under medical or nontechnical persons. *Time perception.*—Mainly past oriented; promptness may not be valued.

Table 4–2   CULTURAL COMPARISONS OF MAJOR ETHNIC GROUPS IN AMERICA *Continued*

Group	Practices and Belief Patterns
Filipino	*Health.*—Acute sick care; health promotion important; mental illness highly stigmatized; some believe evil eye can be cast upon someone through eyes or mouth; "quackdoctor" completely accepted folk health practitioner.
	Approaches to illness.—Biomedical; magico-religious; home remedies, professional providers, and traditional healers consulted; belief in powers of gods, fatalism by some.
	Family structure, roles.—Family dominant; protection, reciprocity, dependency, harmony are group values; shared, rather than private, possessions are valued. Client often protected from being told of poor prognosis to avoid more suffering; family emotional display of grief may come after the death of a loved one.
	Communication patterns.—Touch: some believe evil eye can be neutralized on child by putting small amount of saliva on finger and making sign of the cross on child's forehead when giving child a compliment; touch is stressed; pain: may appear stoic, believing pain is will of God and He will give them strength to bear it; an invitation must be extended more than once and accepted reluctantly, and when offering pain medication, the offer may need to be repeated; eye contact: some may fear eye contact; if established, it is important to return and maintain eye contact.
	Interaction with health team.—Authority and professional time respected, used only if problem considered serious; nurses may carry out rather than question physician order; client very hesitant to give a "no" answer, may remain quiet; intermediary may be used for confrontations; family may want to participate in client care.
	Time perception.—For many, life is lived on day-to-day basis.
Haitian	*Health.*—Passive, acute sick care only; health promotion important; fatalistic attitude may be present; may compare signs and symptoms with those experienced by close relative.
	Approaches to illness.—Biomedical, magico-religious; Western medicine sought more often than traditional; belief in voodoo, prayer, and healing, protective power of God important; ethnomedical beliefs about disease based on maintenance of hot/cold balance within body; herbal treatment of common disorders; specialist called in for treatment of evil eye; religious experiences are integral part of regaining mental health. Culture/folk practitioners: spiritualists assist with financial, personal, spiritual, or physical problems, predominantly in urban communities; voodoo priests(esses) or hougans (mambos) are knowledgeable about herbal properties, interpret signs/omens, cure illness caused by voodoo, use communication techniques to establish therapeutic environment like a psychiatrist.
	Family structure/roles.—Extended family mutually supportive, emphasis on family and kinship more than individuals; a conjugal mate rather than spouse relationship common, and women often bear major responsibility for caring for family members, multiple caretakers common; males often rely on migratory and unsteady work, but still have much pride and sense of obligation to family; siblings close even after marriage; strict treatment of children, asking questions or seeking information from parents can be considered disrespectful of authority; reluctant to discuss sex education or reproduction with non-Haitian health care professionals.
	Communication patterns.—Pain expression: high tolerance for pain, discomfort; eye contact: customary to hold eye contact with all except poor; language: French, Creole, English; barriers may exist.
	Interaction with health team.—Physician primary authority, nurses subordinate in hospital settings; if nurse only health professional available, given more respect; family involved in care given.
	Time perception.—Punctuality not highly valued; society predominantly present oriented, but there is hope for future.
Iraqi	*Health.*—Although acceptance of God's will prevails, Islamic religion influences health behaviors; alcohol and illicit drug use prohibited, cleanliness and moderation stressed, family and elder care and family support stressed.
	Approaches to illness.—Biomedical, one or more persons may accompany client and wish to be present for all exams, and eldest may answer questions for client; demanding behavior, extreme concern for and attentiveness to client are expected family behaviors; special burial rituals, no cremation; exemption from fasting during month of Ramadan is permitted with pregnancy, breastfeeding, old age or illness on advice of physician; Muslim practices and rituals should be incorporated into care if possible (prayer five times daily, facing Mecca, avoidance of pork, fasting, days of observance); hope, optimism, and advantages of treatment are emphasized; negative effects or outcomes are minimized.

Table continued on following page

Table 4–2   CULTURAL COMPARISONS OF MAJOR ETHNIC GROUPS IN AMERICA *Continued*

Group	Practices and Belief Patterns
	Family structure, roles.—Patriarchal; sexual inequities part of legal system, females inferior but exercise power in domestic area; families encouraged to have many children.
	Communication patterns.—Touch: touch, closeness, and embracing on arrival and departure common; pain: expressed quietly to close friend or relative; relief expected immediately and may request relief measures persistently; believe in energy conservation for healing, thus any treatment requiring exertion may be contraindicated.
	Perceptions of health team.—Caregivers/examiners of same gender greatly preferred or demanded; nursing viewed by some as female profession of low status and negative image; reasons for asking personal questions need to be made clear; eldest person present expects to be included in discussion; belief that information may cause needless worry or concern (i.e., prognosis, side effects of drugs, possible risks of therapy, or full disclosure of medical diagnosis) requires appropriateness of routine client education practices be explored with the physician on an individual basis when working with clients of this background; see approaches to illness above.
	Time perception.—Oriented to present, planning ahead may defy God's will; punctuality not important; establishment of relationships before talking business important.
Israeli	*Health.*—Passive beliefs, health self care not prevalent; religion part of daily lives; acute sick care primarily; assertiveness and toughness acceptable health care team behavior.
	Approaches to illness.—Biomedical; holistic; medical and surgical procedures not done on Sabbath or holy days if condition nonthreatening; many prayers for the sick and for hope are in Jewish liturgy and use encouraged; rabbi official representative and counsel may be sought regarding Jewish traditions; strict male observer of faith may wish to keep prayer shawl, cap, and special symbols with him; prayers often chanted and privacy desired during prayer; care of body after death and burial rituals are followed; dietary restrictions (no pork or predatory fowl, milk and meat dishes never mixed, fish only with scales, fins allowed, some special preparations required, kosher foods) followed during illness if possible.
	Family structure, roles.—Attentive, supportive; close family unit; strong religious community support.
	Communication patterns.—Touch: demonstrative; pain: descriptive adjectives used; may be way to get help, sympathy.
	Perception of health team.—Assertiveness and toughness of health care team acceptable; it is expected that medical care be sought when illness occurs.
	Time perception.—Present orientation.
Japanese	*Health.*—May place physical diseases in context of client's social relations.
	Approaches to illness.—Magico-religious; may consult with priests to seek luck and avoid evil before important activities or decisions; biomedical approaches also accepted by some. Family often participate in care of client, family interdependence highly valued, so self-care may not be seen as a valued concept.
	Family structure, role.—Women traditionally passive, domesticated, have power in child rearing, budgeting, achieving educational success; parents expect to be cared for in old age; mother-child relationships strong; respect for authority and collaborative decision making taught; traditional patterns changing.
	Communication patterns.—Touch: handshakes acceptable, pat on back is not; not accustomed to physical contact; greeting often in form of bow, the lower and longer the greeting bow, the more respect conveyed; personal space: increased, more than arm's length; eye contact: direct contact considered a personal affront, lack of respect, invasion of privacy; prefer lateral or shifting gaze; pain: stoically withstand pain; control public expression of grief; language: may divert subject away from embarrassing topic or to avoid direct confrontation; verbal agreement indicates understanding, not agreement; will avoid saying no directly; silence—see Chinese; may use third-party mediator to make complaints or address them indirectly; laughter a common sign of embarrassment, masks bereavement, and conceals rage; happiness concealed with straight face.
	Interaction with health team.—Respect for social rank generally pervasive; titles may be used rather than names; physician expected to know best and use good judgment; thoughts expressed indirectly and listener expected to understand.
	Time perception.—Promptness valued.

Table 4–2 CULTURAL COMPARISONS OF MAJOR ETHNIC GROUPS IN AMERICA *Continued*

Group	Practices and Belief Patterns
Mexican	*Health.*—Passive role, acute sick care only; health often believed to be chance or God's will; disease influenced by hot/cold imbalance; males often perceived as healthier than women or children.

Approaches to illness.—Biomedical; magico-religious; traditional; common beliefs include mal ojo (evil eye); empacho (bolus of food stuck to stomach wall, what may be considered as an intestinal blockage, constipation, bloating, indigestion, other gastrointestinal disorders); susto (results from a traumatic emotional event, fright); mal puesto (hex or illness imposed by another); mal aire (bad air, exposure to drafts, cold air can cause serious illness, death). Self-medication is widely practiced. Curanderas are often seen to assist with healing. These women cure with their minds, their experience, their hands (often massage), and herbs. Warmth and sincere caring for others very important in their work. Migrant worker population faces language, transportation, and access problems when health care is needed.

Often deep mistrust of the system exists, and beating the system can be seen as a diversion and not viewed as wrong. Loyalty to friends and family takes priority over the establishment and adherence to rules. Some believe material success is associated with socioeconomic privilege, good political relations on the job, luck, and favoritism, rather than hard work. This can contribute to stoic acceptance and fatalism.

Family structure, roles.—Family an enduring support system; distinct gender roles based on mix of culture and heritage; patriarchal; father-newborn bonding not always considered appropriate; mother in charge of household; male to be consulted before decisions are made and are included in all counseling sessions; culturally, mother is not allowed authority to give consent for child's treatment but often decides when care should be sought; family decisions can overrule health care provider decisions; women may not be allowed to give care at home that involves touching male genitalia. Women who work are often expected to continue traditional responsibilities at home. Children are expected to respect and obey elders and are shielded from dying and death rituals. Godparents named at child's baptism are very significant in the care of the child, with lifelong bonds. Family members stay around the clock in the hospital with dying family member. Disruption in social relationships or cultural rules can impact physical and emotional health.

Communication patterns.—Consideration of feelings of others and human interaction is most important aspect of a meeting. Touch: often used, especially between those of the same sex; touching people while complimenting them prevents power of evil eye in believers; touching arm or shoulder when making a point is sign of rapport or trust; modesty and privacy valued; handshaking common when greeting or saying goodbye; eye contact: sustained, direct contact considered rude, immodest, or dangerous for some, mal ojo results from excessive admiration and women and children are most susceptible (both may avoid eye contact if believers); personal space: closer than usual; language: English and Spanish very common; pain: both emotional restraint and emotional expression are seen; grief can be very expressive.

Perceptions of health team.—Practitioner may be viewed as outsider; family interdependence may supercede independence, so self-care may not be a valued concept; personal matters handled within the family; curandero or folk healer is often a member of family network; practitioners are expected to be friendly, informal, include family in discussions and explanations, take time to listen and inquire about ill person's health, and if possible in some instances, be the same gender as the client.

Time perception.—Predominantly present oriented, relaxed, flexible concept; interpretation of appointment and arrival times can vary; meetings often have no designated ending times, allowing them to move at more leisurely pace and run their course; if meetings overlap, the first meeting and its process usually take priority; social functions usually have half-hour window for arrival.

Table continued on following page

Table 4–2   CULTURAL COMPARISONS OF MAJOR ETHNIC GROUPS IN AMERICA *Continued*

Group	Practices and Belief Patterns
Native American	*Health.*—Person composed of physical, psychological, and spiritual aspects with powerful sense of real connectedness to the earth and other spirits; balance of these aspects has great impact on one's health and well-being, with spiritual aspect playing a powerful part in illness and healing; health viewed as harmony with the universe.
	Approaches to illness.—Holistic healing; Western and Native American medicine often used to maintain or regain health; hesitance to share folk ways for fear of being misunderstood possible; community members' presence and prayer very important when illness occurs, and open visitation highly valued; ceremonies often carried out to assist client via self-empowerment to restore personal harmony and balance, often done through vibrations (chants and sings), rhythm and sound, prayerful ceremonies, and use of herbs.
	Family structure, roles.—Strong family and tribal ties; special life cycle often marked by specific ceremonies; security and care of the extended family valued more highly than individual success; there is respect for personal choice(s) of an individual; children are valued; elders are respected.
	Communication patterns.—Exploitation of and capitalizing on sacred information shared by Native Americans has led to a more cautious discussion and further sharing of their practices and beliefs; caring, respect, and integrity are just a few of the criteria that must be demonstrated by those seeking such information before revelations are made; periods of silence during communication shows respect. Usually will not ask questions; expect health care members to tell them what they need to know. Eye contact: may be very limited; personal space: often decreased, personal space not considered a need; language: English taught in schools, tribal language.
	Perceptions of health team.—Always a connectedness between the healer and the healed (compassion and empathy), client's own feelings and spirituality, the universe, and higher powers.
	Time perception.—Time orientations not strict; work and productivity are valued.
Saudi	*Health.*—Although the acceptance of God's will prevails, Islamic religion influences health behaviors: use of alcohol and illicit drugs prohibited; smoking prohibited; cleanliness and moderation are stressed; family care, elder care, and family support are religious duties.
	Approaches to illness.—Biomedical; holistic; magico-religious; traditional; Islam beliefs and culture in all aspects of care; active involvement and health promotion seen; many believe invasive treatments (i.e., intravenous infusions and injections) are more effective; health care providers same sex as client in majority of cases; prefer to relate to others of common identity and unlikely to share personal information with care provider who is viewed as a stranger, care is rendered in context of the family.
	Family structure, roles.—Loyalty, dependence, strength, and cohesiveness valued highly; large families common; wife must bear an heir or is divorced from husband; boys and girls educated separately; females wear veils starting at age 12; premarital and extramarital affairs forbidden by Islamic law and punishable by death; extended families in same compound; mother is highly respected, sons seek her advice. Husband is decision maker, wife does not sign consent forms (two males do this for her); family often stay with client, and behaviors are similar to those described in Iraqi information above.
	Communication patterns.—Touch: male may only touch females in family; prolonged handshakes and handholding by males acceptable; modesty highly valued by both sexes; use of palpation with physical exam may be used limitedly or not at all; eye contact: contact by females limited to family and other females; educated respect direct contact as sign of honesty, integrity, casual eye contact often not common practice; personal space: 2 foot distance between persons when talking allows pupils to be seen (pupils dilate with interest, constrict with dislike); pain: expressed verbally and nonverbally, with emotion to family; immediate relief is sought; some may wish to be alert to pray.

Table 4–2 CULTURAL COMPARISONS OF MAJOR ETHNIC GROUPS IN AMERICA *Continued*

Group	Practices and Belief Patterns
	Perceptions of health team.—Care is given within context of family; family relationship, religion, ethnic background, and expertise considered when choosing physician; very reluctant to share personal information (see Iraqi section); informal conversation, pleasantries expected before discussing situation at hand; belief that information may cause needless worry or concern (i.e., prognosis, side effects of drugs, possible risks related to therapy, or full disclosure of actual medical diagnosis) require that appropriateness of routine client education practices be explored with the physician on an individual basis when working with clients of this background. *Time perception.*—Has little meaning except in business, but still as God wills; social rituals continue while appointments go by unattended.

Data and format from Geissler, E. (1994). *Pocket guide to cultural assessment.* St. Louis: Mosby-Year Book. Data also compiled from:

AbuGharbich, P. (1993, December). Cultural norms influencing nursing in Jordan. *Nursing and Health Care, 14*(10), 534–540.

Alston, R. J., & McCowan, C. J. (1994, January-March). Aptitude assessment and African American clients: The interplay between culture and psychometrics in rehabilitation. *Journal of Rehabilitation,* 41–45.

Andrews, M. M., & Boyle, J. S. (1989). *Transcultural concepts in nursing care* (2nd ed.). Philadelphia: J. B. Lippincott.

Axtell, R. E. (Ed.) (1990). Do's and taboos around the world (2nd ed.). New York: John Wiley.

Baugh, J. (1983). *Black street speech: Its history, structure, and survival.* Austin, TX: University of Texas Press.

Bell, R. (1994, May). Prominence of women in Navajo healing beliefs and values. *Nursing and Health Care,* 232–240.

Brownstone, D. M. (1988). *The Chinese-American heritage.* New York: Facts on File.

Cassetta, R. (1994, June). Needs of migrant workers challenge RNs. *The American Nurse, 34.*

Caudle, P. (1993). Avoiding culturally sensitive health care to Hispanic clients. *Nurse Practitioner, 18*(12), 40, 43–46, 50–51.

Davis, D. S. (1994). Dealing with real Jewish patients. *Journal of Clinical Ethics, 2*(3), 211–212.

Heusinkveld, P. (1993). *The Mexican Americans: An inside view of a changing society.* Worthington, OH: Renaissance Publications.

Jarvis, C. (1992). *Physical examination and health assessment.* Philadelphia: W. B. Saunders.

Leininger, M. (1991, April/May). Transcultural nursing: The study and practice field. *Imprint,* 55–65.

Perrone, B., Stockel, H. H., & Kreuger, V. (1989). *Medicine women, curanderas, and women doctors.* Norman, OK: University of Oklahoma Press.

Trafzer, C. (Ed.) (1985). *American Indian indentity: Today's changing perspectives.* Sacramento, CA: Sierra Oaks.

Adisa, O. P. (1990). Rocking in the sunlight: Stress and black women. In E. White (Ed.), *The black women's health book: Speaking for ourselves.* Seattle: Seal Press.

Consider This Scenario

Maria Ruiz runs into the clinic with her sick child in her arms. Speaking in a mixture of Spanish and English, she attempts to relay to the secretary that her child is very "hot and sick." She has him wrapped in several blankets and is holding him tightly. The secretary asks her to sign a consent form for treatment, but Ms. Ruiz says, "No," and, avoiding eye contact, completes her response in Spanish. The only other word the secretary recognizes is "husband." It is very busy, and the secretary is becoming impatient. She puts the form in front of Ms. Ruiz and gives her a pen. "No, husband," says Ms. Ruiz, again without eye contact. "It doesn't matter if you don't have a husband, Ms. Ruiz," the secretary says sharply. The nurse, Miss Smith, walks in. Ms. Ruiz immediately goes to her, talks in Spanish, and shows her the child. "What a beautiful little one, but he looks so sick!" she says to Ms. Ruiz. Ms. Ruiz becomes very upset and looks frightened as she pulls away from Miss Smith. The secretary says, "She won't look me in the eye and won't sign the consent form, so I don't know why she even came here!" Miss Smith asks the secretary to call Mrs. Gonzalez, the social worker, and offers Ms. Ruiz a chair in a quiet cubicle. She then sits down facing Ms. Ruiz and says, "Tell me what is wrong, in English if you can, Ms. Ruiz, so I can understand and help you." Ms. Ruiz starts talking rapidly in Spanish. "Slow down, Ms. Ruiz," Miss Smith says calmly. "Can you speak any English?" Ms. Ruiz nods, and says, "baby sick, hot." Miss Smith holds out her arms, hoping she will be allowed to hold the child. Ms. Ruiz only allows her to touch him. "Oh, my, he is so feverish," Miss Smith says, and she starts to unfold the blankets. "No, no, no!" shouts Ms. Ruiz and immediately wraps him back up. Miss Smith has no idea why Ms. Ruiz is so upset, and although very concerned about the child, she gently touches Ms. Ruiz on the arm for a few seconds and says nothing. Ms. Ruiz talks to and cuddles her child and seems to relax a little bit.

In a few minutes, Mrs. Gonzalez comes in. Miss Smith explains briefly to her what has happened and asks her to find out what is upsetting Ms. Ruiz, to obtain more information about her son's illness, and to explain the need for her to sign the consent forms. She then introduces Mrs. Gonzalez to Ms. Ruiz. Ms. Ruiz is very relieved when Mrs. Gonzalez speaks Spanish.

After a brief conversation with Ms. Ruiz, Mrs. Gonzalez found out she was upset that Miss Smith complimented her child without touching him as she did so, because it put him at risk for evil eye. She was also afraid to let Miss Smith take the blankets off for fear of exposing him to cold air (the air conditioning was on), which could cause him to get extremely ill and possibly die (mal aire). Ms. Ruiz said her husband was always the one to sign the consent forms. He would be there soon and would be very upset if she signed them.

Mrs. Gonzalez then assists Miss Smith in obtaining information about the child's illness by translating information given by Ms. Ruiz. She also explains that eye contact is often limited in the Mexican culture, especially among women and children.

Three major areas for further discussion are:

- Cultural differences: are there keys to appropriate interventions?
- How can language barriers be removed or minimized?
- Who decides which interventions are "appropriate?"

Cultural Differences: Two Keys to Appropriate Interventions

Always treat the client with respect and as an equal partner in care. Never assume that someone who is culturally different is culturally disadvantaged, deprived, or underprivileged. To do so would greatly interfere with developing a positive relationship with clients (Burrows, 1983). Miss Smith addressed Ms. Ruiz in a formal, calm manner. She called her Ms. Ruiz and did not raise her voice. This acknowledged her as an adult and denoted respect. In a comical but true light, sometimes when a person does not understand the dominant language, voice volume and enunciation increase. It is important to realize that volume is not the issue. In the scenario, even though Miss Smith realized they were not communicating, she continued to maintain a consistent tone and demeanor, thus maintaining a consistent status between them. She did not attempt to challenge Ms. Ruiz's behavior until she had more information.

Be aware that behaviors that are not understood may be culturally related. Resistance, withdrawal, anger, or avoidance of questions can be indicators that misunderstanding is occurring and defenses are going up. When this happens, it is important to recognize the behaviors that are contributing to the problem and correct or modify them (Bakker, 1995). Often, behaviors that verbally or nonverbally say "This is the way *we* do it" are the most alienating. Also, any time there are added stressors in the situation, such as unit busyness, understaffing, staff problems, etc., the risk of miscommunication increases. When stressed, a person's tolerance level for any added demands is lowered. In the scenario, the secretary was so focused on getting the form signed that no effort was made to understand what was being said. As a result, total miscommunication occurred. The nurse quickly realized that there was a language problem and requested that the social worker who was fluent in Spanish be called. Miss Smith also provided a quiet, more private place to talk with her client. She sat down with her and calmly attempted to talk with her. These actions provided a more supportive environment in which to talk and reinforced that both nurse and client were on an equal level. When Miss Smith was unsuccessful in understanding Ms. Ruiz, she continued to demonstrate respect and concern for her by remaining calm, staying seated, and touching her arm gently for a few seconds. More knowledge about Mexican culture would have been beneficial to Miss Smith, but she did well by preventing the situation from becoming antagonistic.

Language Barriers: How Can They Be Removed or Minimized?

There is a high risk for miscommunication when working with clients who have English as a second language or no English speaking skills. Differences in attitudes regarding health care and other communication-related misunderstandings often lead to frustration (Haffner, 1992). Personal space, gestures, degree of eye contact, gender issues, and clients' perceptions of the health team and health system can add to an already complicated situation. Being efficient and busy and focusing on tasks can be an approach taken by nurses to limit time spent with clients and result in fewer interactions. This helps limit the frustration that can be experienced when attempting to work with these clients (Chapman, 1980). However, the frustration can escalate for client and nurse, if ongoing communication fails to occur.

Use interpreters selectively. General interpreters who have no medical background may translate inadequately and this may result in client misunderstanding of information (Brooks, 1992). However, use of a professional medical interpreter will facilitate more accurate sharing of information and also provide insights into the complexity of bilingual and bicultural communication in health care settings (Haffner, 1992). When a family member is asked to be an interpreter, be careful to assess what the family dynamics are. For example, if a child or member of the opposite sex is asked to interpret, questions relating to sexual or elimination functions may be embarrassing, and information will be minimal, incomplete, or not sought or given. As mentioned above, the terminology may not be understood or the meanings not easily translated, and accuracy may be a problem. In the scenario, Mrs. Gonzalez provided much assistance by relaying Ms. Ruiz's concerns and also by explaining why Miss Smith's actions upset Ms. Ruiz.

Sometimes attempts are made to communicate using a foreign language dictionary. The concern with this approach is that mispronunciation can convey different meanings and lead to misunderstanding and resentment. Drawing pictures can be inaccurate or embarrassing if the client does not understand what they represent. It is best to delay treatment of noncritical problems until an interpreter can assist with history and assessment with those clients who do not understand the English language (White, 1994). Also, do not try to "fit in" by trying to use the client's language or dialect if you are unfamiliar with it. This can come across as degrading and derogatory.

Who Decides Which Interventions Are "Appropriate?"

For you to establish positive, therapeutic relationships with clients, you must be able to acknowledge that the cultural beliefs and lifeways of clients are valid and valuable and that they must be respected. It is important you appreciate that the way clients view themselves and their relationships with others is determined, in large part, by their culture. From this vantage point, you will be able to see how unique each client's experience of illness, pain, grief, or recovery is. This allows you and the client to be comfortable exploring a variety of interventions and approaches to health concerns.

In the scenario, Miss Smith realized she did not understand all the dynamics going on between her and Ms. Ruiz. Even though she knew the baby needed to be examined, she deferred until more information could be obtained through the interpreter. Also, the consent form had not yet been signed. She reacted to Ms. Ruiz in a positive manner. She was patient and did not become upset when she was not in control of the situation. It is interesting to note that Ms. Ruiz was not in control either. The issue in deciding how to intervene is not about power, but about understanding, or trying to understand, the other's perspective.

What happens when persons do not share a common cultural background and ethical issues arise? Before action is taken, give serious effort to:

1. Thoughtful, careful consideration of one's own position and its basis as well as consideration of the other person's position.
2. Avoidance of imposing the dominant culture's views merely on the basis of power.
3. Interpretation of all viewpoints involved in the situation.
4. Examination of the intent of the interventions.
5. Consideration of possible resolutions of the differences in light of their ethical costs vs. advantages (Carrese, Brown, & Jameton, 1993).

Because these approaches take restraint, patience, and openness, they can be difficult. It is extremely easy for nurses to focus on the technical aspects of care and developing technical expertise, which is vital. However, balance must be achieved between those skills and the communication skills that focus on respect and concern for the individuals on whom technology is used (Rooda, 1992). As we move toward the twenty-first century, more attention will need to be focused on the multicultural, multiracial, and growing diversity of individual and family lifestyles and the impact this will have on health care needs, assessment, and delivery within a community setting (National League for Nursing, 1993). This will require you to care in such a way that will empower, not dominate or control, your clients. Use of a cultural assessment tool can help you gain insight into your clients' cultural backgrounds and health practices. Table 4–3 is an example of such a tool that is short and yet effective in obtaining basic, culture-related information.

Your nurse-client relationship will have to be based on mutual respect and understanding of the client's situation, including cultural background, for almost any intervention to work effectively. True caring for a client cannot be done outside of his or her belief pattern, perceived needs and roles, and life situation (Benner, 1984). Awareness of the diversity of cultural beliefs and health patterns is your first step in becoming sensitive to various client perspectives of wellness, illness, pain, coping, support, comfort, change, the health care team, and effective intervention. It allows for a much broader informational base to work from when communicating with, assessing, planning, and evaluating care with clients. It allows for many more care options and promotes use of interventions designed to meet the individual needs of each client situation. First-hand experience in working with others of various cultural backgrounds will contribute to increased comfort, skill, and expertise in working effectively with them.

Table 4-3   CULTURAL ASSESSMENT TOOL

COMMUNICATION PATTERNS

Language(s) spoken; fluency; choice of words

Eye contact

Personal space needs:

Body posturing, physical distance client assumed during initial contact

Response to handshake

Use of native dress, display of personal items; learn of their significance: "Your clothing is very interesting. Is there special meaning to the way you dress?" "I noticed your personal things on the table. They must be very special to you."

Who speaks for the client; if it is not the client, note who does and the relationship to the client

Emotions exhibited

Expressions of pain, grief

Degree of agreement with what is said; whether questions are asked

Does client follow directions; is there follow-through/compliance with treatment(s), medications

APPROACHES TO HEALTH AND ILLNESS

"What do you do to stay healthy?"

"What health care services are accessible and helpful to you?"

"Tell me about your illness."

"What do you think is causing your _____ (signs and symptoms)?"

"What treatment or home remedies or diets have you tried?" "Did they seem to help?" "In what way(s)?"

Note any signs of prior treatments/home remedies, i.e., dressings, skin alterations, ointments, oils, etc. Ask client to explain unusual findings (what was done, why, how often, results).

"How do you feel we can help you?"

FAMILY STRUCTURE/ROLES

Main spokesperson for client, as above

Note who makes decisions regarding care

Note family interaction patterns

"Will family members be staying with you/heping you while treatment is given?"

"What religious practices need to be followed/respected?"

"How will this illness/treatment/hospitalization affect your role(s) at home?"

INTERACTIONS WITH HEALTH CARE TEAM/PROVIDERS

To what extent does client/family seek out information/ask questions concerning care

Note which health team members the client/spokesperson addresses, seems most comfortable with

To what extent do nonverbal behaviors coincide with what the client expresses verbally

TIME PERCEPTION

Client/family orientation

Past: sense of resignation, lack of control over outcome; compliance often a problem

Present: preventative/acute care focus as it relates to today, short-term goal setting effective (not usually committed to long-range goal setting); promptness highly valued

Future: values/participates in care goal setting, short- and long-term; long-term compliance with treatment usually high

PRACTICAL APPLICATIONS

1. Case Study

   You are admitting Mrs. Jule to the Home Health Care Service for follow-up care at home for her large lower leg ulcer. She has a history of chronic congestive heart failure and lower leg edema. After initial admission information is obtained, she proceeds to show you her affected leg. She unwraps a homemade cloth "gauze." Inside there is a medium-size dressing on top of the wound that is damp with a starch-like whitish substance. You notice the wound is deep, with irregular edges and light yellow drainage. A whitish starchy substance is seen on the wound dressing itself. When you ask her how she has been caring for her wound, she says, "Oh, I'm keeping it clean and then put a special homemade boiled potato starch on it. There's nothing better for getting it to heal than that."

   What questions would you ask to find out more information about Mrs. Jule's wound care? How do you feel about the way she is taking care of her ulcer? Why? How would you introduce the treatment, which includes a special ointment, the physician has ordered for the ulcer? What care options could be explored?

2. Answer the questions in Table 4–1. How would you describe your culture? Discuss with members of the group. Compare your similarities and differences.

3. Pick one cultural group. Discuss how you would incorporate the cultural values and belief patterns of this group into a plan of care that addresses pain control.

REFERENCES

Bakker, L. (1995, January). Communicating across cultures. *Nursing '95, 25*(1), 79–80.

Benner, P. (1984). *From novice to expert: Excellence and power in clinical nursing practice.* Menlo Park, CA: Addison-Wesley.

Bernal, H. (1993, December). A model for delivering culture-relevant care in the community. *Public Health Nursing, 10*(4), 228–233.

Brooks, T.R. (1992). Pitfalls in communication with Hispanic and African American patients. *Journal of the National Medical Association, 84*(11), 941–947.

Burrows, A. (1983). Patient-centered nursing care in a multiracial society: The relevance of ethnographic perspectives in nursing curricula. *Journal of Advanced Nursing, 8,* 477–485.

Carrese, J., Brown, K., & Jameton, A. (1993, July/August). Culture, healing and professional obligations. *Hastings Center Report,* 15–17.

Chapman, C. (1980, August). Nurses are individuals, too. *Nursing '80, 10*(8), 678–680.

Bureau of the Census. *1990 census of the population summary report. Detailed occupation and other characteristics from EEO file for the U.S.* (OP-S-1).

Eliason, M.J., & Macy, N.J. (1992, May/June). A classroom activity to introduce cultural diversity. *Nurse Educator, 17*(3), 32–36.

Haffner, L. (1992, September). Translation is not enough: Interpreting in a medical setting. *Western Journal of Medicine, 157*(3), 255–259.

Hagland, M., Sabatino, F., & Sherer, J.L. (1993, May 20). New waves: Hospitals struggle to meet the challenge of multiculturalism now and in the next generation. *Hospitals,* 22–25, 28–31.

Herberg, P. (1989). Theoretical foundations of transcultural nursing. In J.S. Boyle & M.M. Andrews (Eds.), *Transcultural concepts in nursing care* (pp. 3–65). Glenview, IL: Scott, Foresman.

Jarvis, C. (1992). *Physical examination and health assessment.* Philadelphia: W. B. Saunders.

Leininger, M. (1978). *Transcultural nursing: Theories, concepts and practices.* New York: Wiley.

Leininger, M. (1991, April/May). Transcultural nursing: The study and practice field. *Imprint, 38*(2), 58–65.

Leininger, M. (1994). Transcultural nursing education: A worldwide imperative. *Nursing and Health Care, 15*(5), 254–257.

Malone, B.L. (1993, Winter). Caring for culturally diverse racial groups: An administrative matter. *Nursing Administration Quarterly, 17*(2), 21–29.

Murphy, K., & Clark, J.M. (1993). Nurses' experiences of caring for ethnic minority clients. *Journal of Advanced Nursing, 18*(3), 442–450.

National League for Nursing Publication. (1993). *A vision for nursing education*. New York, National League for Nursing.

Rogers, S. (1988). International opportunities for nurses. *Imprint, 35*(2), 136–137, 139, 141–142.

Rooda, L.A. (1992). The development of a conceptual model for multicultural nursing. *Journal of Holistic Nursing, 10*(4), 337–347.

Rooda, L., & Gay, G. (1993, Nov–Dec). Staff development for culturally sensitive nursing care. *Journal of Nursing Staff Development, 9*(6), 262–265.

Rosella, J., Regan-Dubinski, M.J., & Albrecht, S. (1994, May). The need for multicultural diversity among health professionals. *Nursing and Health Care, 15*(5), 242–246.

Smith, B., Colling, K., & Elander, C. (1993). A model for multicultural curriculum development in bacculaureate education. *Journal of Nursing Education, 32*(5), 205–208.

White, V. (1994, January). Using an interpreter. *Nursing '94, 24*(1), 6.

5

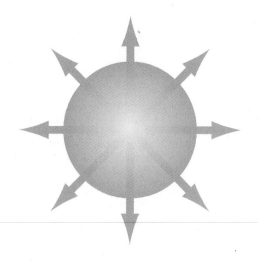

With Clients Across the Life Span

In this chapter, we will discuss:

- Communicating with newborns
- Communicating with preschool children
- Communicating with school-age children
- Communicating with teenagers
- Communicating with elder adults

Do you communicate in the same way regardless of the ages of the persons involved? Or does it vary, depending on the ages of those to whom you are talking? Do you talk the same way to a 10-year-old boy as you would to a 17-year-old young adult? Are you supposed to talk to a 5-year-old child using the same techniques as when talking to a 50-year-old adult? Of course, there are some similarities, but many striking differences must be considered when communicating with people of varying ages.

We often incorrectly assume that everyone has experience communicating with newborns and children. However, many people, especially those that have not had children, may have had little experience with this.

We also assume that everyone knows how to talk to elder adults. Again, this

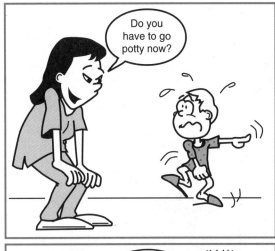

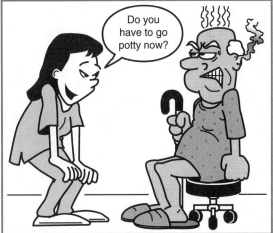

may not be the case. Many misconceptions can hamper accurate communication among different life groups. For example, we often think that all elder adults are hard of hearing and think slowly. This isn't necessarily true. In this chapter, we will examine methods of communicating with children and elder adults.

Children

Consider This Scenario

Connie Somid is a nurse on a pediatric unit. Her assignment today includes:

- LaToya Simms, age three, pneumonia
- Mikel Chuck, age six months, sickle cell crisis
- Martina Smith, age fifteen, fractured femur
- Denise Mali, age ten, chemotherapy for leukemia

As Connie begins her day, she considers the needs of each child. During report she could hear crying coming from a nearby room. She knew that it was Mikel, who had been crying on and off much of the night. The midnight nurse reported that Mikel was quiet when they were holding him. Connie went in and picked him up and sure enough, his crying stopped. She held him for a few minutes, talking softly to him. He seemed to enjoy it when Connie patted his back. Because Connie had other children to assess, she asked a "foster grandma" to sit and hold Mikel.

Connie went in to see LaToya, who had pneumonia. "Hello LaToya, I am Connie and I am your nurse today. You have a nice doll. Is that the doll that cries when she is hungry?" LaToya nodded her head shyly.

"LaToya, I am going to use this stethoscope to listen to your breathing." Connie listened for a while and then did the rest of the assessment. "I want to show you some pictures, and you can show me which of them looks the most like you." Connie showed her the pictures of children's faces, and LaToya picked the face of a child that was sad. "I see that you picked this face as the most like you. Are you feeling a bit sad?" LaToya nodded her head. Just then, a woman walked in.

"Hello, I am Connie Somid, and I am LaToya's nurse."

"I'm Stephanie Simms, LaToya's mother. Is she doing better today?"

"Her breathing is OK now, and the physicians have said that she might go home today."

"That would be great! I really miss having her at home."

Connie and Ms. Simms decided that Ms. Simms would give LaToya a shower while Connie checked on her other clients.

The last two clients were roommates. Martina had just been admitted to the pediatric unit after a car accident. Denise was what the pediatric nurses called "a frequent flyer." This phrase was a way of saying that a child was in the pediatric unit often. Denise was in the hospital every six weeks for several days as a result of her chemotherapy.

As Connie went in to see them, she could quickly see that Martina wasn't happy having a younger child for a roommate. Martina said loudly, "Hey, are you the nurse around here? I need a new roommate. This kid is listening in on all of my phone calls, and while you are at it, I want something to eat!"

"Yes, I am a nurse here. My name is Connie and I will be taking care of you today." Connie went on to explain to Martina that she couldn't have anything to eat because she was going to surgery later in the day. She could not have a new roommate because the pediatric unit was functioning at top capacity.

Connie could see that Denise was listening to every word spoken. "Denise, why don't you come with me to the playroom for a while. I think you need to find something to do."

In deciding on an appropriate way to communicate with children, nurses must take into consideration the child's developmental stage, which could be:

- Newborn
- Preschool
- School-age
- Teenager

Other criteria to consider are the maturity of the child within his or her developmental stage and the number of times a health care provider has provided care.

Remember, too, when talking with children you often will be communicating with their parents or guardian. For infants and preschool children, nearly all the information will come from the parent or guardian. For school-age and older children, the child can provide some, if not all, information.

When talking with the child's parents, it is best to refer to them by name (if you know it), instead of by title. For example, you could say, "Is Mr. Brett here?"

instead of "Is your husband here?" or "Is the baby's father here?" It is common for the person at the child's bedside to be the boyfriend or girlfriend of the parent, not the child's father or mother. Often, the terms "husband," "wife," "father," or "mother" may be inaccurate.

It is important to establish a rapport with the child. This can be accomplished by talking directly to the child instead of channeling questions through the adults. Start the interview by introducing yourself to the child first and then to the parent or guardian. Ask the child his or her name, or ask if the child has a nickname. If possible, make a positive statement to the child, such as, "That is a really nice doll you have" or "What an interesting haircut!"

Does it matter what you wear when you provide care to children? The answer is a resounding "Yes!" Children are the most comfortable with health care providers who wear street clothes or white pants and a colored top (Meyer, 1992).

Most often, but not always, a parent or guardian accompanies the child to the hospital. To help with child-parent relations, many pediatric units have unlimited visiting hours for parents and guardians. When the child is hospitalized, the parents and the nursing staff might need to negotiate their roles as Ms. Simms and Connie did in the scenario. Some parents may want the nursing staff to do all the child's care, whereas other parents might want to provide as much of the child's care as possible. Ask the parents what aspects of care they would like to perform and incorporate their wishes into the plan of care to the extent possible.

Remember that having a sick child can be a very stressful event for both the parent and the child. The parent might be exhausted from providing care for the child and because of this stress, be less tolerant of the situation. Sleep deprivation, worry over the child's condition, and concern over the home situation have impact. If the parents are upset, these unsettling emotions will be transferred to the child. Assess the parents' stress level by talking to them. Encourage them to express their feelings about what is happening in their lives (Brown & Richie, 1989).

It is vital to maintain a nonjudgmental attitude when communicating with parents and their children. If the parent or child perceives that you are being critical of them, they may not share information with you.

Many of the children seen in the pediatric units of hospitals have chronic illnesses. Many of these children and their parents know a great deal about their illness, which can be intimidating for a student nurse. Look at this type of encounter as a learning situation and ask the child and parents for information about the illness and how they have coped with it (Clubb, 1991).

Being with the parents is an excellent way to assess the interaction between parent and child. It is also a good time for teaching the parent, if needed, about parenting skills, growth and development, and the child's illness.

Newborn

How Do Newborn Children Communicate?

Because they are unable to talk, infants depend on nonverbal communication. They are calm and quiet when their needs are met, and they cry when they are hungry, tired, or uncomfortable. After spending time with an infant, you may be able to detect differences in the child's cry, which could range from high-pitched screaming to low moaning. Many experienced parents can listen to their child's crying and decipher what the child wants. "I think he wants to eat," said a father as he heard his child's loud cries.

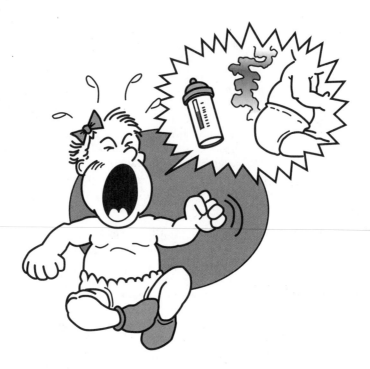

How Do You Communicate With Infants?

Because nonverbal communication is so important to infants, they respond well to a calm caregiver. Of course, it can be difficult to remain calm when providing care to a child who has been crying for long periods of time. (You may need to remind yourself continually that the infant does not feel well, which is why he or she is in the hospital. Crying is an infant's way of saying "I feel sick.")

Many infants respond well to a low comforting voice, no matter what the words. Newborns respond better to a higher-pitched voice than to a low-pitched voice. Sometimes a nurse can be seen sitting at the nurses' station holding a crying child while giving report to the oncoming shift. Hearing the nurse's reassuring tone calms the child. If you are at a loss as to what to say to an infant, you can use a comforting voice to describe your surroundings: "It's snowing outside, but it's nice and warm in here."

Holding infants and gently patting their backs or bottoms also helps to calm them. Repetitive motions are interpreted by an infant as comforting.

In the scenario, Connie comforted baby Mikel by holding him and patting his back and by providing him with a hospital volunteer to hold him.

Older infants will be anxious around strangers. They may respond better when their parents are near. It is helpful for the parents to provide a list of words the child might know. The nursing staff could use these words when providing care.

Preschool

How Do Most Preschool Children Communicate?

Because preschoolers believe that the world revolves around them, it is important to understand their perspective. Their communication is direct and literal. Because

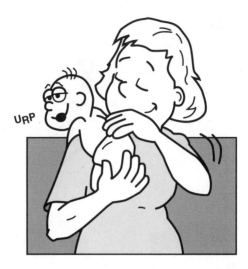

of this, avoid expressions such as "I need to take your temperature," which could be interpreted as someone removing something from the child. Other common expressions to avoid are "that just kills me" or "you are driving me crazy."

How Do You Communicate With a Preschool Child?

Small children express their feelings through play. Because of this, pictures can be an excellent tool to use when communicating with preschool children. These pictures could be the child's own drawings or pictures and photographs that help you communicate with the child. For example, you could show the child pictures with a happy face or a sad face (Fig. 5–1) and ask the child to point to the one that is most like the child, just like Connie did in the scenario with LaToya.

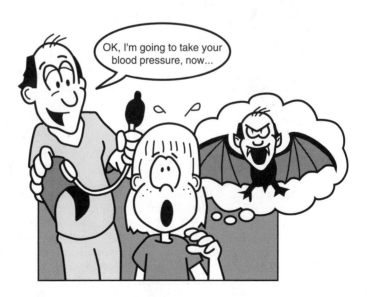

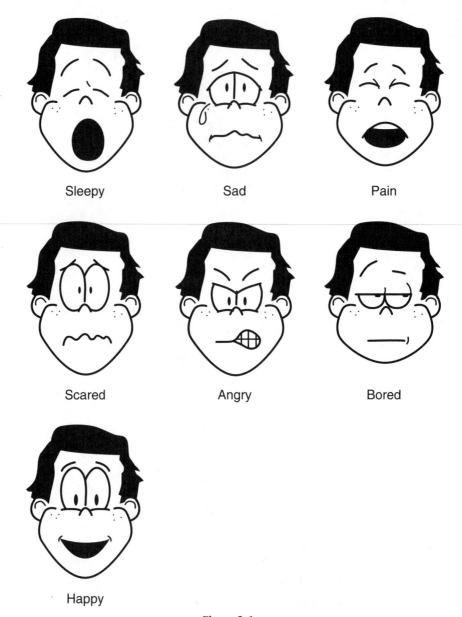

Sleepy   Sad   Pain

Scared   Angry   Bored

Happy

Figure 5–1

Pictures can also be used to help the child communicate the extent of illness or pain. The child is shown illustrations of facial expressions, ranging from extreme pain to no pain at all. Ask the child to point to the face of the child that represents the way he or she feels.

Even though preschool children communicate better with nonverbal expression of their feelings, do not forget to encourage them to ask questions. Just keep the answers simple and concrete. Many times, preschoolers ask questions that show the unique perspective of a child. For example, when a nurse started an IV on a preschool child's sibling, the preschooler wanted to know why the IV solution "looked like pee."

School Age

How Do School-Age Children Communicate?

School-age children are capable of understanding cause and effect and usually want to know why something is done and how things work. They understand the concepts of life and death.

Because school-age children want information, they often try to listen to adult conversations. Problems can arise when they overhear only part of a conversation or perhaps don't understand what they have heard. It is common for a school-age child to try to fit parts of an overheard adult conversation together to draw a conclusion, perhaps an incorrect one!

How Do You Communicate With a School-Age Child?

It is important to provide information in a manner the child can understand. The child can be included in most discussions with the parent(s). The use of simplified anatomical drawings can be the basis for explaining procedures (Vessey, Braithewaite, & Wiedmann, 1990). Written materials can be very helpful if they are simple enough for the child to understand. Verify that the child really understands what was read by asking the child to repeat or explain what was read, in his or her own words.

After you have explained something to the child, ask what the child believes will happen during the event. This will be very helpful to clarify incorrect information (Broome, 1990).

If you are providing information to the child's caregiver that you do not want the child to hear, make sure your conversation is held in a private place.

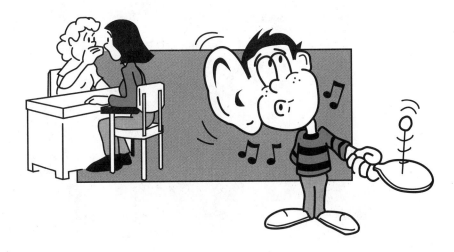

Teenager

How Do Teenagers Communicate?

A better term for teenagers is "tween-agers," because they are no longer children and not quite adults. The behavior of most teenagers ranges from childlike to very adult, sometimes in a matter of minutes. Teenagers believe that their friends are vital and that their opinions are valued. On the other hand, adults (especially the parents of the teenagers) are seen as out of touch and therefore their opinions and ideas are not as valued.

It is common for teenagers to use colloquialisms or slang when talking about or to their peer group. This can certainly be a source of communication difficulty!

How Do You Communicate With a Teenager?

It is vital to talk to teenagers like adults, even if they are not adult yet. Use their title and last name instead of just calling them by their first name. For example, use "Ms. Talifarro," instead of "Maggie." Addressing them formally shows that you view them as adults. If they ask you to call them by their first name or a nickname, then do so.

Whether to use street slang with an adolescent is controversial. If you believe you must, use only slang with which you are very familiar, and use it in an appropriate context. (Do not use profanity or other offensive terms, however.) Using street slang inappropriately will make you look foolish in the eyes of the teenager. If the client uses slang and you do not understand the terms used, be sure to have the client clarify exactly what is meant.

Ensure privacy during any intervention with a teenager, including the physical

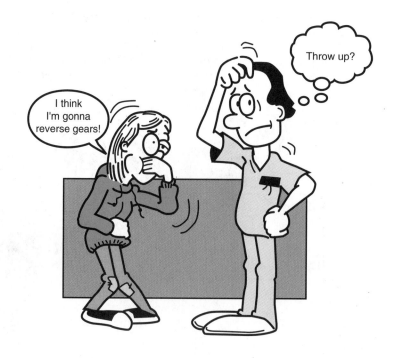

exam and history taking. You can expect the teenager to be awkward when discussing personal physical functioning. Because the teenager might be too embarrassed to really listen to you, also provide written information during verbal discussions.

Consider This Scenario

Martina, age fifteen, was admitted to the pediatric unit several hours ago after a car accident that injured three other teenagers. Her parents were at her bedside when the anesthesiologist discussed the types of medications used in anesthesia during the proposed surgery. In their presence, the anesthesiologist asked Martina if she had taken any recreational drugs within the last two or three days. Martina hesitated to answer because she knew that her parents were angry with her for getting into the car accident, and they would be even more upset if she admitted to smoking pot. So she told the anesthesiologist, "Oh no, I don't even smoke cigarettes."

Martina was taken to the surgical preoperative holding area. While they were starting her IV, she was again asked "Do you smoke pot or take any street drugs? We need to know because they can interact severely with the anesthesia we are going to give you." Realizing the seriousness of the matter, Martina said "OK, OK, I smoked pot in the car right before the accident. Are you going to tell my parents? I don't want them to know."

The nurse told Martina that this information would need to be given to the anesthesiologist and surgeon, but her parents would not be informed, if she didn't wish it to be. The nurse cautioned Martina that this information would be available to her parents in an indirect fashion, because they could obtain a copy of her medical records since their insurance was paying for the hospitalization. Martina said that she understood this. She was taken to surgery and given an alternate anesthesia medication.

Is communication between a teenager and a health care provider confidential? Should parents be told that their teenager admits to drug use if the child does not wish the parents to be told? This controversial subject is becoming an increasingly common problem. Some people believe that there cannot be information withheld from the parents or guardians of children below the age of legal adult status. Others believe that if a child is capable of understanding the idea of confidentiality, then confidentiality can exist between a child and the health care provider, no matter what the age of the child. In any case, the adolescent should be informed about what will be disclosed to the parents.

Elder Adult

Consider This Scenario

"You are getting a new client. She's ninety-six years old and coming from a nursing home. They think she's had a stroke because they found her underneath her bed at the nursing home." An hour later, she arrives via an ambulance. As you go in to greet her and perform her admission assessment, you find an elderly woman trying to hit the ambulance attendants. They tell you, "She's a real fighter. Be careful."

You place your hand gently on her shoulder and say, "Hello, I'm Tenika Smith, the registered nurse who will be taking care of you. I see that your name is Fredrika Steinbock." You note that she appears to be distraught, and she is yelling that she cannot see what is going on because she is not wearing her glasses. The room lights are on and so you dim them slightly to decrease the glare. The door of the room is open and noise from the busy nursing unit filters in. You get up and close the door.

As you begin to do the admission assessment, the thought that runs through your head is, "I wonder what symptoms of the stroke she is demonstrating?" Knowing that emotional outbursts are symptoms of a stroke, you note that she appears to be very angry.

You start the interview but Mrs. Steinbock shouts at you, "Look, I don't want to be here. There is nothing wrong with me. No one listens to me. You aren't listening now."

"I *am* listening to you. Now I would like to ask you some questions. I need this information to understand your health condition."

"No! I don't want to answer any questions! Let me out of here!" Mrs. Steinbock starts to climb out of the bed.

"Mrs. Steinbock, you can't get out of bed." You think to yourself, "I think we are going to need some soft restraints on her arms." But as you talk to her, Mrs. Steinbock begins to calm down somewhat.

"Don't you see? I need to get out of here. Jessie needs me."

"Who is Jessie?"

"Why, she's my daughter! She lives with me."

"I thought you lived in the nursing home, not with your daughter."

"I live with my daughter in the nursing home! She had a stroke and I live in the nursing home to help take care of her. I told you that you weren't listening!"

"OK, OK, just tell me what happened to you today."

"I dropped my glasses and crawled under the bed to get them. That danged aide found me there and yelled for help. Then they pulled me out from under the bed. All the time I was telling them to let go of me, but no one listened. They kept saying that I had a stroke. I didn't; I was just getting my glasses. I was so mad at them for not listening to me, I spit at them. Then they called for the ambulance. All the time we waited I told them that I was fine, but no one listened to me."

"Now I understand why you are so upset. Please answer a few more questions and then I need to listen to your heart and lungs. After that, I'll call your physician and discuss it with him. I understand that you want to get back to your daughter as soon as possible."

"It is OK if you ask questions, but I want to know something. Why don't you wear your white uniforms and caps anymore? They looked so nice, and I could tell who the nurses were. I don't have my glasses here and I can't see you. But if you were wearing a white uniform and had a nursing cap, I would know you were a nurse even without my glasses. And you don't look old enough to be my nurse anyway."

In this scenario, the nurse had to use communication skills to calm an elder adult who was angry because no one listened to her. Three things to keep in mind are:

- How do you communicate with elder clients?
- How do you assess their cognitive function?
- How do you deal with elder clients with special needs?

How Do You Communicate With Elder Clients?

Elder adults, just like any other age group, need an individualized approach to communication. Start your interaction by addressing the client by title and last name. Never use terms like "Gramps," "Granny," or "honey" to refer to an elder client. Introduce yourself, including your first and last names, along with your title. Use the words for your title, not the initials because the initials may be unfamiliar. Speak slowly and clearly. You might need to repeat your name several times.

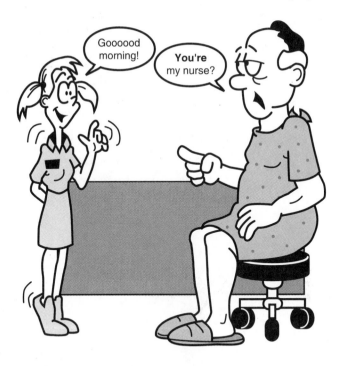

Remember that many elder adults may be unable to read the nametags that health care providers wear.

You need to provide all the indicators of your position because elder persons might not think you look like a nurse. They may be unaccustomed to the practice of health care providers wearing street clothes or scrubs. Elder clients prefer a professional nurse to wear a white uniform and nursing cap. Without them, they might not think you are a nurse (Kucera & Nieswiadomy, 1992).

Because of the striking age difference between some elders and their health care providers, the elders might lack confidence in the abilities of the health care provider. In the scenario, the client thought that the nurse did not look old enough to be a nurse. If you are a younger person, it might be helpful to arrange your hair or makeup in as mature a style as possible.

Early in the interview, it is important to identify the client's cognitive ability and level of orientation. Other factors to consider are sensory deficits such as sight, hearing loss, and decreased sense of touch. Consider medications that can affect cognitive functioning, such as pain medications, sleeping medications, and sedatives. If your conversation includes sensitive topics, you must clearly explain the reason for the information you need. Many elders have become conditioned to their privacy and are hesitant to provide personal information without a good reason for doing so. "Sensitive" topics could include financial or sexual information, or any information held very personal by the elder adult.

Talk slowly and clearly. Allow sufficient time for elder adults to answer questions. It may seem like they take a long time to answer, but to rush them gives the impression that they are unable to function as you wish them to.

It is vital to remember to use plain English, with no medical or street jargon.

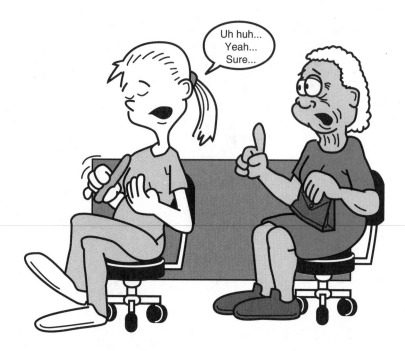

This can be difficult for a health care provider to do, because one's manner of speaking can become very ingrained in a person.

Do elder adults enjoy humor? Of course they do! Elders value humor if it especially relates to the events of their everyday life. The trick to using humor effectively is to laugh *with* people, not *at* them. Make sure that the humor is appropriate for the situation and the persons within the situation. Remember that cognitively impaired clients may not understand the humor and may interpret it incorrectly (Davidhizar & Shearer, 1992).

Remember, too, that many elder adults speak English as a second language or may have a low educational level, thus requiring the use of simple educational aids (Lusis, Hydo, & Clark, 1993)

Focus detailed conversation during peak times, such as midmorning. You will have to observe your clients to find out when their peak times are. Allow for slowed response time and avoid information overload. It is helpful to keep information sessions short and to the point. If any visual aids are used, they need to be in large print and as simple as possible.

Consider placing a notebook at the bedside of the elder client to enhance retention of information (Fig. 5–2). Visitors and health care personnel can write in the book, in large print, as needed.

Cognitive Level

To learn the level of cognitive function in elders, it is important to do a mini-mental exam. This could be done as a baseline and then as needed to point out changes in the client's condition.

Before conducting the mini-mental exam, ensure that the client's sensory

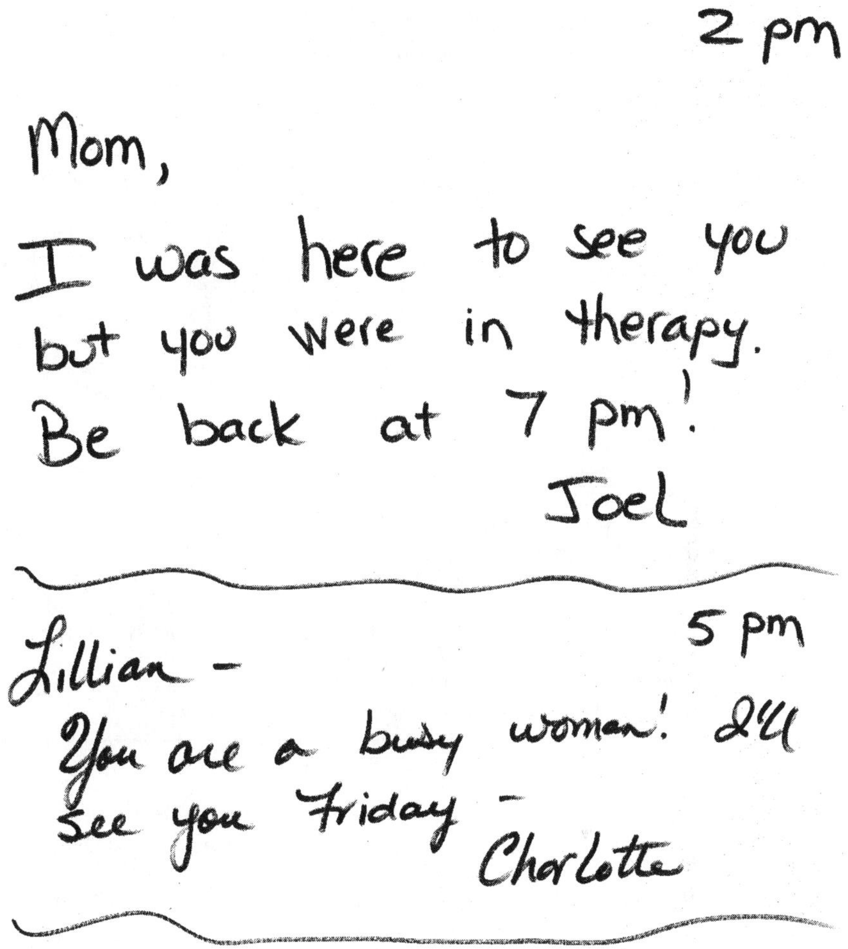

2 pm

Mom,

I was here to see you but you were in therapy. Be back at 7 pm!

Joel

Lillian —   5 pm
You are a busy woman! I'll see you Friday —

Charlotte

Figure 5–2

abilities are maximized. For example, glasses should be on and hearing aids in place. Questions may not be answered accurately if the client cannot hear or see you. The client should be alert and paying attention. Try to decrease the external stimuli as much as possible to decrease distractions. In the scenario, Tenika closed the door of Mrs. Steinbock's room to lessen external stimuli while doing her admission interview.

There are several types of mini-mental exams, but all have similar components. They focus on level of orientation, ability to retain new information, and ability to follow simple directions. Table 5–1 shows an example.

The Elder Client With Special Needs

Impaired Hearing

Because it is estimated that 90% of nursing home residents suffer from impaired hearing, you can see that hearing loss can be a major factor in an elder client's

Table 5–1   MINI-MENTAL EXAM

Although there are several versions of a mini-mental exam, the following could be used in assessing the cognitive ability of elder clients.

Directions: Choose an appropriate time so that the client is rested and has few distractions. The lighting in the room should allow the client to see the examiner. To obtain accurate results, it is important to use a tone of voice that will allow the client to adequately hear you. If the client wears a hearing aid or glasses, have the client wear them during testing. It may be helpful to sit where the client can see your face.

Ask the client the following questions. Ask each question slowly, and wait for the response. The questions are such that you will be able to determine if the client has the correct answer.

Remember that the testing may not be accurate if the client has recently taken any consciousness-altering substance such as pain medication or sedatives.

1. What is your name?
2. Where are we located?
3. How long have you been here?
4. What season are we in?
5. What is the year?
6. Who is the president of the United States?

Rating: How many questions did the client answer correctly? If the answers are 100% accurate, it is most probable that the client is mentally alert.

If the client has less than 100% correct, then the client should be tested further to determine the causes of the confusion.

ability to communicate (Taylor, 1993). You might find that hearing impaired clients speak in a loud tone and closely watch others for clues about the conversation. Of course, the most accurate method to detect hearing loss is to have testing done by an audiologist, but a simple test to assess the ability to hear is to ask the client if he or she can hear you. Another method is to stand out of the client's line of vision and ask him or her to perform a simple task. Did the client do it? (Remember to consider cognitive impairment also.) If you believe that the client has significant hearing loss, consult with the physician about formal hearing testing. Table 5–2 provides some additional management strategies for the client with hearing loss.

Does your client have a hearing aid? It is estimated that only 18% of hearing impaired clients do (Taylor, 1993). If the client has a hearing aid, is it being worn? Because of problems with manual dexterity, many clients are unable to insert the hearing aid. It may need to be inserted by the nurse or the client's family. Another factor to consider is whether the battery is working. Most hearing aids have an off/on control. When you turn it on, do you hear any noise coming from the hearing aid? If not, the battery might not be working. Contact the audiology department or the client's family for a new battery.

Visual Impairments

Many elder clients have visual impairments. This could lead to a decreased interest in their environment and thus an increased safety risk. Does the client wear glasses? If so, a simple but often overlooked method to improve vision is to have the client

**Table 5–2 MANAGEMENT STRATEGIES FOR CLIENTS
WITH HEARING IMPAIRMENT**

1. Provide good visual contact with clients. Hearing impaired individuals need to supplement hearing with lipreading
2. Avoid glare or shadows on the speaker's face.
3. Reduce background noise.
4. Speak at a normal rate and volume.
5. Use short sentences and pause between sentences.
6. Use gestures or visual aids.
7. Have client repeat information so that you know that he or she understands.
8. Keep your hands away from your mouth while you are speaking. This allows the client to lipread.
9. Do not exaggerate lip movements when speaking.
10. Face the client when speaking.

Data from Taylor, K. (1993, March/April). Geriatric hearing loss: Management strategies for nurses. *Geriatric Nursing,* 74:676. Used by permission.

wear the glasses. Clean them before placing them on the client. It is helpful to place a note in the Kardex and make a sign for the client's bedside to say that the client wears glasses.

The room lighting can make a big difference for clients with visual impairments. Keeping the room well lit will enhance the client's ability to see. Consider keeping a light on, even at night (although the light should be dimmed).

Another good idea for visually impaired clients is to keep the room arrangement the same. The client may not be able to see an obstruction such as a chair if it is left in the client's path.

Confused/Agitated Clients

If clients are confused and unable to tell you what they need, respond to the feeling tone, not to what is said. Speak in a calm voice, using only a few simple words. Nonverbal techniques are also very useful when providing care for confused clients. Pat a confused client's shoulder gently or try to hold the client's hand. Use slow, flowing movement; try to avoid sudden movement because it might be perceived by a confused client as a violent act toward him or her. Environmental stimuli can affect the confused client. It is very helpful to reduce background noise and extremes of light, just as Tenika did in the scenario.

Isolation/Loneliness

As people age and their situations change, they may lose contact with the people they love and with their cherished possessions. Hospitalized clients are removed from their familiar surroundings and also from their routines.

The strongest predictors of loneliness for hospitalized elders are physical isolation from loved ones and the absence of items that are meaningful to them (Proffitt & Byrne, 1993). If you think that your client is lonely, there are actions you can take to help. Sitting with an elder client and listening to the client talk about his or her life and loved ones will be helpful. The sense of touch can also decrease

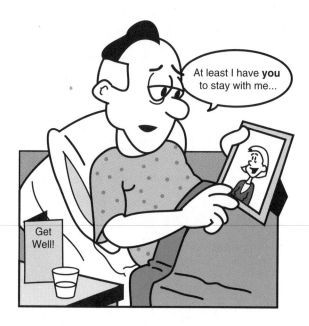

feelings of loneliness. It is helpful to hold the client's hand or pat his or her shoulder. If you don't have the time, a volunteer, the chaplain, or a family member could be asked to sit with the client.

To personalize the environment, have family members bring a few items from home that the client likes, and keep these personal items within the client's sight. (Remember that the client's vision may be very limited.) However, on short-term hospitalizations this may not be practical.

In addition to assessment of the client for feelings of isolation and loneliness, it is also useful to assess the spouse and family. The spouse and family might be lonely and isolated because the client is not able to communicate or help them with chores. In addition, they might be fatigued as a result of the actual work of getting to the institution to visit the client. It is common for the spouse of an elder client to also be in ill health.

Conclusion

It is important to vary communication methods according to the ages of those involved. For children, the most important factors are related to their developmental stages. For elder adults, maximizing sensory and cognitive abilities will enhance communication.

PRACTICAL APPLICATIONS

You are assigned to the emergency department for a clinical rotation. Your first client is a 4-year-old girl who is crying continuously. You try to ask her questions, but she just cries. Her mother is present, but speaks very roughly to the child. "She has been crying for hours! I haven't had any sleep. I haven't eaten!" says her mother. The little girl cries even harder.

1. What can you do to get the little girl to talk?

2. How could you decrease her crying?

3. How could you decrease the frustration of the mother?

The next client is a 76-year-old man who is being admitted from a convalescent center. The staff at the convalescent center believe that the client has had a stroke. Although he is on a stretcher, he is combative and yelling for "Mona." You come toward him and he yells at you, "Mona, get over here! The cops have got me in handcuffs!"

1. What limitations might he have that would impair his ability to communicate with you?

2. What interventions could you use to calm him?

3. What voice tone would be helpful to use with him?

REFERENCES

Baillie, V., Norbeck, J., & Barnes, L. (1988). Stress, social support and psychological distress of family caregivers of the elderly. *Nursing Research, 37*(4), 217–222.

Broome, M. (1990). Preparation of children for painful procedures. *Pediatric Nursing, 16*(6), 537–541.

Brown, J., & Ritchie, J. (1989). Nurses' perceptions of their relationships with parents of hospitalized children. *Maternal-Child Journal, 18*(2), 79–96.

Clements, D., Copeland, L., & Loftus, M. (1990). Critical times for families with a chronically ill child. *Pediatric Nursing, 16*(2), 157–161.

Clubb, R. (1991). Chronic sorrow: Adaptation patterns of parents with chronically ill children. *Pediatric Nursing, 17*(5), 461–465.

Davidhizar, R., & Frank, B. (1992). Understanding the physical and psychosocial stressors of the child who is homeless. *Pediatric Nursing, 18*(6), 559–562.

Davidhizar, R., & Schearer, R. (1992). Humor: No geriatric nurse should be without it. *Geriatric Nursing, 13*(5), 276–278.

Deevey, S. (1990). Older lesbian women: An invisible minority. *Journal of Gerontological Nursing, 16*(5), 35–37.

DiFlorio, I. (1991). Mother's comprehension of terminology associated with the care of a newborn baby. *Pediatric Nursing, 17*(2), 193–194.

Gregory, D., Peters, N., & Camerson, C. (1990). Elderly male spouses as caregivers: Toward an understanding of their experience. *Journal of Gerontological Nursing, 16*(3), 20–23.

Hamilton, B. & Vessey, J. (1992). Pediatric discharge planning. *Pediatric Nursing, 18*(5), 475–478.

Hoffman, S. (1992). Elder beliefs: Blocks to pain management. *Journal of Gerontological Nursing, 18*(6), 19–23.

Kucera, K., & Nieswiadomy, R. (1992). Nursing attire: The public's preference. *Nursing Management, 22*(10), 68–70.

Lusis, S., Hydo, B., & Clark, L. (1993). Nursing assessment of mental status in the elderly. *Geriatric Nursing, 14*(5), 255–259.

Meyer, D. (1992). Children's responses to nursing attire. *Pediatric Nursing, 18*(2), 157–160.

Nelson, P. (1990). Religious orientation of the elderly. *Journal of Gerontological Nursing, 16*(2), 29–34.

Parette, H., Hourcade, J., & Parrette, P. (1990). Nursing attitudes toward geriatric alcoholism. *Journal of Gerontological Nursing, 16*(1), 26–30.

Phillips, L. (1987). Respect basic human rights. *Journal of Gerontological Nursing, 12*(3), 36–39.

Proffitt, C., & Byrne, M. (1993). Predicting loneliness in the hospitalized elderly: What are the risk factors? *Geriatric Nursing, 14*(6), 311–313.

Ryan, M., & Robinson-Smith, G. (1990). What does it mean? Making sense of the hospital experience. *Journal of Gerontological Nursing, 16*(9), 17–20.

Taylor, K. (1993, March/April). Geriatric hearing loss: Management strategies for nurses. *Geriatric Nursing,* 74–76.

Vessey, J., Braithewaite, K., & Wiedmann, M. (1990). Teaching children about their internal bodies. *Pediatric Nursing, 16*(1), 29–33.

Weinrich, S., & Boyd, M. (1992). Education in the elderly: Adapting and evaluating teaching tools. *Journal of Gerontological Nursing, 18*(1), 15–19.

Whall, A. (1986). Overlooking the emotional needs of older adults. *Journal of Gerontological Nursing, 12*(4), 37

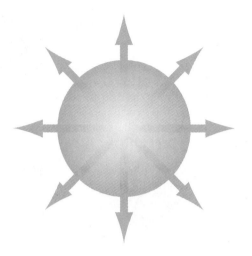

6

With Distressed People

In this chapter, we will discuss:

- What is behavior?
- What is distressed behavior?
- Environmental concerns
- Client behaviors
- Staff behaviors

As a nurse, you will be providing care to clients in a variety of situations, ranging from joyous, such as the birth of a child, to heartbreaking, such as the unexpected death of a young man. Many situations will fall somewhere in between.

One common theme among all the clients you will see is that they are under stress. Because of the circumstances that brought them into the health care system, the clients and their families might be sick, frightened, sleep deprived, in pain, nauseated, or otherwise vulnerable. The clients we see are sick, and because of this, they are simply not at their best, nor are they capable of displaying their best behavior.

Nurses provide care for a variety of clients, each of whom lives a unique life and responds differently to adverse circumstances. When faced with extreme stress, some people get angry and very verbal, whereas others become depressed and quiet.

Providing appropriate nursing care to clients who exhibit distress can be a big challenge. Many nursing students do not feel confident when providing care for clients who exhibit symptoms of emotional distress in addition to physical distress. It is important to recognize that nurses encounter many clients on general nursing units who have mental health problems as well as physical problems. These psychiatric problems can range from mild anxiety to outright psychosis. Yet, no matter how extensive or how minor the problem, the nurse needs to know how to deal with it.

This chapter is meant to provide some practical applications for caring for distressed clients. We will look at some of the common distressed behaviors that clients and their families may exhibit.

What Is Behavior?

Behavior is our response to events. Something happens, and we react to it. From childhood, we are taught how to respond and interact with our environment. Of course, behavior is altered depending on the situation and your physical condition, culture, and experiences. Behavior can be viewed as a continuum—it is not all good or all bad. We all have the capacity for distressed behavior, depending on circumstances.

What Is Distressed Behavior?

Behavior is our response to events and to the environment. Distressed behavior can be defined as any behavior that falls outside the realm of "normal behavior." Although there is certainly a great deal of variation as to what "normal behavior" is, some distressed behaviors such as anger or violence are usually obvious to the observer. Other distressed behaviors are more subtle.

There are many ways of categorizing distressed behavior. In this chapter, we group distressed behaviors into two general categories: anger that is directed outward and anger that is directed inward.

Examples of anger directed outward are aggressive behaviors such as swearing or physical violence. More subtle types of anger that are directed outward are controlling behaviors such as being highly demanding or manipulative. Sexual, racial, and verbal harassment are other examples of anger directed outward.

When a person is angry but unable to express this anger directly, he or she may turn the feelings inward. Examples of anger turned inward are depression and substance abuse.

What Causes Distressed Behavior?

Distressed behavior can be caused by a variety of events involving physical, emotional, or environmental stressors (Table 6–1). Often it can be caused by simply too many stressors occurring at once—the straw that broke the camel's back. People usually can cope with a certain number of stressors, but everyone has a limit, and

Table 6–1 WHAT ARE SOME OF THE COMMON STRESSORS FOR A CLIENT WITHIN THE HEALTH CARE SYSTEM?

Physical stressors
Pain and discomfort
Lack of sleep
Alcohol or drug use or withdrawal
Impaired hearing or perception
Head injury
Any physical illness

Emotional stressors
Resentment
Feeling lost, insecure, forgotten
Feeling out of control of the situation
Mental illness
Loneliness
Insecurity
Helplessness

Environmental stressors
Sensory overload
Change in schedule or routine
Poor parking, small rooms, roommates
Long waits to be seen, not enough health care staff
Apparent inhospitality of health care system
Culture: may not like or respect a health care worker because of race/sex/age/physical appearance/expectations or demands
High-tech equipment

when additional stressors occur, they simply become overwhelmed. When the stressors occur suddenly, serious problems can result.

Expectations Within the Health Care Environment

We base our interactions with others on expectations or perceptions we may have of the person. William James suggests that when two people meet, there are really six people present:

- The person each perceives himself/herself to be
- The person that the other person perceives him/her to be
- The person each really is

Most people have rather strong feelings about how others should act and feel. These perceptions are rarely based on rational analysis, but rather on "gut feelings" that may defy description. Where do our perceptions come from? Experiences, culture, socioeconomic factors, the media, and your upbringing all affect how you view others. Often these influences can be so subtle that you are not even aware of them; you come away from interactions feeling anger or disgust, but not really knowing why.

Although there are many reasons people become health care providers, it is common to hear that people become nurses because they want to "help people" or perhaps because they "want to make people better." When this is the motivation

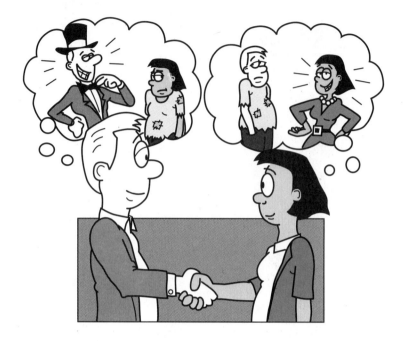

for entry into practice, what happens when the client doesn't want to be helped or perhaps doesn't want to get better? How do nurses cope with a client who has a terminal illness? Nurses can get angry with the client for not fulfilling their needs, grow discouraged with themselves for having these emotional requirements, or become frustrated when cure is not an option.

Of course, the client has expectations of the health care system, too (Table 6–2). These expectations might be based on previous encounters with the health

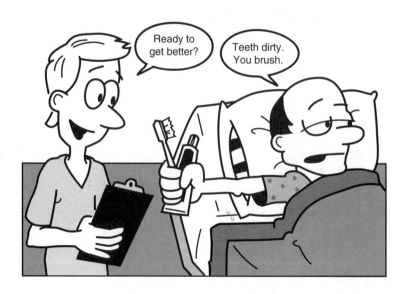

Table 6–2   EXPECTATIONS

Optimal Health Care Environment
Quiet, pleasant, and private surroundings
Nonintimidating surroundings, low tech
Enough staff members who speak the same language that you do
Good food
Nonpainful, inexpensive treatment that is available when you need it; no waiting
Quick cures
Optimal client
   Grateful for the care they receive
   Treats nurses and other health care workers with respect
   Follows recommended plan
   Respectful of others' property
   Polite, doesn't use curse words
   Wants to get better
   Lives a "normal" lifestyle
   Pleasant appearance: clean, neat, tidy, normal body weight, no body odor
   Has a job
   No drug or alcohol abuse
Optimal family
   Wants the best outcome for the client
   Willing and able to help with home care
   Speaks and reads English
   Grateful
   Polite
   Doesn't use swear words
   No alcohol or drug abuse
Optimal staff
   Can apply theory content to the client's condition
   Good interpersonal skills
   Able to do all psychomotor skills after they have seen them once
   Never afraid, nervous, nonconfident

This table was developed using some common themes that seem to recur in health care. Read the list and think about whether you agree with it. You may not agree with all the items, and you may disagree with a few. This list of expectations is meant to be thought-provoking. You need to think about how you perceive others before you can understand how your attitudes can influence the behavior of distressed clients.

Questions to ponder regarding expectations:
1. Do I agree with all these expectations?
2. Would I disagree with any of these expectations?
3. If so, which ones?
4. Would any of my colleagues or family disagree with any of these expectations?
5. Do any of your professional feelings differ from your personal feelings regarding these expectations?
6. Is it possible to meet these expectations?

care system. Because there have been massive changes during the past few years, clients may encounter a health care system that is very different from the one when they were last hospitalized. The media also influences the client's beliefs, with television shows such as "Marcus Welby," "St. Elsewhere," "E. R.," and "Chicago Hope" often providing a very inaccurate glimpse of health care providers.

What Happens When These Expectations Are Not Met?

Usually people are dismayed or very upset when their expectations are unfulfilled. The emotions they experience can range from mildly irritated to absolutely homicidal. Anger, hostility, sadness and depression, or physical illness can occur.

Nurses also can report disequilibrium when their expectations for clients and their family members do not happen. Many nurses report that providing care for clients and family members with distressing behaviors is the most difficult part of their jobs. Many times, the distressing behavior is one that is "frowned upon" in American society, and thus we look at clients exhibiting such behaviors as less than normal or acceptable.

Anger, violence, depression, manipulative behavior, and drug use are certainly topics that many people have strong feelings about. You probably do too. Some of these topics may be very important to you, whereas other topics in this chapter might not provoke much emotional reaction. When you provide care for clients who exhibit these problematic behaviors, you need to provide professional nursing care and keep your personal feelings to yourself. It is very important to note the difference between personal feelings and professional actions. As a private person, your feelings and actions are your own. But as a professional, you must provide each client with courteous, appropriate care.

Throughout the chapter, examples of the nurse's personal feelings are discussed in each scenario. You might find that you agree or disagree with these possible nurse reactions to client behavior. Remember that it is very normal to have feelings about the client's distressed behavior. The important thing is to separate the personal feelings from the professional actions. Of course, it isn't always easy to do when your personal and professional feelings do not coincide.

Environmental Concerns

Consider This Scenario

Mrs. Ranee brought her 6-month-old daughter into the emergency department because of a rash on the baby's stomach. The nurse at the admission desk took one look at the rash and said "You need to go to the Sick Child Clinic on the 6th floor." Mrs. Ranee redressed her crying baby and walked to the elevator. As she got in the elevator, she noticed that it went only to the 4th floor. So she got out and asked for directions. She found a man sweeping the floor.

He told her, "Take this hallway until it deadends. Then take a right turn. Go to the second set of elevators and then go to the 6th floor." Mrs. Ranee tried to do this but she must have made an incorrect turn, because she wound up in the cafeteria. So again she asked for directions. This time she made it to the 6th floor. She saw signs directing her to the Sick Child Clinic. This was good, because she was tired and her crying baby was giving

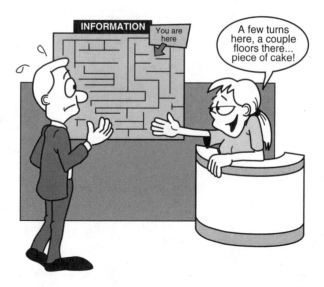

her a headache. When she found the Sick Child Clinic, she stopped dead in her tracks. There must have been 50 women and children waiting to be seen. Many of the children were crying, and most of the women looked like they wanted to cry, too.

Mrs. Ranee filled out the registration forms and found a place to sit. She was glad that she had brought a baby bottle and some diapers. They waited for 2 hours, during most of which the baby cried. It was a warm day and the air conditioner wasn't working well. Boy, the room was hot!

Finally, they were ushered into an examining room. About 15 minutes later, a woman entered the room and said "I'm Dr. Sandra Pierce. How are you today?" At that, Mrs. Ranee started to cry.

This scenario shows how the environment can affect behavior. Although our health care system is evolving, some aspects are slow to change. The physical environment of many institutions can be difficult to deal with. The institution itself may have been built many, many years ago and may not be very functional or physically attractive. Many hospitals are overcrowded and have long waiting times and overflowing waiting rooms. Because many people continue to use the hospital emergency department as their primary source of health care, the waiting time to receive health care can be extensive. For example, an emergency department in a typical inner-city hospital provides care for 80 to 90 clients in a routine 8-hour shift. In this emergency department, it is common for a client with a nonemergency problem such as an ankle sprain to wait 5 or 6 hours to receive treatment. Waiting this long can certainly make tempers flare!

Some emergency departments in large cities are issuing waiting numbers to clients with nonemergency problems. The clients go back home and call a hotline to find out when they will be seen. With this system, the client may not receive treatment for several days, which certainly isn't the ideal, but it is a reality for our current health care system.

The location, layout, and size of many hospitals can also create environmental problems. The area that they were built in may have deteriorated over the years. People may be frightened to even visit that part of the city. Also, the layout of the

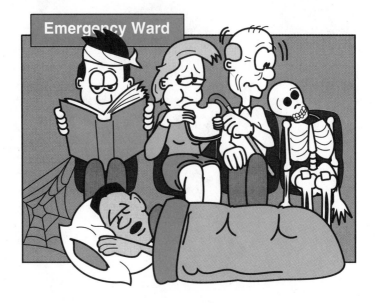

institution can be confusing. The buildings may have been built over many years, with buildings and floors that do not directly connect to each other. Because of this, it may be difficult to get from one area to another. Have you ever heard the phrase "you can't get there from here"? It probably seems this way to many people trying to find their way in a large medical institution.

The size of many medical centers can also be intimidating. One large medical center has 29 nursing units, 11 critical care units, and more than 50 elevators.

Another institutional barrier is the impersonality of the environment. People prefer to deal with other people who care about them. In a chaotic hospital environment, this may not be evident. Many clients state that they feel reduced to a name band or a number.

Some behaviors to help clients cope with the institutional environment include helping them find their way and intervening for them. It may be helpful to provide a map, write out directions, or actually take them to where they want to go. Many institutions have volunteers, and this would be a good job for a volunteer. Intervening on the behalf of clients requires you to get involved, which could include making phone calls for them or telling them about opportunities of which they may not be aware.

Client Behaviors: Anger Directed Outward

Aggressive Behaviors

Consider This Scenario

John DeMarco was brought to the emergency department by two of his friends. It was obvious that all three men were intoxicated. During a fight in a bar, John had been stabbed twice. Fortunately, neither of his wounds was serious. As they approached the emergency department admission desk, they saw that there was a long line of people waiting to be triaged. (Triage means assessment to figure out severity of injury; usually the sickest people are seen first.) John and his friends rather grudgingly waited in line a few minutes, then one of John's friends started to talk loudly about having to wait in line with a "bunch of do-nothing blacks." He talked so loudly that a security guard overheard him. The guard came over and told them that they needed to quit making racial statements. He also told them to talk more quietly or they would have to leave the emergency department. This made them even more angry, because the bar owner had told them to be quiet also.

Finally, the nurse was available to triage John. She saw that John's stab wounds were not serious; in fact, both had already stopped bleeding. She told John and his friends that they would have a short wait to get medical treatment. Because the emergency department was so busy, the "short wait" turned into 6 hours. During this time, every 10 minutes or so, John or one of his friends would go to the desk and ask when they would be seen. On his last trip to the desk, John said "Hey, bitch, what's a guy got to do to get help around here?" The triage nurse said, "It's really hard to wait so long, but we are really busy tonight. But don't call me 'bitch.' Call me 'nurse,' or I don't answer you. We see people according to how sick they are. We will call you when it is your turn." John's friends were getting angry, but John told them to calm down "'cause I got to get stitched up."

The three men walked outside to have a cigarette. This seemed to calm them down. After a while, they went back into the emergency department. "Mr. DeMarco, we were looking for you. Come into this examination room." After he went in, the emergency department nurse practitioner came to see him. John and his friends couldn't believe it! Not only was the nurse practitioner a woman, but a black woman at that!

"Hey, I don't want no black woman to take care of me. Get me a man and make sure that he's white!" John yelled.

"Sir, my name is Mirabile Sovee, and I'm a nurse practitioner. I would like to look at your wounds, but if you want someone else, it's your choice. There are two physicians here tonight. One is black and the other is a woman. Would you like to have one of them see you? If you do, you'll have to wait until one of them is available."

"Damn it all! I guess I'll have to make do with you."

Ms. Sovee put on gloves and began to examine his wounds. "I can see that you'll need stitches on both of these. I'll get a suture kit."

Just then, an ambulance arrived with three auto accident victims. After John waited for about 10 minutes, he went to look for Ms. Sovee and found her as she was coming out of a supply room.

"Hey, what's the deal?" he said. "I'm sick of you ignoring me! Look, bitch, I want you to get your ass over here and take care of me *now*!"

Ms. Sovee started to tell him that he would have to wait, but he drew up a fist and hit her in the face. A security officer was nearby and came quickly to her aid. The security guard told John that he could either wait for the treatment or leave. If he chose to wait, the security guard would sit with him to ensure that he wouldn't hurt anyone else. John and his friends chose to leave, saying, "Let's get out of this hole!"

This scenario demonstrates how swearing and violence can affect a situation. It is important to learn how to handle:

- Socially inappropriate language
- Anger and violent behavior

Socially Inappropriate Language

American society has classified words as appropriate or inappropriate to use. You might find that individuals take the classification system further and distinguish between moderate swearing and extensive swearing. For example, "damn" might be considered by some people as a moderate swear word and find that it is moderately offensive. Many people would consider other swear words as extremely offensive and thus never appropriate in communication.

The use of profanity is variable, depending on the situation and the people involved. For example, a construction worker may swear more than would an office worker. The use of socially inappropriate language generally falls into three categories.

EVERYDAY LANGUAGE   For many people, using socially inappropriate language is part of their everyday speech pattern, as in the case of John and his friends in the scenario. Most people, however, attempt to curtail their swearing in situations in which it is obviously inappropriate.

INTIMIDATION   Using socially inappropriate language can also be a form of intimidation. Using words such as "bastard" or "bitch" shows contempt for the other person and uses the words as if they were weapons.

LOSS OF INHIBITIONS CAUSED BY INJURY   After a stroke or head injury, a client may have suffered damage to the part of the brain that regulates appropriate behavior. Without this control mechanism, the client may use inappropriate language.

If a client is using socially inappropriate language, you will need to consider its cause and also the depth of your interaction with the client. After all, if you are going to be with the client for only a few minutes, you probably will not be able to succeed in getting the client to change his or her language pattern. On the other hand, if the client is going to be in the institution for an extended length of time, you may try to address the issue.

Is the language part of the client's everyday speech pattern? If so, the client may not even be aware that what is being said is offensive. If the client's language is offensive, try to set limits on this behavior. Instead of globally asking the client not to swear in your presence, get specific. Tell the client the word or words that you find offensive and suggest another word to use.

Is the client using socially inappropriate language to make a point or to intimidate you? Try to get the client to modify his or her behavior by indicating that you hear the client's feelings of anger, and then offer another word to use. In the above situation, John called the triage nurse "bitch," indicating his anger with the situation. The triage nurse told John not to call her "bitch" and said she would not talk to him unless he used an appropriate title for her. She told him to call her "nurse," and he complied.

After a stroke or head injury, many clients use profanity, which can be very distressing for the client and the family. Recognize that in this situation, the client's word choice may not be voluntary and thus not controllable. Consult with a speech or rehabilitation therapist to explore ways to deal with this behavior, and be prepared to accept that it is not always extinguishable.

Remember that as a professional health care provider, it is never appropriate for you to swear, even if the client is being extremely profane. Always talk in a professional manner.

Anger and Violent Behavior

Most people function rationally. We are able to make our needs known and act reasonably. We handle problems and irritations in an acceptable way. Of course, this doesn't mean that we don't ever get angry; it simply means that we have developed coping mechanisms that are considered acceptable, such as leaving the situation or problem solving to help deal with life's problems. We try to relate to others generally in an appropriate way.

What Causes People To Act Inappropriately?

Some people may react differently to problems and irritations. They may not have learned positive coping mechanisms and may have limited ability to tolerate frustration or delayed gratification. When irritations pile up or a specific incident occurs to provoke them, they may feel powerless and use anger and hostility as a coping mechanism. Aggressive behavior also may give them a sense of power, which in reality they lack.

Violent or hostile behavior can be rooted in a physical or mental disorder or both. Stroke, Alzheimer's disease, and head injury are common physical causes of behavior alterations. Drug use and antisocial personality types can cause psychological alterations in behavior (Gorman, Sultan, & Luna-Raines, 1989).

It is important to realize that even people who react appropriately under normal circumstances can become angry or even violent under extreme stress. Think about this example: The parents of a critically ill child have been awake since the child's accident 3 days ago. They are eating their meals from candy machines and drink jugs of coffee to stay wake. An hour ago, the physician told them the child is brain dead. When an overzealous security guard tells them to leave the unit because visiting hours are over, the father's emotional keel just snaps. He yells at the security guard, "I'll leave when I am damn ready to! Get out of my sight!" Then he begins to cry.

Extreme stress has made him act in ways that were not typical for him. Is the father's anger appropriate under the circumstances? Most of us would say that it certainly is, and many nurses would say that such expression of grief should be encouraged rather than discouraged.

You need to recognize, though, that anger is an uncomfortable feeling, and many people are uncomfortable around angry people. You might feel this way as well. If you are uncomfortable around angry people, you might find that you try to placate them or do other actions to try to make the anger go away, instead of allowing them to vent their feelings.

As a first-line health care provider, nurses feel the brunt of many angry and violent clients. How pervasive is the problem? The answer is that the prevalence is frighteningly high. Health care workers are verbally threatened or physically abused on a regular basis. The prevalence of abuse varies according to the type of nursing unit as well as the physical location of the hospital. The emergency department is the most common site of encounters with violent or hostile clients and their families. Other high violence locations are mental health units and substance abuse units. In a large study of emergency department nurses in Pennsylvania, an astounding 98% of the nurses stated that they had been physically or verbally abused during their careers (Mahoney, 1991).

Location of the institution also makes a difference when it comes to violent clients. An emergency department in a large inner-city hospital reported approximately 60 incidences of physical abuse to their health care providers per month. Some of these incidences were severe enough to require medical treatment and

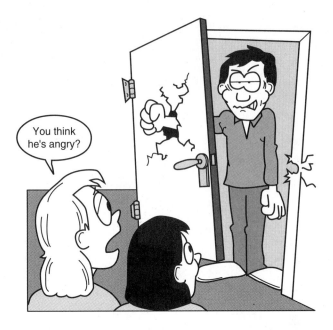

time off from work. The occurrence of violence usually is much greater at inner-city facilities than at suburban hospitals.

Another factor to consider is the gender of the nurse. Male emergency department nurses reported more frequent incidences of physical assault and verbal abuse than did the female nurses (Mahoney, 1991). This might occur because male nurses may appear more intimidating than do the female nurses.

After the assault on Ms. Sovee, the emergency room staff decided to review their policy on violence and assault. They realized that they needed to be able to anticipate problems and have an action plan to prevent violence or to intervene appropriately if violence does occur. They began by looking at characteristics of the type of client who is the most likely to become violent (Table 6–3).

John and his friends fit the majority of high-risk descriptors. One of the nurses pointed out that this table lists only those at highest risk. Other types of people can also become hostile or violent. One of the hospital security officers stated that

Table 6–3   WHO IS MOST LIKELY TO BE VIOLENT OR HOSTILE?

1. A male, under age 25, who dislikes authority figures.
2. One who exhibits signs of increased agitation:
   a. Restlessness
   b. Tense and angry
   c. Loud voice, uses profanity
   d. Argumentative
3. One who becomes defensive when someone comes near.
4. One who uses alcohol or street drugs or is withdrawing from them.
5. One who has a history of violence or hostility.

Data from Lewis, S., & Blumenreich, K. (1993). Defusing the violent patient. *RN, 56* (12), 24–29.

many emergency departments are reporting an increase in women and teenagers displaying violent behavior. He also said that his colleagues who work in security at suburban institutions are seeing an increase in hostile and violent clients, although it still was not as large a problem as with the urban hospitals. He reminded them that violent behavior toward health care providers does occur more frequently in large cities, but it can happen anywhere. Also, he wanted them to remember that violence can occur on any unit of the hospital, not just the emergency, mental health, or substance abuse departments.

The staff members began to discuss their feelings regarding caring for clients who might be hostile or violent. Ms. Sovee stated that now she was becoming afraid of any client who looked the slightest bit angry. Several other staff members echoed this feeling. One nurse said that she was really insecure about setting limits with hostile people because this just made them angrier. After much discussion, they agreed that it was good that they recognized their feelings, but they also needed to be able to adequately care for all the clients that came into the emergency department. And this meant that they needed to provide care without retaliating against or avoiding these types of clients. They decided that a good skill to learn when dealing with hostile clients is to hear criticism without becoming defensive yourself. This would help gain control over the situation.

To help the staff understand how an assault commonly occurs, a chart demonstrating a typical situation was presented and discussed (Table 6–4).

The security officer discussed actions the nursing staff members could use to lessen their risk of being assaulted by a client or a client's family member.

Table 6–4 A TYPICAL SITUATION

Something happens that irritates the client. This could be:

Situational
Long wait
Staff conflict
Fear of illness

Mental Health
Mania
Borderline personality disorder
Drug use or withdrawal
Age-related brain dysfunction

Because of poor coping skills, the client is unable to deal with this problem in a positive way.

The client becomes angry, which makes the other people in the situation irritated.

The irritated behavior of others (as perceived by the client) makes the client angrier.

The situation escalates. . .

Violence erupts

With intervention at the appropriate time, the client's anger may de-escalate.

BODY LANGUAGE AND SPEECH PATTERNS   Speak slowly and use a calm voice. People prone to violence are very quick to pick up on the feeling tones of other people in the environment. Move slowly and with a purpose that is obvious to the viewer. Otherwise, the client may misinterpret your motives. Remember that if the client thinks you look and act threatening, it may escalate the situation. If you act calm and collected, you may be able to keep the situation under control.

Of course, it may be difficult to act calm when you really want to scream and run the other way, but it is important to maintain your composure. In the scenario, John became upset when the security guard moved quickly and came close to him.

PHYSICAL SPACE   If you believe that a person is at high risk for violence, don't turn your back on that person, and don't let that person move between you and the door. When someone is getting agitated, keep your distance and stay an arm's length away.

Monitor for intrusion of the client's personal space, which can easily happen during many nursing interventions such as taking vital signs or starting an IV. If the client is agitated, try to leave these activities until the client calms down.

ENVIRONMENT   To reduce violent behavior, you need to be able to decide if objects within your environment could be used as weapons against you. Are there materials that could be thrown, such as IV poles or medical supplies?

Don't wear things around your neck such as a stethoscope or jewelry such as large hoop earrings; these could be easily grabbed. Don't wear your hair in a ponytail because it is also easy to grab.

CAUSATION   Consider the cause of the client's anger. Has an event occurred to anger the client? We cannot prevent every person from becoming angry, but knowing the cause can be helpful to de-escalate it.

Is the Situation Escalating?

Although not all angry or hostile people become violent, you should be prepared for those who do. What are some signs that a client may be losing control? The client may express aggressive statements or threats (which should never be ignored). Pay attention to tone and pattern of voice. Does the client sound as if he or she is getting out of control? Physical signs to watch for are clenched fists, rigid posture, or increased activity, such as pacing the floor (Kinkle, 1993).

Listen to your instincts. If you feel uncomfortable with a client or a situation, something may indeed be wrong.

There are four options available when a client becomes violent (Lewis & Blumenreich, 1993). Because every situation is unique, the appropriate handling of each will vary. Your overall goal should involve the least amount of force, and safety for all persons involved should be maintained.

VERBAL INTERVENTION   This can be the most valuable tool to use with agitated people. Many people become angry when they lose control over a situation. Your goal with verbal intervention is to acknowledge this and help the person to reestablish some degree of self-control.

It is important not to deny the client's anger. Simply telling the client "Now, don't get upset" will not make the anger go away and might enrage the client further. Instead, acknowledge the angry feelings by saying, "I see that you are angry."

PHYSICAL INTERVENTION   Clients who are dangerous to themselves or others may require physical intervention by the health care team to prevent injury. This is definitely a step-up in the seriousness of the situation. In most institutions, physical interventions to subdue clients are done by a team of four or more specially trained people. This is sometimes called a "show of force." Simply seeing the staff assemble in such a way might be enough to help a person regain self-control.

A student nurse normally wouldn't be expected to subdue a client. Some agencies are training their personnel in personal safety skills. Check with your school or institution to find out if this might be helpful to you.

RESTRAINTS   Clients who present a danger to themselves (perhaps by pulling out their tubes as a result of their confusion) or to others might need to have their hands (and perhaps feet) restrained.

There are two types of restraints: soft restraints and leather restraints. Soft restraints are used with the majority of clients who need to be restrained. Leather restraints are used when the client is especially strong and might break soft restraints.

The use of restraints requires a physician's order and frequent, documented client assessments. Your institution's policy will guide you.

MEDICATION   Medications can be given to calm or sedate the client. Because the medications are usually given in an IM or IV injection, their administration can be difficult and must be done with assistance. Remember that these drugs take time to work, so the client must be protected from injury until the medication takes effect.

If You Are Assaulted

You certainly have the right to protect yourself from further harm. But be careful to keep your own anger under control. This can be really hard to do when someone

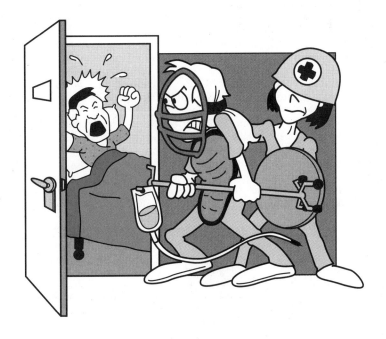

is assaulting you. Most people become very upset when assaulted, and health care providers do too. Remember that you can't hit the client in return just because you are hurt and angry. Getting angry in return could turn a small fight into an all-out war. You may need to blow off steam, but do it in private after the situation is over.

After the assault, when the client is in a position to not hurt others, find out the extent of your injuries. You may need to seek treatment. In the majority of institutions, you must fill out an incident report. (See Chapter 10 for suggestions on filling out an incident report.) If continued violence is an ongoing or frequent occurrence at the hospital, consider forming a support group.

Keep in mind that nurses do not lose their civil rights simply because they are health care workers. If you believe that the client was acting in a malicious manner, consult with your nurse manager and the institution's public safety department about calling the local police and filing charges of assault and battery. Many nurses do not do this because they believe that it will not help the situation. It certainly won't take away your feelings about the incident, but filing criminal charges will help to show the severity of the problem.

Controlling Behaviors

Controlling behaviors are those that lead people to act as you want them to act, instead of them doing as they wish.

Consider This Scenario

Harrison Alfred III was admitted to your unit last week with another bout of pancreatitis, a disease in which the pancreas malfunctions and thus digests itself. It causes a great deal of abdominal pain, which can become chronic pain over time. This is Mr. Alfred's fourth admission this year. In fact, he has been in the hospital more than he has been home during the past 6 months.

Mr. Alfred is a stockbroker and likes to have things done just so. He believes that his wants and needs come first, above those of everyone else, just like they do at home. If he doesn't get *what* he wants *when* he wants it, he makes sure that everyone hears about it. You remember him from his last admission, when he called the hospital CEO because he didn't think that he was receiving adequate care.

Most of the time, Mr. Alfred is a charming man, and yet at times he complains bitterly about his care. He is very good at manipulating the staff into doing what he wants by telling each nurse that he or she is his favorite. He often tells the staff of his personal friendship with the medical chief of staff and the hospital CEO, Mr. Hadst, and he gives the strong impression that if you did not do what he wants, he could have you fired.

Mrs. Alfred is another story. When she is at home, she worries about Mr. Alfred constantly. When she is at the hospital, she worries about her children and the dog constantly. She is very familiar with many medical words, yet the nurses have learned to always use the same terminology with her, because she panics whenever a similar though different word is used. She takes these similar words to mean that something new and bad had arisen.

The nursing staff knows when Mrs. Alfred is visiting because the call light goes on about every 10 minutes. When the nurses answer the light, Mrs. Alfred provides a nonsensical reason for needing the nurses, such as "Do you think it will rain?" or "What do you think the President's chances are for getting reelected?" She cannot sit still and so she paces the floor. Whenever her husband disagrees with the staff, which is often, she becomes even more anxious. Her husband appears to ignore her anxiety and just tells her to go home.

The client assignments are made and you notice that Mr. Alfred is among your assigned clients. You cringe because you know that although Mr. Alfred doesn't require a lot of physical care, it is mentally taxing to provide care for him. This is the fourth day you have been assigned to him.

You start your client care and notice that several call lights are on. You hurry to answer his light first, because you have found that it is easier to treat him like a king than it is to fight with him. He asks you for more ice water and you quickly comply. When you come back, you complete his physical assessment. His abdomen seems more distended and he tells you that it hurts.

You know that his pancreatitis is getting worse and that he seems to be in more pain every day. His pain medication, Demerol, can be given only every 3 hours, yet he begs for more medication 2 hours later. He tells you that the other nurses give it to him every 2 hours, but the medication records show that it has been given every 3 to 4 hours. The physicians are aware of his continued pain and have changed his pain medication accordingly. You note that it is time for his new pain medication and give it to him.

Later in the morning, he puts on the call light to ask for his pain medication. The unit clerk tells him that you are busy but will be there shortly. "Hey, you find her *now*! If you don't, I'll call Mr. Hadst and tell him to fire you!" Ten minutes later, you finish what you are doing and prepare his pain medication. "Well, thank you for gracing me with your presence," he says sarcastically. You ignore this comment and prepare his medication. Before you give it to him, he tells you that it won't work either. "Mary, did they stop my Demerol? Can I get both medications?" When told that he cannot have both medications, he looks angry but just asks to be left alone. A few minutes later, you smell cigarette smoke. You know that smoking is not allowed in the hospital, but there sits Mr. Alfred smoking a cigarette. "Now, Mary, Mary, Mary. Don't get so huffy about my smoking. I'm just in so much pain, I can't be expected to follow the rules. I've been smoking and the other nurses let me. I didn't think you'd mind either." You sternly tell Mr. Alfred to put out his cigarette and he tries to convince you that it is all right for him to smoke. "Come on, I really need this."

After report one day, the nursing staff talked about their feelings about caring for anxious persons such as Mrs. Alfred. One of the nurses said that she found that she would get anxious herself just being around such an anxious person. Another nurse said that she just couldn't be as empathetic as she wanted to be because Mr. Alfred's condition didn't warrant the amount of anxiety Mrs. Alfred delivered. Several nurses commented on how they had done their best to help Mrs. Alfred, but they felt "burned out" because her anxiety didn't go away. Many of the nurses said they were angry with her for the amount of time she consumed "for just silly things."

In this scenario, a client and his wife were masters at the art of controlling others through their behavior. You will need to recognize and deal with:

- Highly anxious behaviors
- Manipulative clients

Highly Anxious Behaviors

Anxiety involves feelings of nervousness, tension, or impending doom. Anxiety is the body's way to engage our defense systems via enhanced use of the sympathetic nervous system. The anxious person has an increased pulse and blood pressure, dilated pupils, and a heightened sense of awareness.

We all feel anxiety during our lives. Hospitalized clients feel it every day. (Nursing students feel it too!) These clients have been effectively removed from their family and occupation and placed in a large institution where people poke them and prod them. They don't feel well, and many support systems have been taken from them. No wonder they are anxious.

Many times, anxious feelings, however unpleasant, contribute to our well-being. Consider how you feel before taking a test. Your pulse and blood pressure are increased, and your alertness is heightened. If not taken to an extreme, this should help you concentrate on the test.

Being in an anxious condition can be acute or chronic. Many people have not learned methods of coping, and they live in a chronic condition of high anxiety.

How can you tell if a person is anxious? Some of the signs and symptoms are readily visible even to the untrained eye:

- Personal statement of anxiety, fear
- Looking apprehensive
- Pacing the floor
- Having a narrow or scattered focus of attention
- Finding fault with everything
- High pitched or rapid voice
- Fidgeting

How can you help the anxious person? One of the easiest and best ways is to simply sit when interacting with him or her. This tells the anxious client that you have the time and the interest to be helpful. It is very important to monitor your voice tone, attitude, and pacing of activities. Pacing can be a particular problem in a health care setting, where many events occur rapidly with very short notice. Nevertheless, no matter how hurried you are, the anxious person should feel that you have all the time in the world to complete your activities.

Avoid reassuring the client that his or her anxiety is useful, because it certainly

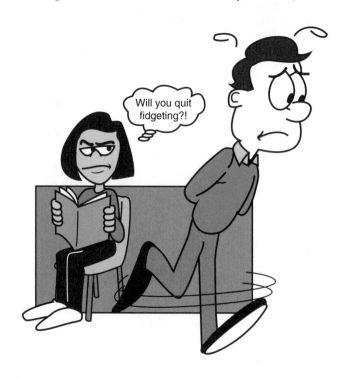

doesn't feel useful to the client. Even though the client's anxiety might have basis in reality, don't try to provide empty explanations as to its cause. Telling someone "I'd feel anxious too, if I were waiting for my biopsy results" won't make the person feel any better.

You must be extremely cautious of what you say to anxious clients because they may incorrectly interpret the information. An anxious client became panic stricken when a nurse referred to her tumor as a "mass." "You mean that I have a mass as well as a tumor?" she asked. To prevent this type of problem, use the same words as the other nursing staff. To find out what the client already knows, you could ask. In addition, it might be helpful to ask the other health care providers what they have told the client.

Try not to add to the stimuli by using a loud voice or talking quickly. Instead, try being quiet and peaceful around them. If you bounce into their room with a "Hi! How are you today?," this could simply rev them up. In addition to being quiet, it is also good to decrease external stimuli, such as dimming the room lights or decreasing the TV sound. Also, lowering the pitch of your voice could be soothing to the client.

It is helpful to encourage the client to express what he or she is feeling. Many times, clients will do this without prompting. But if not, you could simply say, "Tell me about how you feel . . . ."

Most anxious clients prefer to have someone stay with them. Because frequently it is not always possible to have nursing personnel sit with a client, encourage clients to have a family member sit with them. (As long as this doesn't increase their anxiety!) You could also tell them that you will check on them several times an hour. Because the nurses in the scenario recognized that Mrs. Alfred needed reassurance, they tried this. Because they checked on her three times an hour, she quit putting on the call light so often.

Remember that the perceptions of clients may be narrowed when they are anxious. They may have difficulty with problem solving, paying attention to the situation, or remembering things (Lewis, Grainger, McDowell, Gregory, & Messner, 1989).

Manipulative Clients

People interact with each other in a variety of ways. They can be open and honest about their feelings or they can be covert and try to get others to do their bidding in a not-so-obvious way.

As children, we begin to learn how to interact with others. Some children discover that they can get what they want by openly asking for it. In asking for things and receiving them, children learn that they have at least partial control over their environment. Other children learn that the best way to get their needs met is by subterfuge and manipulation. They appear to have no obvious control over the events that happen within their environment, and the only way they can get anything is by manipulation of others.

These manipulative skills are practiced over the years, and some people are so very good at manipulation that those being manipulated don't even know it. This can happen because the manipulator knows how to behave as the situation requires, rather like a chameleon. They can act charming, demure, bold, uncertain, or whatever they need to be to get what they want. Because manipulative clients may act radically differently with each staff member, the staff may have differing perceptions of the client. Some of the staff may believe that the client is pleasant, and others find the client to be extremely offensive. A favorite activity of manipulative clients is to pit the staff against each other. This type of behavior can create havoc within a working group.

How can you tell when clients are manipulating the situation to meet their own needs? It is not always easy to tell, but even clients whom you do not know well may be identified by the following behaviors:

- They think the rules don't apply to them and break them without apparent regret.
- They are demanding, but they are always unsatisfied with the results.
- They can be charmers, able to easily find your "weak spots."
- They are noncompliant with the health regimen.
- They make comments such as "You're the best nurse here. The other nurses are really mean to me," or "You're nice . . . you'll give me my pain shot early." Although it's good to take pride in compliments, this type of comment may not be sincere.
- They attempt to divide the staff into groups—the good nurses and the bad nurses. If you hear comments by other nurses about the client such as "You just don't understand him," or "I think you don't like him," consider whether the client may be acting differently to each staff member. Talk to the other nurses about this.

As the nurses began to talk with each other about their feelings regarding Mr. Alfred, it became painfully obvious that he was a master at manipulating them. A team meeting was held to decide how to help Mr. Alfred. This included all staff members, nurses (even those on second and third shifts), physicians, the unit social worker, and ancillary staff that worked regularly on the unit.

During this meeting the staff expressed their feelings regarding caring for Mr. Alfred. Some of them were angry about being manipulated. Others found that they engaged in power struggles, which wasn't productive for either party. Several staff members said that they found the health care environment stifling, and they identified with the client when he complained about the quality of his health care. The majority of the staff stated that they did not want to provide care to Mr. Alfred, because it was simply too emotionally draining for them. "When I am Mr. Alfred's nurse, it feels like we are in a battle. It's him against me."

The staff thought about the problem and developed a plan of action. They were very careful to make the care plan so detailed that everyone (staff and Mr. and Mrs. Alfred) understood what was expected of them.

After the plan was developed, it was shared with the client and his wife. At first, he was outraged that others thought he was manipulative. Mr. Alfred believed he was simply standing up for his rights as an American health care consumer. After the staff cited specific examples of his behavior, Mr. Alfred conceded that he did like to have his own way about things. With a few minor changes, he and his wife agreed to follow the plan.

The plan went into action that night. The staff knew that it was vital for them to be consistent in its use. To encourage consistency with the plan, the unit manager assigned the same nurses to Mr. Alfred as much as possible. When he did not follow the plan, the nurse was careful not to argue with him, but simply stated the infraction and the consequences.

Because of an illness of one of the nurses normally assigned to Mr. Alfred, a nurse who was unfamiliar with him was assigned. The nurse manager spent 20 minutes explaining Mr. Alfred's care plan. The next day, when the nursing instructor was making assignments, he inquired about Mr. Alfred having a student nurse. It was decided that he wouldn't be an appropriate assignment for a student.

Client Behaviors: Anger Directed Inward

Some clients are unable to directly express their feelings and turn their unhappiness inward at themselves. There are two common types of distressed client behaviors that fall within this category: depression and substance abuse.

Consider This Scenario

Ms. Young, a medical-surgical nurse, sat in the break room trying to balance her checkbook. As her coffee break drew to a close, it was obvious she was overdrawn again! With a sigh, she went back to work.

She went to check on Mrs. Latney, who was hospitalized with a deep vein thrombosis of her right leg. She had been in the hospital for nearly a week now. It seemed to Ms. Young that Mrs. Latney had become quieter over the past few days than she had been previously. Mrs. Latney's physician was aware of her emotional outlook and asked a psychiatrist to see her. A diagnosis of depression was made and medication was started.

While she was helping Mrs. Latney move her leg, Ms. Young thought "I just don't see what she has to be depressed about. She has a loving husband and three good-looking kids. She lives in a big house in the suburbs and she doesn't even have to work. I just don't get it." After Ms. Young helped her, Mrs. Latney asked to have the window shades lowered and the door shut.

Ms. Young also was providing care for Mr. Reyes, who had broken his leg and arm in a motorcycle accident while driving under the influence of alcohol. Even though his leg was getting better, he still wanted his Demerol every four hours. When his Demerol was late, he became very angry.

One day Ms. Young came into Mr. Reyes' room and noticed an unusual smoky odor in the room. She recognized it as marijuana and confronted him. "Sure, I'm smoking pot. You won't give me anything for my leg."

He was told that he couldn't continue smoking marijuana and he just smiled. "OK, I'll take care of it."

The next day, Ms. Young found him drinking whiskey. "You can't drink that either!"

"Look, I need something. If you won't help me, I'll help myself."

The nurses knew that Mr. Reyes had a significant substance abuse problem but did not know what to do about it.

You will need to learn how to recognize and provide care to clients with

- Depression
- Substance abuse problems

Depression

Depression can be described as a feeling of melancholy. Sadness, inactivity, and self-depreciation all accompany depression. Depression can range from mild sadness to full-blown major depression in which the client is consumed with feelings of hopelessness.

Depression is a very common problem in both the hospitalized and nonhospitalized client. It is estimated that 15% of the public will have a problem with depression during their lifetime. This number increases to 20% to 30% for the African-American population. Lewis et al. (1989) suggested that depression is the most common of all psychiatric conditions for the hospitalized client.

Depression can be classified as an appropriate or an inappropriate response. It is certainly appropriate to be sad when experiencing loss. A person will go through grief stages and experience quite severe depression. Although it certainly can be therapeutic to counsel a person who is grieving, the client must still go through the grief process. The therapy or counseling cannot change this. With time, the depression usually lessens.

A major depression that seriously interferes with normal functioning and that lasts longer than two weeks is considered to be pathological. This type of depression requires treatment.

How can you tell when a person is depressed? One way is to look at his or her environment and general attitude.

- Is the environment altered to reflect the person's emotive mood?
- Is the room dark, quiet?
- Is the person's clothing appropriate for the time of day?
- Is the person's general appearance reflective of his or her emotive mood?
- Is the person's body language or voice tone altered?

When caring for a depressed client, realize the importance of simply "being there" for the client instead of "doing something" for the client. This can be very difficult for a dynamic objective-oriented nurse to do. We are very accustomed to *doing things* for our clients. Unfortunately, there is little one can *do* to take away depression. Do not try to "cheer up" the depressed client. The most important intervention is to spend time with the client and listen to his or her concerns.

It might be helpful for you to point out positive attributes in a gentle manner.

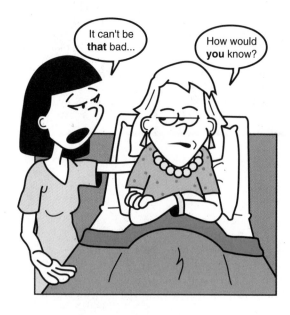

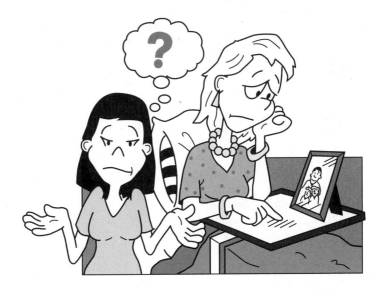

Don't be forceful, because this won't help. Usually depression is not a "rational" disease, and it doesn't lessen the depression to make a point of the obvious. Avoid clichés such as "it can't be that bad," because to the client it may be very bad. Talking to the client in this manner trivializes the condition, as does suggesting that there is a cookbook remedy. Activities such as exercise (if allowed) and interactions with other people should be encouraged. These actions have proved to lessen depression. If the problem is severe or chronic, the client may need counseling or medication.

The nursing staff may think the client is a chronic complainer or may not understand the depression, especially if the nurse perceives that the client has a "good life." Other comments you might hear nurses say are that the nurses might get depressed just being around the depressed client. They also might get angry that the client won't cheer up, because after all, the nurses are doing their part of the job! These feelings, although common, are not helpful for depressed clients.

In the scenario, Ms. Young needed to address how her own feelings affected her ability to be therapeutic with a depressed client.

Substance-Abuse Problems

Many nurses find caring for clients who abuse drugs to be quite a challenge. It is quite common to find clients who abuse drugs to be admitted to medical-surgical units for reasons other than drug abuse.

Actually, substance abuse is a disease with which many nurses are quite familiar. Research has shown that a significant number of nurses come from backgrounds in which at least one family member abused drugs (usually alcohol). The research also suggests that many nurses marry people who are alcoholics or are prone to the disease. This puts a different slant on nurses providing care for substance-abusing clients. The nurse might have significant firsthand experience (Summers, 1992).

This firsthand experience might affect how the nurse views clients with drug-use problems. Because the nurse might remember how he or she was treated by a family member, the nurse might believe the client will treat the nurse in the same manner. Many nurses with drug-abusing family members report that it is extremely difficult for them to be compassionate toward drug-using clients.

How can you detect if a client abuses drugs? Watch your clients for these symptoms:

- Personal statement of drug use
- History of drug use
- Intoxication
- History of legal problems from drug use
- Preoccupied with drug use (prescription or street drugs)
- Dependant on prescribed drugs in institution
- Resentful of authority
- Manipulative behaviors
- Demanding behaviors

The nursing staff drew together to develop a plan of care for Mr. Reyes because of his drug-seeking behaviors. To help them with this process, the substance-abuse nurse practitioner, who also was Mr. Reyes' therapist, joined them.

She suggested that the nurses monitor for illicit drug use while Mr. Reyes is in the hospital. Visitors might bring in street drugs or Mr. Reyes might be taking extra drugs that he brought with him. From now on, when he had visitors, the nurses were to leave his door open and make frequent checks. When one of the nurses suggested searching his belongings, the nurse practitioner cautioned her that unless they have probable cause to believe that Mr. Reyes has something illegal in his belongings, they cannot be searched without his consent.

As they talked, one of the nurses commented on how difficult it was for her to provide care for clients who abuse drugs because she came from a family with many drug abusers. She knew that she needed to come to grips with her own feelings about drug users. For her, one of the most troubling aspects about her family becoming drug-free is that they needed repeated attempts to detoxify. It seemed that they would become drug-free for a while, then slip back into their old ways. It wasn't an easy process.

The nurse practitioner encouraged the nurses to listen to Mr. Reyes' feelings about drug use. When a nurse laughed, "I think he just wants more drugs," the nurse practitioner asked her to consider if Mr. Reyes thought there were any negatives to his drug use. This made the nurse stop and think about it. Most substance-abusing clients wish they could stop.

The nurses developed a care plan that described how Mr. Reyes would receive his medications. It was written in a very specific way. This way, both the client and the nurse knew what was expected of them. A substance-abusing client may need the structure of limit setting to ensure compliance. (This information should be written in the care plan.) When you are using a very detailed care plan, it is important to take the time to inform nurses who may be unfamiliar with the client's background or the treatment plan. Otherwise, the client may view a new nurse as a good way to get increased medications.

Many nurses feel antagonistic toward a person who abuses drugs, and these feelings can affect the nurse's care of the client. Some may believe the client is a weak person who could stop abusing drugs if he or she just wanted to. Others may

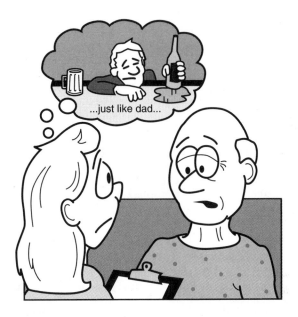

react angrily to the client's manipulative behaviors and so may be over-controlling in return. The nurse might intentionally withhold prescribed medications because he or she "doesn't want to contribute to the client's habit." The drug-abusing client may remind nurses of a person in their lives who is a drug user. The nurse might develop a rescue fantasy and think, "Down deep, this client is a good person who just needs a person like me to help him" (Summers, 1992).

Staff Behaviors

Nursing today is very different from the health care delivery system of earlier days. Although nursing has always involved stress, many nurses believe that stress is increasing along with nursing's increased responsibilities. Many factors affect how the health care staff members will be able to function, including being overworked and feeling a lack of control over their professional day. They are commonly faced with difficult circumstances, such as trying to prioritize their time. When under a severe time-crunch, should they sit with the parents of a child who has just died or get another child ready for surgery? Sometimes nurses are faced with decisions for which there is no good answer. Also, many nurses report feelings of uncertainty resulting from changes in the health care delivery system. Their jobs may be changing and may not even exist in 10 years.

The behavior of the client and family will impact the nurse in varying degrees and various ways, depending on the situation and the general stamina of the nurse. It is certainly easier to deal with a hostile person when you are feeling rested than when you are tired.

A distressing and potentially illegal behavior that nurses may encounter within the health care environment is harassment, which can be verbal, sexual, or racial in nature.

Consider This Scenario

Denise Nowland is a new staff nurse at GetWell Medical Center. During her first week of work, she met Dr. Matthew Farrier, an orthopedic resident. She thought he was pleasant, and perhaps even cute, but her mind was focused on learning her role as a new staff member and so she thought no more of him. The next day when she saw him again he came up to her, made some small talk, and then asked her to go out on a date with him. When she told him "No, thanks," Dr. Farrier just laughed and told her that she would probably change her mind about it in the future.

The next week, she encountered Dr. Farrier again. While she was sitting in the nurses' station, he put his arm around her, gave her a squeeze, and said, "How's my woman?" Denise was quick to get out of his reach and said to him "I'm not your woman." Again he said, "Well, you will be. Don't fight me, you'll never win."

She saw him again a few days later, and once more he came up to her. "I've got tickets to a concert tonight. How about I'll pick you up around 7:00?" Denise recognized that she needed to make her intentions perfectly clear to Dr. Farrier. "Look, I am not interested in dating you. I don't even want to talk to you unless it's about client care. Please leave me alone." Dr. Farrier grabbed her arm, "You better understand something. I have a lot more power around here than you do. I mean, you're just a nurse and I can have you fired if I want to. So use your head and be nice to me." Denise was visibly shaken and just walked away.

For the first time, she saw Dr. Farrier as something other than a would-be persistent suitor. What should she do?

There has been a great deal of attention in the media about harassment in the workplace. Harassment can be:

- Verbal
- Racial
- Sexual

The laws regarding harassment stem from the Civil Rights Act of 1964. Since then, the court systems have continued to work on the definition of and penalties for harassment. Because racial, sexual, and verbal harassment are illegal and not in keeping with appropriate treatment of people, they must not continue to occur.

Although studies show that the majority of adults understand that harassment is illegal, it still occurs with an alarming frequency. Forty percent of nursing students in one study reported being sexually harassed during their clinical rotations (Kettl, Siberski, Hischmann, & Wood, 1993). Another study reported that 60% of the nurses claimed to have been sexually harassed during the previous year (Creighton, 1987).

Verbal abuse of nurses is also alarmingly frequent. In one study, two thirds of nurses stated that they were verbally abused at least once every 3 months. Half stated that they were often verbally insulted by physicians.

The frequency of racial harassment of nurses is harder to pinpoint. Few studies have been done. But when discussing this issue with minority nurses, they speak of subtle and perhaps not-so-subtle racial harassment occurring often.

Why does harassment occur? Although there are several reasons, one stands above the rest. People harass and demean other people because doing so makes them feel powerful. To make it obvious that one person is subordinate to another, the harassing person may use verbal, racial, or sexual harassment. The harassing person may have underlying personal beliefs that he or she is superior to other persons, and the harassment is simply an indicator of this superiority. Conversely, some harassers have low self-esteem and harass others as a way of handling this.

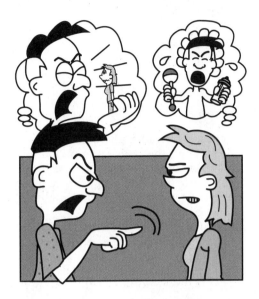

Verbal Harassment

Verbal harassment can be defined as raising one's voice when speaking to a person or verbally insulting a person. As compared with racial or sexual harassment, both of which can be very subtle, verbal harassment is usually clear. In one study of relationships between nurses and physicians, 40% of the nurses reported being yelled at in front of other people. They reported often being yelled at in front of the client or the client's family.

Racial Harassment

Racial harassment is any physical or verbal behavior that would subject an individual to an intimidating or hostile environment as a result of race or ethnicity. Racial harassment may be subtle or obvious and occur with any race as the target.

Sexual Harassment

Sexual harassment is defined as unwelcome sexual advances, requests for sexual favors, and other forms of sexually related conduct when:

1. It is a condition of employment
2. Acceptance or rejection of the conduct affects employment status
3. Such conduct creates an intimidating, hostile, or offensive working environment (EEOC, 1980).

Sexual harassment can take many forms. It can be overt or very subtle. Despite the legal definition, it can be difficult to prove that one is being sexually harassed.

Feelings About Being Harassed

Because harassment is about power, it should be no surprise that most people being harassed feel intimidated and perhaps powerless. Some may even feel that they deserve to be treated this way. Others may feel frightened that they may lose their job and respect from their coworkers and family. Many people worry that others think they "asked" for the harassment because of the way they acted or dressed.

If You Are Being Harassed

The harasser must be told explicitly to stop his or her behavior. Give some thought as to the location for this conversation. You could talk to the harasser in private or in public. Speaking in private allows the incident to remain private, but with this method you are deprived of witnesses to your request that the harassment stop. Speaking in public will bring the situation to the attention of others and, of course, this creates witnesses.

If more than one person is the subject of the harassment, you might try a group confrontation with the harasser. If the harasser realizes that the group will no longer tolerate the behavior, the harasser may be forced to alter it. This method is commonly used by nurses to contend with verbally abusive physicians.

It is vital that you document the harasser's behavior, your reaction to it, and your requests that the behavior be terminated. Get a small notebook and keep it in your pocket. (Make sure that it never leaves your hands!) If a situation arises, make a notation in your book. Describe the incident and the names of any witnesses.

If you are being harassed, it is important to not lose your cool. Even though someone is harassing you, it does not give you the right to verbally or physically attack that person in return. There are legal methods to handle the situation.

If the harassment does not stop after you have asked the person to alter his or her behavior, tell your supervisor about the problem. They will discuss the situation with the affirmative action officer for the institution and take action, if necessary. At this point, if the harassment still does not stop, go back to your supervisor and the affirmative action officer.

Conclusion

Health care workers must help others handle stress and address ways to help clients function when their coping mechanisms are not adequate. Because a client may be so distressed, the entire health care team will need to work together to help the client cope. Although this can be a challenge, it is a very important part of the nurse's role.

PRACTICAL APPLICATIONS

Consider the following scenarios and answer the questions that follow:

Scenario 1

A client on your unit has had multiple hospitalizations for a nonhealing wound on his leg. He has diabetes, does not follow his diet, and takes his insulin sporadically. He is verbally abusive to many members of the nursing staff. He has called several of the staff members racial slurs and has made comments on their physical appearance. You are making the assignments for the next shift. Each of the nurse's aides has asked that he be assigned to someone else.

1. How do you expect clients to act?

2. Do any of your professional feelings differ from your personal feelings regarding these expectations?

3. Is it possible to meet these expectations?

4. How do you feel about clients who are noncompliant with their medical regimen?

5. Can you change his behavior?

6. How can you affect this situation to allow the staff to provide care for this client?

Scenario 2

While on duty one day, you notice a small group of people in the hallway. They look lost. You talk to them and, indeed, they *are* lost. You start to give them directions to where they are going, but you stop when you see the look of confusion on their faces.

1. How can you get these people to where they are going?

2. What can you do to change the environment to help others find their way?

REFERENCES

Antai-Otong, D. (1988). What you should and shouldn't do when your patient is angry. *Nursing '88, 18*(2), 44–45.

Bradley, V. (1992). Workplace abuse: Unrecognized emergency department violence. *Journal of Emergency Nursing, 18*(6), 489–490.

Burgess, A. W., Burgess A. G., & Douglas, J. (1994). Examining violence in the workplace. *Journal of Psychosocial Nursing, 32*(7), 11–15.

Casey, D. (1992, November). Billy wouldn't budge . . . until the hard truth hit him. *Nursing '92, 26–48.*

Cox, H. (1987). Verbal abuse in nursing: Report of a study. *Nursing Management, 16*(11), 47–50.

Creighton, H. (1987). Sexual harassment: Legal implications. *Nursing Management, 18*(5), 18–22.

Daum, A. (1994). The disruptive antisocial patient: Management strategies. *Nursing Management, 25*(8), 46–51.

Diaz, A., & McMillin, J. (1991). A definition and description of nurse abuse. *Western Journal of Nursing Research, 13*(1), 98–109.

Gorman, L., Sultan, D., & Luna-Raines, M. (1989). *Psychosocial nursing handbook for the nonpsychiatric nurse.* Baltimore: Williams & Wilkins.

Gomez, G., & Gomez, E. (1993). Depression in the elderly. *Journal of Psychosocial Nursing, 31*(5), 28–32.

Horrigan, K. (1993, February). Judy was an expert on diabetes...and noncompliance. *Nursing '93, 62–64.*

Kettl, P., Siberski, J., Hischmann, C., & Wood, B. (1993). Sexual harassment of health care students by patients. *Journal of Psychosocial Nursing, 31*(7), 11–13.

Kinkle, S. (1993). Violence in the ED: How to stop it before it starts. *American Journal of Nursing, 93*(7), 22–24.

Kirschner, G. (1989). If you scream, I'll kill you. *RN, 52*(3), 35–40.

Lewis, S., & Blumenreich, K. (1993). Defusing the violent patient. *RN, 56*(12), 24–29.

Lewis, S., Grainger, R., McDowell, W., Gregory, R., & Messner, R. (1989). *Manual of psychosocial nursing interventions: Promoting mental health in medical surgical settings.* Philadelphia: W.B. Saunders.

Mahoney, B. (1991). *Victimization of Pennsylvania emergency department nurses in the line of duty.* Pennsylvania State University. PhD Thesis.

McConnell, E. (1987, April). Does your patient seem too cheerful? *RN,* 23–24.

McKinney, B. (1994, April). COPD and depression: Treat them both. *RN, 20*(4), 48–50.

Medved, R. (1990). Strategies for handling angry patients and their families. *Nursing '90, 66–67.*

Parker, B. (1992). When your medical/surgical patient is also mentally ill. *Nursing '92,* 66–68.

Renz, M. (1993, October). The trouble with sister. *Nursing '93,* 58–60.

Rosenthal, T., Edwards, N., Rosenthal, R., & Ackerman, B. (1992). Hospital violence: Site, severity, and nurses' preventive training. *Issues in Mental Health Nursing, 13*(4), 349.

Rucitti, C. (1992). Caring for a combative patient. *Nursing '92, 22*(9), 50–51.

Summers, C. (1992). *Caregiver, caretaker.* Mt. Shasta, CA: Commune-A-Key Publishing.

Teaching patient relations in hospitals: The hows and whys. (1983). The American Hospital Association.

U.S. Department of Health and Human Services. (1993). Depression in primary care: Detection, diagnosis and treatment. *Journal of Psychosocial Nursing, 32* (6), 19–28.

Vincent, M., & White, K., (1994). Patient violence toward a nurse: Predictable and preventable? *Journal of Psychosocial Nursing, (32)*2, 30–32.

Warren, B. (1994). Depression in African-American women. *Journal of Psychosocial Nursing, 32* (3), 29–33.

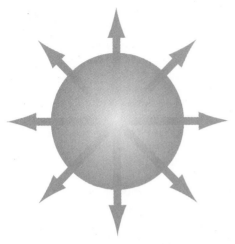

7

With the Critically Ill Client

In this chapter, we will discuss:

- Basic theory relating how severity of illness can affect communication
- The stressors of critical care
- So many machines/such high technology care
- Limited visiting hours
- Teaching the family how to visit
- Coping within a state of crisis
- Level of awareness
- Roller coaster effect
- Transition from critical care to a general nursing unit
- Code blue
- Verbal speech limitations
- So little hope
- Deterioration in health condition

Hearing the words "you are going to be admitted to the critical care unit" strikes fear into many people's hearts. Yet, this action happens often, because the number of hospital admissions to critical care units is steadily increasing. We are providing health care to clients who are much sicker than in the past. Because of current technology, we keep people alive who years ago would have died.

While visiting in the critical care unit, visitors walk past rooms that seem to be filled with beeping machines. There is so much equipment that one might wonder if there actually is a client in each bed. The clients appear to be so sick! And the rooms seem small because of the equipment and the number of the health care personnel going in and out of the rooms. Because the nurses need to be in constant view of the clients, doors are kept open and curtains are pulled back. This contributes to the lack of privacy. Many visitors report that they don't like to be in the critical care waiting room because families of other critically ill clients talk about how sick their loved ones are.

Yet, in the midst of this high-tech environment, we cannot overlook the human element. From the client's perspective, it is very frightening to be this sick. The stress of being in such an environment and the stress of serious illness may be overwhelming. For the family, the intensive care environment can add to the stress of having a seriously ill family member. For students, the responsibility of helping provide care to critically ill clients is stressful and often magnified by the demands of the critical care environment.

This chapter will provide information on communicating within the context of the critical care unit. We will look at factors affecting communication with the critically ill client and the family. Then we will look at three scenarios that are common to the critical care environment and how communication is accomplished within each of these.

Basic Theory Relating Severity of Illness to Alteration in Communication Skills

It is well known that an alteration in health status can result in an increase in the amount of stress a person experiences. This stress level can become even higher when a person has a serious illness that requires the intervention of highly educated health care personnel and the high-tech equipment found in a critical care unit.

Many factors affect the ability of the client, family, and friends to cope with a severe illness. One is the ability or inability to communicate effectively with each other and with the health care providers. Titler (1991) looked at the perceptions of critically ill adults and their families. Although the client and family reported good communication skills before the client's illness, after the illness there was poor communication among family members. Family members reported that home routines were disrupted during the time of illness, and there were changes in role relationships. Clearly, the critical illness impaired or contributed to the altered ability to communicate because of this disruption and the resulting role changes.

Other factors influencing the ability to cope with a critical illness are as follows:

SEVERITY AND LENGTH OF CRITICAL STATUS   During a critical illness, a client's health care status can range from an acute, short-term illness to hovering near death for a long period.

SUDDEN ONSET OF CRITICAL ILLNESS   A person could have been healthy yesterday and today is comatose.

PRESENCE OF CHRONIC ILLNESS   Chronic Illness is a stressor in itself for the client and family. The occurrence of an acute, severe illness can add demands on an already strained family system.

CRITICAL CARE ENVIRONMENT   Intensive care areas are full of unfamiliar machines and other high technology equipment. These machines have many blinking lights and make a great deal of noise. The overwhelming physical presence of the machinery can cause clients and their families undue concern.

POOR PROGNOSIS   Many clients and families often must deal with the client's poor prognosis.

FINANCIAL PROBLEMS   The financial impact an acute illness may have on a family cannot be overlooked. The client may not return to work for a long time, if at all.

A serious illness can be a crisis situation. Any stressful event that threatens a client's sense of biologic, psychologic, or social integrity can result in disequilibrium and crisis. Becoming critically ill can certainly be classified as a stressful event or crisis.

The first stage of crisis is the phase of shock and denial. This is the most common stage of crisis seen in the hospital. During this time, client and family or friends are overwhelmed by stressful stimuli and exhibit high anxiety and helplessness. They may lack reasoning skills and problem-solving abilities. They often have trouble organizing their thoughts and feelings and may be highly emotional. Many studies have shown that individuals react in a similar pattern to a crisis. This has led health care providers to identify helpful behaviors to help the client cope with a crisis. An awareness of the emotional state of the client and family will guide appropriate nursing interventions.

It is helpful for clients in crises to verbalize their perceptions of their condition, procedures, and environment. With this information, the nurse can correct any misperceptions they may have.

What Are the Stressors of Critical Care?

Although the critical care unit environment is certainly intimidating, what is it that really adds to the stress of hospitalization? To find an answer to this question, a survey of critical care clients and nurses was undertaken, the results of which are found in Table 7–1. Although there are many similarities between the two lists, there are also differences. This is important to note, because nurses have an important responsibility in helping clients cope with stressors effectively. To ensure

Table 7–1   COMPARISON OF WHAT NURSES AND CLIENTS DEFINE AS STRESSFUL IN A CRITICAL CARE SETTING

Client	Nurse
Having tubes in your nose or mouth	Being tied down
Being stuck with needles	Not being in control of oneself
Being in pain	Having tubes in your nose or mouth
Not being able to sleep	
Being thirsty	

Adapted from Cochran, J., & Ganong, L. (1989). A comparison of nurses' and patients' perceptions of intensive care unit stressors. *Journal of Advanced Nursing, 14*(12), 1038–1043.

that critical care stressors are correctly identified, appropriate assessment must take place. In doing so, the nursing staff may realize that their definition of stressors may be different from that of the client and family. Ongoing nurse-family interaction enhances client and family coping. It is only through effective communication that client needs are identified and strategies are chosen.

Monitoring a client after a major surgery is a common type of admission to a critical care unit. Although this type of hospitalization is certainly stressful for the client and family, it often is uneventful, and the client recovers.

Consider This Scenario

CLIENT WITH MAJOR SURGERY—SHORT STAY

Jamilia Stevens, age 14, was born with a cyst between her heart and lungs. For many years, it did not cause any health problems and so it was simply monitored regularly. In the past year, it started to grow, putting pressure on her heart and lungs. Consequently, it was decided that the cyst needed to be removed.

The surgeon explained that the surgery would take about three hours and that Jamilia would go to pediatric intensive care after surgery. To become familiar with the setting, Jamilia and her parents toured the pediatric intensive care unit two weeks before the surgery. They met several nurses, and one took them into an empty client room to show them the equipment and discuss its usage.

"My name is Chen Lu and I am a registered nurse in this unit. Let me tell you about the equipment we will use to help you after surgery. The machines on the IV pole help us to count the IV rates and keep the IV fluids accurate. They sometimes beep to let us know to check the IV machines. This does not always mean that anything is wrong with the machine or with your IV. There will be sticky pads on your chest called electrodes that attach to wires and connect to the heart monitor. The heart monitor tells us how fast your heart is beating. You may find that it makes a loud beep at times. This beep is to tell us to check on you. It does not necessarily mean that something is wrong with your heart. It could mean that something else happened, such as one of your sticky pads came loose or you turned in bed. You will also have two tubes coming out from your chest wall attached to a plastic box that helps keep your lungs expanded. What questions do you have about the equipment? (Pause) The nurses will explain this equipment again to you on the day of surgery."

Jamilia and her parents asked a few questions and then went to the laboratory to have her preoperative blood work drawn.

Jamilia's surgery went as planned, and she came to the pediatric intensive care unit afterward. After Chen Lu assessed her and found her condition to be stable, she went to the waiting room to find Jamilia's parents. "You can come in to see her now. I want to remind you that she is still very sleepy from the anesthetic. You will see that there is a lot of equipment in the room, just like we talked about two weeks ago. If you want to know more about what the machines do, just let me know. Let's go see her now."

When Jamilia's parents first came to see her, they stood in the far corner of the room. With encouragement from Chen Lu, they soon learned to stand on the left side of Jamilia's bed, because much of the equipment was on the right-hand side. While they were in the room, they looked decidedly uncomfortable with the surroundings. Chen Lu asked if they wanted to help with Jamilia's care, and taught them how to encourage Jamilia with her coughing and deep breathing each hour.

Jamilia's parents stayed in the room with her for most of the day. Later in the day, Mrs. Stevens asked Chen Lu, "Is there something wrong? I've noticed that you check on her all the time." "No," Chen Lu replied, "it is part of our routine nursing care to do this kind of checking. We measure her pulse, temperature, blood pressure, and breathing frequently. By having this information, we can keep a close watch on how she is doing. Do let me know of any other questions you may have."

The pediatric intensive care unit visitor guidelines allowed one person to stay in the child's room around the clock, except during procedures and during shift report. Jamilia's parents took turns in her room and both commented on how nice it was that they could be with her. Mr. Stevens told the nurses that he had recently been in an accident at work and spent three days in intensive care. There, they allowed only two visitors to come in every hour for 10 minutes. Mr. Stevens said the short visiting period really made him feel cut off from the rest of his life.

In the scenario, several factors added stress to the family:

- Fast pace and multitude of machinery
- Family's unfamiliarity with the environment

So Many Machines/Such High Technology Care

The amount of technology needed to provide care for a critically ill client is astounding. We are using technology that may not have existed 10 years or even 10 months ago. In a typical critical care client room you may find:

- Ventilator
- Dialysis machine
- Five or six IV machines
- Arterial line
- Cardiac monitor
- Chest tubes
- Tube feeding pump
- Pulse oximeter
- Cardiac output monitor
- Pneumatic stockings
- Temporary pacemaker
- Patient-controlled analgesia (PCA) machine
- Automatic blood pressure machine
- Suction equipment

Depending on the circumstances, you may find even more equipment than is listed above. In the scenario, Jamilia had IV lines that were attached to IV machines, cardiac monitors, and chest tubes. To the patient and family, these machines can be intimidating because of their size, blinking lights, and loud noises. Many clients find it frightening to have to rely on machinery. They may believe that the more machines that are in the room, the sicker they must be. (This isn't always true!) You might find that the family watches the cardiac monitor instead of talking to the client.

To help you communicate with the client, consider how overwhelmed you were the first time you saw a critical care nursing unit. Then, explain things to the client and family in way that they will understand. It is helpful to explain the purposes of the equipment in as simple terms as possible. In most circumstances, you need to tell what the equipment is used for, what sounds it may make, and briefly what these sounds might mean, just as Chen Lu did in the scenario concerning the IVs, cardiac monitor, and chest tubes.

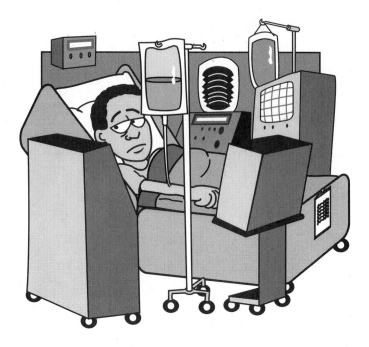

It is also helpful to explain why physical assessments are done so frequently. Again, clients and families may perceive that checking vital signs and other assessment parameters means they are getting worse. A simple explanation often alleviates unnecessary anxiety. It may also put a family at ease knowing that someone is watching the client so closely. It would make it easier for the family to go home periodically. This was illustrated when Mrs. Stevens asked Chen Lu why Jamilia was being checked so often. Mrs. Stevens thought something was wrong. Chen Lu simply explained the routine and explained why the routine was being followed.

Limited Visiting Hours

An added difficulty to communicating effectively with critically ill clients is the limited visiting hours found in most intensive care units. A common type of visiting restriction would be to allow visiting for 10 minutes every 2 to 3 hours. These visiting restrictions are much more stringent than those in the general hospital units. This means the family and friends try to pack as much communication as possible into a short time frame. Also, many intensive care units allow *only* immediate family members. Sometimes significant others are excluded.

Another problem caused by limited visiting hours is that they provide limited opportunities for family and friends to interact with the health care workers. They might not have the time to get to know you, and you might have little time to talk to them.

Observe the client and family interaction during visiting hours. Do they talk to each other? Do you hear comments like "I never get to see him long enough!"? Does it seem that the client and family need more time together? If so, the visiting restrictions may be problematic for the client and family. Consider how the visiting hours could be altered to suit the needs of the client. In the scenario, the 24-hour visitation was very helpful to Jamilia and her parents.

This type of problem can sometimes be alleviated by the nurse talking with family and friends during times other than visiting hours in the hallway or waiting room. It is helpful to maintain contact with the family by talking with them every hour or so. This may not always be possible, especially if the nurse is unable to leave the client's bedside. If this is the case, perhaps the charge nurse or another nurse can give the family a brief progress report and see if there are any questions.

Does the Family Know How To Visit?

Because of the intimidating environment and the severity of the client's illness, the family and friends may need to be taught how to visit the client.

It would be helpful to know if they have ever visited the client before. Observe the family when they are visiting the client. When in the client's room, where do they stand? Are they standing in the doorway, as if afraid to come any closer? Or do they confidently move to the client's bedside? In the scenario, it took much encouragement to get Jamilia's parents to come close to her bed.

Before you bring the family to the client's room for the first time, provide a basic description of what they will see. Include any noises the machines will make and anything they may smell. Also explain what the client looks like—does he or she have dressings, nasogastric tubes, endotracheal tubes, or IV lines? This was helpful for Jamilia's parents because they knew what to expect when they saw her.

Often, the family will not want to touch the client because they are afraid of disturbing the equipment or harming the client. Once the family and friends are in the client's room, tell them where they can stand and what they can touch.

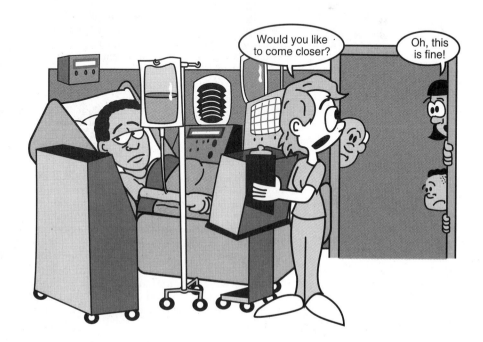

Encourage them to touch the client and talk to him or her. Also, tell them what *not* to touch (usually the tubes and machine settings).

The nurse might need to monitor what the family says to the client. For example, this would *not* be the correct time to talk about financial problems, stressful events, or hardships incurred related the client's hospitalization.

In some situations, you may want to include the family and friends in the care of the client, just as Chen Lu did by teaching the family how to help Jamilia with her coughing and deep breathing. It's quite common for the family to say that they wish they could be of assistance to the client. In addition, the client may benefit from having the family near. With supervision, the family can:

- Comb hair
- Apply body lotion
- Do range of motion exercises
- Sit quietly at the bedside without talking; their presence alone can be very reassuring
- Supervise coughing and deep breathing

Consider This Scenario

A CAR ACCIDENT

Juan Garcia, his wife, and three children were in a serious car accident. As they entered the emergency department, Mr. Garcia was obviously seriously injured. He was taken immediately to surgery because of acute abdominal injuries. His wife was conscious and had a broken arm, which was placed in a cast. The three children were shaken and bruised, but otherwise uninjured. As might be expected, they were very anxious, which may have been compounded by the fact that they had never been in the hospital before.

After a 4-hour surgery to repair internal injuries, Mr. Garcia was returned to the surgical intensive care unit. The surgeon discussed his injuries with Mrs. Garcia. The nurse providing his care met briefly with Mrs. Garcia in the waiting room after assessing Mr. Garcia and checking that all the equipment was working properly. The nurse said, "He is still unconscious, so he can't talk to you, but do talk to him anyway. You will notice that there are a lot of machines in the room. We're using them to help us provide care to him. Are there any questions I can answer?" When Mrs. Garcia indicated that she didn't have any questions, the nurse said, "Let's go in to see him."

Later in the day, the nurse said to Mrs. Garcia, "I've written out a list of the physicians that are providing care to him. Also, I've included the booklet that tells you about the surgical intensive care unit. Let's go over this information."

After a few days, Mrs. Garcia started to ask questions about Mr. Garcia's care. The nursing staff took this as a cue to start to provide more in-depth information.

Mr. Garcia was unconscious for about a week after the accident. During this time, Mrs. Garcia just sat in his room and didn't speak to him at all. "Do you think he can hear us?" she asked one of the nurses. With some encouragement, Mrs. Garcia began to talk to him.

As Mr. Garcia began to recover from his injuries, he became more alert. When he became stronger, the physicians decided to transfer him to a surgical unit because of his progress. Mr. Garcia and his wife were told of the reasons for his transfer, and they thought it was a good sign. The nurse encouraged Mrs. Garcia to visit the surgical unit before Mr. Garcia's transfer.

Several days after Mr. Garcia was transferred to the surgical unit, he complained of dizziness and pain in his head. Later that day, he became difficult to arouse. It was determined that he had suffered a massive stroke. Because of the stroke, he had difficulty with swallowing and a tube feeding was started.

During the next several weeks, he would improve, and then he would relapse again into unconsciousness. Although the family received support from the nursing staff and from their priest, it was a very difficult time for them.

Two months after his accident, Mr. Garcia had a cardiac arrest. All the people in the waiting room, including Mrs. Garcia, heard the overhead announcement "Code Blue: 7-Main." With this, the anxiety level in the waiting room rose considerably. The visitors watched as people wearing scrubs rushed down the hallway toward the unit. Each person in the room thought that their loved one had the cardiac arrest. The nurse manager came into the waiting room and asked Mrs. Garcia to come into her office. The nurse manager told her that her husband suffered a cardiac arrest. The nurse manager held Mrs. Garcia as she cried. The two women sat and waited until word came that Mr. Garcia's heart rhythm was normal again.

Many clients are admitted to critical care because of a serious accident or injury. Some of the factors that affect communication in this type of situation are:

- Is the family in a state of crisis?
- What is the client's level of consciousness?
- Roller coaster effect (getting better, getting worse)
- Transition from critical care to a general nursing unit
- Code blue

Is the Client or Family in a State of Crisis?

When an illness occurs over a long period, people have time to practice their coping skills and perhaps develop an effective coping pattern. But when illness has an abrupt onset, such as an auto accident, there is not time to learn coping skills. When a car accident occurs, the client and family are probably still in a state of shock and disbelief one day later.

Consider how much information the client and family can handle at the time of the discussion. This amount can vary greatly. For example, the type and amount of information provided to a client who is unresponsive to stimuli will be very different from the information given to a client who is alert and on a ventilator. Usually, during the first few days of a crisis, the client, family, and friends want to know only simple, important facts. In the following days, they will want to know more details. In the scenario, the nurse gave Mrs. Garcia only the needed information. Not only did she explain the information, but she also gave written information. Having written information can be very useful in a crisis situation.

Assess what the client, family, and friends already know and add to it. Listen to them and allow them to ask questions before you talk. Ask them what they want to know. To keep your information at the appropriate level, approximate their general educational level. This will direct the descriptors used in your conversations. Assess their emotional state. Are they calm and able to follow what is being said, or are they anxious and having difficulty remembering what they have been told? Remember, though, that *appearing* calm does not always mean they are *actually feeling* calm.

Do not be surprised if the family repeats questions or asks questions that you have just answered. Short-term memory is usually very poor in a time of crisis.

The most helpful methods of communication during a crisis period include:

- Offering concrete, basic information

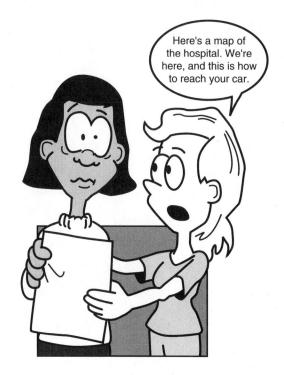

- Telling the client, family, and friends only what they need to know. Don't tell them things that are just "nice to know" at this time.
- Being supportive of their feelings. Let them direct the conversation.

Crisis intervention research has shown that information needed on the day of an emergency surgery includes:

- Names of the nurses providing care for the client
- Names of the surgeon and other physicians providing care
- Location of the intensive care unit, waiting room, cafeteria, and rest rooms
- Visiting hours for the intensive care unit and the phone number for the unit
- Basic descriptions of the disease process
- Brief description of what the next 24 hours will entail

It would be helpful to write down the above information for the client, because research has shown that little verbal information is retained during a time of crisis. Providing written reminders will improve retention and accuracy of the information.

By the second and third day of hospitalization, the client, family, and friends will want to know more detailed information. Reasons for equipment usage, the basic jobs of the personnel, places to spend the night, restaurants in the area, and more detailed descriptions of the disease process may be welcomed at this time.

Alterations in Level of Consciousness

How can you tell if a comatose client can hear you? It is very difficult to know if a client can hear if he or she is unable to tell you or do something to suggest that he or she may have heard you. Although it is possible to test comatose clients for hearing disorders, it is not commonly done because the problem most often results from the client's inability to process data, not from the ability to hear.

Many nurses can relate stories of clients that were comatose while the nurse provided care but later recognized the nurse's voice as familiar. Were they able to hear the nurse, but unable to respond while they were comatose or does it simply seem familiar for another reason? There is no way of knowing which of these is true.

No matter what the client's level of consciousness is, you need to talk to the client, watching for any sign that he or she may have heard you. Remember to consider hearing loss, medication usage, and unwillingness to communicate before you decide that a client is unable to communicate with you.

Some suggestions for communicating with comatose clients:

- *Always* assume the client can hear you. Never say anything within the hearing range of a client that you wouldn't want the client to hear.
- Families will ask you if you think the client can hear. A good answer is, "We are unsure if he/she can hear you, but talk to him/her anyway just in case he/she can. Tell him/her whatever you want him/her to know." This was demonstrated in the scenario.
- Tell family and friends not to say anything within the client's hearing range that they don't want the client to know.
- Explain to the client on a regular basis what is happening to him or her.

Roller Coaster Effect (Getting Better, Getting Worse)

The pathway for a critical illness is marked by hills and valleys. Clients get better, then sometimes they get worse. This is especially true with a lengthy, serious illness such as a severe head injury or cancer.

The getting better, getting worse is difficult for the client, family, and friends. When the client gets better, the family might regain hope in the client's recovery. But when the client gets worse, sadness and anger aimed toward the client, family, and health care staff may be evident.

Monitor the general emotional attitude of the client and family. As the days pass, how are they dealing with the stressors of hospitalization? Do they seem tired and quiet? Do they take time out for themselves to rest, eat, and take care of things? Or maybe they talk of gaining weight and being angry with the world.

Nurses help people through these difficult times when they:

- Explain what is happening and what is being done to improve the situation.
- Are supportive of the feelings of friends and family.
- Continue to verbalize hope about the situation, if this is realistic.
- Encourage family and friends to be helpful to the client. An example of this would be to teach the client *and* the family how to perform a simple nursing intervention for the client, such as coughing and deep breathing. Ask the family to encourage the client to do it hourly.
- Give the family "permission" to take breaks, go for a walk, or get away for a little while.
- Allow the family time to verbalize anxiety, questions, and fears.

- Tell the family that setbacks are not uncommon. Doing this will help them not be so surprised when a setback does occur.

Client Transition From a Critical Care Setting to a General Nursing Unit

When it is decided that a client no longer needs the services of a critical care unit, the client will be transferred to another unit. This could happen because the client's condition has improved or because it has been determined that his or her health status cannot be improved despite the high-tech care provided by the critical care unit.

In a critical care unit, the nurse-to-client ratio is usually one or two patients to one nurse. However, a typical nurse-to-client ratio on a medical floor may be six patients to one nurse. The client may have become accustomed to the monitors

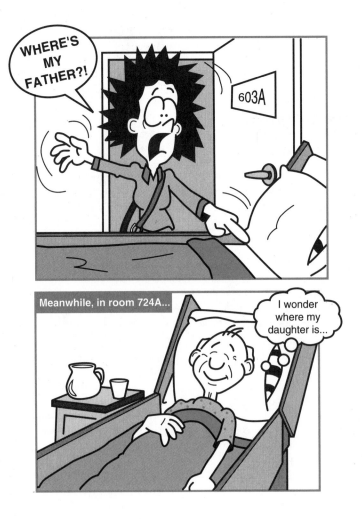

and equipment and found it comforting to be so closely monitored. Going to another type of nursing unit can be stressful and frightening for the client, family, and friends. Careful planning and good communication will make this transition easier.

Does the client and family know of the proposed transfer? How do they perceive the move? Do they think this transfer is a step in the right direction or does it have negative connotations? Some suggestions to make the move easier:

- Discuss the reason for the transfer with client, family, and friends. Is it because the client is getting better? If so, perhaps this could be viewed as making progress. Reassure the client that "they will take good care of you also. Look at this move as a graduation." Sometimes, though, the client is transferred out of critical care because of a lack of clinical progress. Acceptance of this depends on acceptance of the client's condition.
- Go over the medical and nursing orders and plan of care with the nurse from the receiving unit.
- Include the family as much as possible in the transfer plans. The family should be called if the transfer occurs when they are not at the hospital. It is very frightening for families to see an empty bed where their family member was.
- Inform the family about visiting policies on the client's new unit.
- Assess the family's expectations of the care on the general floor to see if they are realistic. If not, more teaching may be necessary.

Code Blue/Cardiac Arrest

One of the worst possible fears for a family member sitting in an intensive care unit waiting room is to hear "Code Blue—ICU." Even if the family knows that the client is not in critical condition, the family member fears that perhaps it is their loved one who has suffered a cardiac arrest.

If the cardiac arrest *is not* their family member, simply say, for example, "No, your father is fine." For confidentiality reasons, you cannot tell which client has suffered the arrest if it is not their family member.

If the cardiac arrest *is* their family member, tell them, "Yes, it is your father. We are doing everything possible for him" (providing this is the case). Could the family be allowed to wait during the arrest in a private area away from the other visitors? This would serve two purposes. The first is that it will allow the family privacy, and the second is that the families of the other ICU clients will not have to witness the family's grief, wondering if it will be their loved one next time.

During a time of crisis, it is very helpful to have someone stay with the client. Does the client have any family or friends who may be in the hospital at the time of the arrest? If possible, have someone from the hospital sit with the family and friends. Perhaps the hospital chaplain could stay with the family during this time. If possible, bring information to the family and friends during the arrest situation, especially if it is a lengthy one.

Consider This Scenario

THE CLIENT WITH A COMPLICATED INTENSIVE CARE STAY

Mrs. Thomas was absolutely tired. Her husband Franklin had chronic obstructive pulmonary disease (COPD), and this was the fourth time he had been in the hospital this year. As she left the hospital, she wondered if Franklin would ever make it home again, but she doubted it. He had been too sick for too long.

The next day when she came to see him, she saw that his breathing was difficult, and within an hour, he was placed on a ventilator to help him breathe. Mrs. Thomas was saddened that Franklin wasn't getting better, but he had been on a ventilator many times before so it wasn't a new experience. She discussed methods of communication with the nurse that Franklin could use now that he was on the ventilator. They decided to use paper and pencil, as this had worked well in the past.

Mr. Thomas remained on the ventilator in a semicomatose state for several months. One afternoon, Mr. Thomas's blood pressure began to fall. Little was done to correct this, as everyone agreed that Mr. Thomas had been through enough. A do-not-resuscitate order had been discussed with the client and his family, and a client order for this had been written. The nurse taking care of him called Mrs. Thomas. "This is Megan Zammy calling from GetWell Medical Center. Is this Mrs. Thomas? Mrs. Thomas, your husband's condition is getting worse. Could you please come to the hospital?"

The Thomas family came to the hospital to be at his bedside when he died.

Some critical care clients are extremely ill upon admission to the unit and continue to have serious physiological problems throughout their intensive care stay. These clients may have had a very extensive trauma or physiologic illness such as a heart attack. They may also have other chronic conditions such as lung disease or diabetes. They could be in the intensive care unit for weeks or perhaps even months. Their hospital stay is marked by slow or marginal improvement, with many complications along the way.

Some common problems seen with this type of hospitalization include:

- Verbal speech limitations
- So little hope
- Deteriorating health

What Is the Client's Ability to Communicate?

It is common for a critically ill client to be mechanically ventilated and have tubes coming out of every natural orifice and even some man-made ones. The presence of the machinery and the stress can make it very hard to communicate. But even with these tubes that may impair communication, people still have concerns, cares, and feelings. We need to be able to assess for potential communication barriers for a client in the intensive care unit (Williams, 1992). Assess your client for the following:

- Impairments such as paralysis and altered level of consciousness
- Medications such as sedatives and narcotics that may alter the level of consciousness or cause paralysis
- Lack of physical strength resulting from severity of illness
- Endotracheal/tracheostomy tubes
- Surgical procedures that alter one's ability to speak (glossectomy, laryngectomy)

If your client has one or more of the above, his or her ability to easily communicate may be altered. These barriers to communication can sometimes be alleviated through the proper communication method.

Verbal Speech Limitations

Many clients in critical care areas have an impairment of verbal function. This could be the result of altered physical condition (such as removal of the larynx or trauma), medications (such as paralyzing agents), or the use of machinery (such as mechanical intubation). The most common reason for temporary verbal impairment is needing mechanical help to breathe. Requiring ventilatory assistance means that the client will have either an endotracheal tube or a tracheostomy. Although the endotracheal tube is considered to be a short-term measure, a tracheostomy may either be temporary or permanent. With an endotracheal tube in place, the client is unable to talk. Clients with most types of tracheostomies also cannot talk. (There are types of tracheostomies that allow a client to verbally communicate, but they are not as common.)

Having a surgical procedure such as a glossectomy or laryngectomy means that the client will need to learn a permanent new method of communication, because he or she will have lost the ability to produce verbal speech. After the client has recovered from the surgery, an electric voice synthesizer may be used, but until this time, an alternative communication device will be needed.

When it is detected that the client is unable to verbally communicate, an alternate communication system must be established as soon as possible. Ideally, a communication system should be established before the communication alteration takes place. While this may not be possible in instances such as trauma, it could be done for clients with scheduled surgeries who will have these alterations postoperatively. Alternate communication methods are presented in Table 7–2.

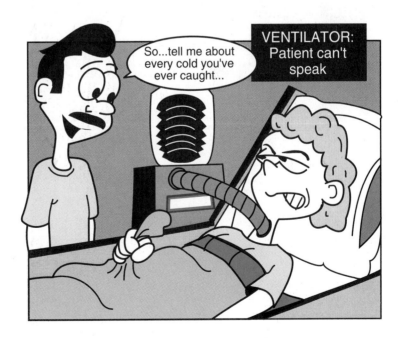

Table 7–2 ALTERNATIVE METHODS OF COMMUNICATION

Method	Advantages	Disadvantages
Lip Reading The client uses lips to mouth words. Encourage the client to say each word slowly and distinctly. The client may need to repeat the words several times. Verify with the client he or she is mouthing English words.	Useful for clients with immobile arms. Do not need any special equipment.	Can be very difficult to understand what the client is trying to say. This can be very frustrating for the nurse and the client. Not useful for clients who are orally intubated. Cannot be used for clients with little English usage.
Picture Board A large poster board with pictures of typical client needs is shown to the client. The client points to the item required.	Easy for the client to point to the item needed. Can be used by a client who cannot read, write, or speak English.	Must be able to use arms. Only able to use the pictures on the board. How would you express "I'm afraid" via the board?
Paper and Pencil/Magic Slate Give the client paper and pencil or pen, a clipboard, or a magic slate. Encourage client to write clearly.	Able to write out whatever the client wishes to express. Could be used for non-English-speaking persons if you have someone available to translate the writing into English.	Not useful if can't move arms. Hard to write while on back. Have to be able to read and write. Writing is exhausting, so encourage the client to write only the main words.
Eye Blinks The usual method is for the client to blink once for "yes" and twice to indicate "no." An easy reminder for this system is to remember that "no" has two letters in it and thus has two blinks.	Useful for clients who may be paralyzed from the neck down.	Able to answer only "yes" or "no" questions. This limits the client's ability to express him/herself. However, for a intubated or trached quadriplegic client, this may initially be the only communication method available, and it is a starting point for communication.
Written Words/Pictures on Note Cards Use 3 × 5 cards with pictures or words on them. These are commercially available or you can make your own. Give the client the cards and have him or her sort them into sentences or phrases to indicate what is needed. For clients who do not speak English, make cards with both the English words and the equivalent words in the client's language.	Simple to use. Do not need to be able to write. Do not need to be able to read (if only pictures are used). Can be used for clients who don't read or speak English.	Able to use only the cards available (unless you make more, which is easily done).
American Sign Language This is a method of hand and finger signals to indicate letters and words. It is a standard method used throughout the world to communicate with deaf people.	Universally understood.	Too complicated to learn while in a crisis situation.
Computer-Aided Communication A computer keyboard is used to type out messages.	Able to type any type of message.	Time consuming. Must be able to type. Expensive—must have access to a computer.

Table 7–3   HOW TO CHOOSE THE BEST COMMUNICATION SYSTEM

To choose the best communication system, assess clients for the following:
Consciousness
   Are they alert and oriented?
   Are they under the influence of sedatives or narcotics?
Language
   What is their primary language?
Fine motor skills
   Are they able to use a pencil and paper?
Gross motor skills
   Are they able to squeeze your hand?
Paralysis
   Are they chemically or physiologically paralyzed?

Data from Williams, M. (1992, July/August). An algorithm for selecting a communication technique with intubated clients. *Dimensions in Critical Care Nursing, 2*(2), 293–298.

There are a variety of alternate communication methods that may be used for the verbally impaired client. It is common to use several alternate communication methods with a verbally impaired client. Each method has its advantages and disadvantages; you should assess the client and choose those that may work (Table 7–3).

To use these communication systems, it is important for the caregiver to remember which methodology the client can use to respond to a query. For example, if eye blinks are being used, you must remember to ask the client a "yes" or "no" question. You can't ask the client, "How do you feel today?" when he or she is expected to answer via eye blinks. In addition, the family and friends will need to be able to use the communication system. Remember to teach them how to use it and encourage its use. If the client has a limitation in the ability to speak, explain the reason to the family and friends. Show them how to use an alternate communication method (such as the picture board).

Tell them to talk to the client, whether the client is alert and oriented, disoriented or comatose. It may be that the family doesn't know what to say to the client when the client can't communicate verbally. Encourage them to talk to the client as they normally would before the illness. You could suggest that they talk about what is happening at home and what the children are doing (as long as this doesn't add more stress to the client!). Other activities for improving client/family communication could include reading the newspaper to the client or reading the get-well cards received. Provide as much privacy as the client's condition allows.

Because of the client's difficulty with verbal expression, the nurse must use the client's nonverbal behaviors to provide insight into the client's thoughts and feelings. Visually assess the client's body language and verify its meaning with the client. Correctly interpreting nonverbal behavior can be very challenging. However, it can become easier if the nurse tries to place himself or herself in the client's place. What would the nurse want done if he or she were intubated and on a ventilator? Try to think like your client. Could he or she be in pain? Is he or she cold? Does the client want to be turned over? Is the client frightened and lonely? What could he or she want? If your client can move his or her arms, you could ask the client to point to what he or she wants. This information could be a good starting point to help the client get what is needed.

Although it is always important to make sure the call light is within reach of the client, this is *vital* for a client with a verbal impairment. A variety of call light devices are available to meet varying degrees of client coordination and movement. If these would be useful for your client, contact the unit nurse manager or perhaps the speech therapy department. The biomedical department of the institution will also be helpful to obtain a useful call light device.

If the client has verbal limitations, place a note at the call light answering station, indicating that the client is unable to verbally communicate over the conventional system. When the call light goes on, the nurse must go into the client's room to see what the client needs.

A major problem with using the alternate communication systems is that for several systems clients must be able to use their arms or hands to make them work. This creates a problem for clients with upper body paralysis and for clients who may have their wrists restrained or encumbered by intravenous or arterial lines. It is common procedure to apply soft restraints to the wrists of mechanically ventilated clients to prevent them from pulling out their endotracheal tubes. The clients must be restrained because these tubes are frequently very uncomfortable, and many clients attempt to pull them out. It can be dangerous to remove the wrist restraints to allow a client to point to a picture board or to use a paper and pencil. To remove a restraint to improve communication may be just enough time for the client to quickly pull out a tube, requiring it to be quickly put back in. This risk must be weighed carefully.

Besides interpreting the client's nonverbal language, remember to recognize the feelings of frustration the client, family, and friends may have during this period of difficult communication.

Many institutions have speech therapists on staff. If you are having difficulty communicating with a verbally impaired person, consult the speech therapist for suggestions.

So Little Perceived Hope

Many clients in critical care units are severely ill and have been told that they may not recover from their illness. The client and family may need the support of the nursing staff to help them come to terms with this information. Although you don't want to encourage false hope, you also don't want to rob them of their beliefs. What can you do or say that will accomplish this?

How much does the family know about the client's illness or injuries? To assess this, you could ask them "What has the physician told you about your husband's condition?"

Remember to consider the emotional and spiritual needs of the client and family. When they are speaking of hope for the client's recovery, they may intellectually know that the client may be dying, yet emotionally and spiritually they must still hope for recovery. Clergy can be extremely helpful in these circumstances.

It can be emotionally draining to be supportive of a family member who continues to insist that a dying person will recover. However, it is rarely useful to demand that the person accept the situation as it really is. You will need to be sensitive to the person's hopes and dreams, yet try to inject a small amount of reality into the situation.

Respond to the family's hopes, yet don't make statements about the client's condition that may not be true. When a family member expresses hope that a brain-

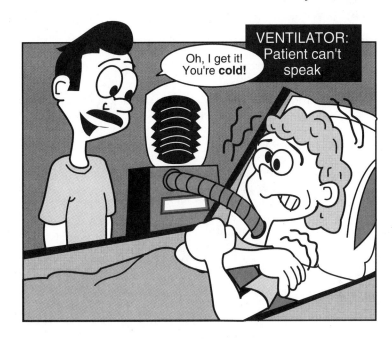

dead woman will recover because her chest is moving (the ventilator will make the chest move) you could say, "I hear you tell me how much you'd like her to get better, but I don't know if that will happen."

In the scenario, Mrs. Thomas hoped her husband would recover. The nurse responded: "I can tell that you want him to get better. I do not know if he will recover. I hope he can."

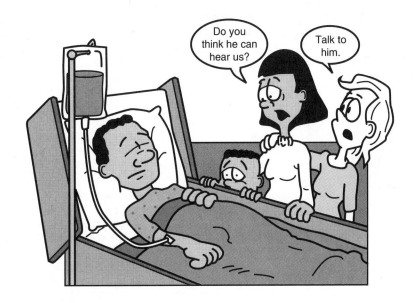

The Client With a Lengthy Downhill Course

A client may sometimes linger near death for days or even weeks. Although this period of time may provide needed time to get affairs in order and to say good-bye, it also can be extremely fatiguing for the family, friends, and staff. The Family Leave Act of 1993 allows an employee to take a leave of absence for family illness, which can be very beneficial to allow the family member to spend time with the client and also keep his or her job. But even with an official leave of absence, other stressors may still be present. Laundry still has to be done, groceries have to be bought, children have to go to their ball games, and bills have to be paid. How does one do these things and still be able to be with the client as much as possible? The answer to this must rest with each individual client and family.

How are they holding up with the stress of a lingering illness? Talk to the family and friends about their coping abilities.

By providing appropriate information, the nurse can help family and friends in deciding when to stay at the hospital and when to leave.

The nurse can also provide a sounding board for client, family, and friends. They may need someone to talk to about how this whole process is dragging on for a long time. Both client and family may feel guilty for wishing that death would come sooner. The client, family, and friends may be at different stages of the grief process. The client may be ready to let go, but the family may not be able to accept this. Sometimes the client may seem to be trying to stay alive just for the sake of the family. Sometimes the family may tell the client, "You don't have to keep trying. It's OK for you to let go and die." The client may just need to know that the family is ready for them to die.

Try to encourage family members to talk about their feelings regarding the illness and the changes that have resulted. The hospital chaplain can be a very valuable resource to work with clients and families on coping skills.

The Client With a Deterioration in Health Care Status

When a client's condition is deteriorating, it is very important to keep the family informed. This is an especially difficult issue if the client has just been transferred to the intensive care unit from another area of the hospital or has just been admitted to the hospital.

What does the family know of the client's condition? You need to know this to provide appropriate information. How well do you know this family? Your intervention will be different for a family who knows that their family member is dying than it is for a family who is unaware that their loved one died shortly after admission.

If the family is not at the hospital, it is common to telephone them to notify them of the client's condition and to ask them to come to the hospital. The policy and procedure vary from hospital to hospital about who phones the family and what is the proper thing to tell the family and friends. In some institutions, the charge nurse calls the family, and in other institutions, the nurse working with the client makes the phone calls. Follow the guidelines for your institution. Some general suggestions:

- Make sure you are calling the correct person. It would be devastating to receive a phone call telling you that a loved one's condition is deteriorating and find out later that it was a wrong number.
- If possible, find out ahead of time which member of the family to call. This is an especially good idea if the next of kin is elderly or ill. In this case, it might be better to call another family member.
- An example of what to say is, "This is Shakira Branch calling from GetWell Medical Center. Is this Mrs. Alkenes? Mrs. Alkenes, your husband's condition is getting worse. Could you please come to the hospital?"
- Have someone watching for the family when they arrive so that they do not walk into the room unprepared.
- Call the attending physician to let him or her know of any change in the client's condition even if the consultant physicians are handling the problem. Otherwise, the family may call the attending physician who would know even less about the situation than the family does.
- Telling someone over the phone that a loved one has died is a controversial subject. Many nurses believe this is better done in person than on the telephone. Although nurses usually do not volunteer this information on the phone, they will answer truthfully if the family or friend asks a direct question such as "Has my mother already died?"

We have described how the critical care environment can affect communication patterns. Let's pull it all together by looking at two examples of communication within the critical care setting.

PRACTICAL APPLICATIONS

The **WRONG** Approach

Andre Ringwold, RN, is providing care for Mr. Waldon Singer, a man admitted yesterday because of an industrial accident. Mr. Ringwold has been a critical care nurse for several months, and it seems that he has not mastered the skill of communicating effectively with critically ill clients and their families. He explains the equipment in the room to Mr. Singer as follows:

"Mr. Singer, I want to talk to you about the machines. This is a ventilator and that is an IV machine. I won't bore you with the details of what they do. You've got that tube in your mouth so you can't talk, Mr. Singer. I see that you are trying to say something but I can't lip read very well, so I'll just ask your wife what you want. Or you can wait to talk to me when the tube comes out." Mr. Ringwold is speaking rapidly, with his face turned away from the client.

Mrs. Singer is standing in the doorway of Mr. Singer's room. She says in a low tone of voice, "Waldon, the kids are driving me crazy. Sheri has wrecked the new car and Franklin has been arrested again for shoplifting. Nurse, what's wrong with my husband? His face is really red and he's pulling on those arm tie-downs. Do you think he's upset?"

What do you think Mr. Ringwold and Mrs. Singer are doing wrong in the art of communication?

1. Andre Ringwold, the nurse, needs to speak slowly and explain the purpose of the equipment. Clients may not need to know the name of the piece of equipment, but they do need to know its purpose.

2. Mrs. Singer should be encouraged to stand closer to Mr. Singer's bed and speak more loudly.

3. The nurse should have discussed suitable topics of conversation with Mrs. Singer. If this isn't possible, Mr. Ringwold might have attempted to indicate to Mrs. Singer that car crashes and being arrested are not good discussion topics for a critically ill person. The wife also verbalizes that she doesn't understand about her husband's condition.

The **CORRECT** Approach

"Mr. Singer, I want to explain to you about the machines we are using to provide care for you. The tube that is in your mouth connects to this machine, which is helping you to breathe. With the tube in your mouth, you can't talk. You can talk again when the tube comes out. We will need to come up with a way for you to tell me what you want. Do you think you could write out your messages on paper? Nod your head 'yes' or 'no.'" Mr. Singer nods his head "yes." Mr. Ringwold brings him a pencil and tablet of paper. Mr. Singer writes, "I want to see my wife." "I'll go get her, and be back in one minute," says Mr. Ringwold. As he leaves the room to get Mrs. Singer, he notes that the machine settings are correct, the machine alarms are all set, and Mr. Singer's hands are restrained to prevent him from pulling out his tubes.

He goes to the waiting room and asks for Mrs. Singer. "Mrs. Singer, I'm Andre Ringwold, and I'm a registered nurse in the intensive care unit. I'm providing care for your husband today. Could you come into the unit so that I could talk to you further? I can leave him alone only for a very short period." They walk into the unit, stopping outside Mr. Singer's door. Mr. Ringwold glances into the room, making sure that everything is functioning normally. "Mrs. Singer, have you spoken with your husband's doctors today?"

"Yes, I have," she replied. "They tell me that he's doing better. I'm so glad! I need him to come home and straighten out our kids. They are in trouble again."

"Mrs. Singer, I hear you saying that you need your husband to help you with your children, but do you think you could wait a day or two to talk to him about it? Although his condition is improved, he needs to be restful and calm. Wouldn't it be upsetting to him to hear about his children?"

"Well, you're probably right, I'll wait until tomorrow to tell him about the kids. Can I go in to see him now?"

They walk into the room, but Mrs. Singer stops just inside the doorway and begins to speak, "Hello, Waldon, how are you feeling?" Mr. Ringwold intervenes, saying, "Mrs. Singer, come on over here so that your husband can hear you better. It's all right. You can stand right here and not hurt anything. Please don't touch any of the machines in the room. Also, I would like you not to untie his hands because he might pull out his tubes. He really needs all these tubes right now, so we can't let him pull them out. He can't talk because of the tube in his mouth so we have this message board that he's using. Do either of you have any questions?"

REFERENCES

Cochran, J., & Ganong, L. (1989). A comparison of nurses' and patients' perceptions of intensive care unit stressors. *Journal of Advanced Nursing, 14*(12), 1038–1043.

Crickmore, R. (1987). A review of stress in the intensive care unit. *Intensive Care Nursing, 3*(1), 19–27.

Chyun, D. (1989). Patient's perceptions of stressors in intensive care and coronary care units. *Focus on Critical Care, 16*(3), 206–211.

Lewis, D., & Robinson, J. (1992). ICU nurses' coping measures: Response to work-related stressors. *Critical Care Nurse, 12*(2), 18–25.

Kupferschmid, B., Briones, T., Dawson, C., & Drongowski, C. (1991). Families: A link or a liability? *Clinical Issues in Critical Care Nursing, 2*(2), 252–257.

Mallett, K. (1988). The relationship between burnout, death anxiety and social support in hospice and critical care nurses. *The University of Toledo.*

Titler, M. (1991, March). Impact of adult critical care hospitalization: Perceptions of patients, spouses, children and nurses. *Heart and Lung,* 174–182.

Williams, M. (1992, July/August). An algorithm for selecting a communication technique with intubated clients. *Dimensions in Critical Care Nursing,* 222–228.

Winacek, J. (1991). Promoting family-centered visitation makes a difference. *Clinical Issues in Critical Care Nursing, 2*(2), 293–298.

Wlody, G. (1984). Communicating in the ICU: Do you read me loud and clear? *Nursing Management, 15*(9), 24–27.

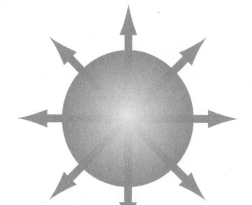

8

With Chronically Ill Clients and Their Families

In this chapter, we will discuss:

- How chronic illness is different from acute illness
- Client and family issues and interventions
- Care environment issues

How Chronic Illness Is Different From Acute Illness

When persons experience an isolated acute illness or health problem and seek treatment, the plans of care often focus on client understanding of and preparation for diagnostic tests, medical and/or surgical intervention(s), and recovery activities. Acute illness is a limited event with onset, treatment, and recuperation phases, and clients return to their usual lifestyles with little, if any, changes required. When persons experience a chronic illness, however, plans of care must shift from a focus on cure to a focus on disease/symptom control and lifestyle changes. There is no

156

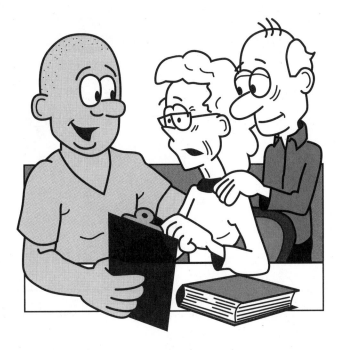

complete recuperation phase, and lifestyle changes are inevitable as the disease progresses. Clients with a chronic illness and their families must learn to work through periods of transition as the illness demands changes in various aspects of their lives. These can include changes in identities, roles, relationships, abilities, and behavior patterns (Schumacher, 1994). Chronic disease can follow three courses (Wright & Leahey, 1987):

1. Progressive: increasing degree of disability occurs, with minimal periods of relief; adaptation to the illness and the role changes it demands are often continuous; rapidly progressive disease requires increasing adaptation within shorter periods of time (example: cancer that does not respond to treatment); slowly progressive diseases require a greater emphasis on stamina in dealing with the disease as it slowly progresses (example: emphysema, adult-onset diabetes).

2. Constant: after an acute injury (example: stroke or spinal cord injury) a period of physical stability follows and adaptation to physical deficits or limitations occurs; overall, this is a period of stability, and care needs are fairly predictable.

3. Relapsing or episodic: these illnesses (example: migraine headaches, multiple sclerosis) have "quiet" periods of varying lengths with minimal to absent signs or symptoms and normal lifestyle that are interrupted by flare-up periods of acute illness that require care and often demand family role changes; the unpredictability and frequency of flare-up periods cause strain on the client and family.

To assist chronically ill clients and their families as they face the course of their disease, attention must be given to their physical and psychosocial needs and their ability to adapt to the changes demanded of them. Their needs and abilities change

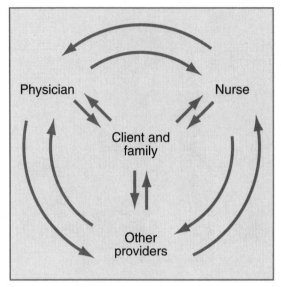

Figure 8–1   Adapted from Siegler EL, Whitney FW: *Nurse-Physician Collaboration, Care of Adults and the Elderly.* Springer Publishing Company, Inc, New York 10012, 1994, pp 4–5. Used by permission.

over time and are impacted by age, grief caused by illness-related losses, belief patterns and personal goals, role changes, financial factors, coping methods, and knowledge and use of support systems. Effective care planning requires clear, open, ongoing communication with the client and the family as center of the health care team (Weaver & Wilson, 1994). Figure 8–1 shows a collaborative, client-centered practice model. The interdisciplinary team members work with each other and with the client, and no care provider dominates continuously. The circular design emphasizes ongoing and mutual give-and-take communication patterns and collegiality (Siegler & Whitney, 1994).

Client- and Family-Related Issues and Interventions

When you work with chronically ill clients, ongoing assessment of key areas will assist you in identifying their psychosocial and functional abilities, strengths, and weaknesses. This is important as the course of the illness changes and clients and families face periods of transition. Factors have been identified that affect how well these transitions are made (Schumacher, 1994).

- What meaning does the transition have to the client and family?
- What are the client and family's expectations as they anticipate and deal with the changes?
- What is the client and family's emotional and physical state?
- Does the client and family have the level of knowledge and skills needed to successfully work through the transition?
- Is the environment supportive?
- How thorough is the planning to assist the client and family as they work through the transitions as they occur?

These factors serve as a guide to assess clients and their families as they face these transition periods. Table 8–1 offers an assessment tool that combines these factors with questions that will assist you in obtaining related client and family information. Examples of nurse interactions helpful in obtaining the desired information are also included.

Table 8–1   ASSESSMENT OF CLIENTS AND FAMILIES FACING TRANSITIONS RELATED TO CHRONIC ILLNESS

What meaning does the transition have to the client and family?

Where are the client and family in the process of adapting to the change(s)?

"I know you have to make/have made some changes in your lifestyle, Mr. Ho. What do you think is/will be easy? What do you think is/will be difficult?"

Consider: Is the change sudden or will it evolve over a period of time? What does it mean to those involved? Is it a positive, negative, or neutral experience?

"I realize how quickly your condition has changed. How do you feel about all that has happened?"

"You seem to be on top of getting things ready for your mother at home, but you have never indicated how you felt about all the upcoming changes in her care. How are you doing with all this?" or *"Do you see this as a good move?"*

"I know it must be difficult to face ongoing changes in your son's condition. You seem calm (or angry) so much of the time. What have those experiences been like for you?"

How do they interpet the change(s) or situation in light of their culture or religion?

"Mrs. Lister, you mentioned that your husband must repent before things can change for the better for him. Is it your belief that very little can be done to help your husband until he makes his peace with God?"

What are the client's and family's expectations as they anticipate and deal with changes?

Do they know what to expect as they work through changes?

"How different do you think your home routines will be when you start caring for your father at home?"

"How do you see yourself handling your family's demands for your time and attention along with the demands of your new treatment schedule?"

Consider: Is this situation similar or different than previous experiences they have worked through?

"Think about your last round of therapy that involved two afternoons a week and how you managed your work and home schedules. This round of therapy will be stronger and involve three afternoons a week. Also, some clients often need a few hours to allow the side effects that we talked about to wear off. Do you think the same strategy for handling everything will work again this time or will you need to make some changes?"

As they work through the transition, are their expectations realistic?

"Mrs. Smith, I can tell you have been giving your daughter excellent care. You, though, seem very tired and overwhelmed. It seems that the plan just isn't realistic. Maybe we need to revisit her needs, your needs, and the resources available and then explore different approaches that will allow you to meet both sets of needs."

What is the client's/family's physical status?

Is physical discomfort interfering with their ability to take in and use new information and to learn a new skill?

"I need to review your medications with you today. When do you feel most alert and rested?"

The more comfortable the client and family feels about physical changes that occurred or are occurring, the more positive their feelings will be during the transition.

What are the client's and family's emotional states?

What emotions or feelings of distress are the client and family experiencing? Anxiety, insecurity, frustration, depression, apprehension, loneliness, and ambivalence are common.

"How do you feel about the way things are going?"

"You seem _____. How do you feel?"

Note behaviors that indicate *anxiety* (crying; increased muscle tension; pacing; wringing of hands; difficulty expressing thoughts and feelings); check out headache, dizziness, nausea, sleeplessness; increased pulse or respirations; *depression* (increasing difficulty with concentration and memory; appearance or expression of sadness, worry, or emptiness; negative dispositon or expression; social withdrawal; decreased energy level; appetite changes; decreased interest in personal hygiene; lack of eye contact), or *grief and loss* (see chapter 9).

Is there role conflict or change?

"Tell me how your role(s) at home have changed. How do you feel about these changes?"

"You mentioned how you have taken on a lot of the household responsibilities that your wife used to do. How has this been working out?"

Table continued on following page

Table 8–1   ASSESSMENT OF CLIENTS AND FAMILIES FACING TRANSITIONS RELATED TO CHRONIC ILLNESS *(Continued)*

Do the client and family have the level of knowledge and skills needed to successfully work through the transition period?

Identify what skill and knowledge are needed and what timeline you have to work with.

"Mrs. Kim, you have been working with us and taking good care of your husband and are familiar with a lot of his treatments. However, there have been a few changes made during this hospital stay. To feel secure about taking care of him, what information and additional practice do you need with the new treatments before he goes home?"

Consider: how predictable are the client's needs and the timeliness? Is uncertainty a problem? (How defined can the change be?) If uncertainty is a problem, here is one approach to serve as an example:

"There are several care problems that are not an immediate concern but most likely will occur sometime in the near future as you care for him at home. I want you to be aware of them, to understand why they occur and what to do, and how to seek our assistance when they do occur."

Be sure to also provide written information for future reference.

Is the environment supportive?

Are social supports and resources in place and utilized?

"Tell me how you manage your care at home? Does it seem to be working well?"

"Here is a list of support services that are available to you. Have you had any contact with any of them? If so, which one(s)? How were they helpful?"

"Do you feel that the resources/services are coordinated?"

Are cultural and religious practices supported whenever possible in the health care environment?

"Are there any cultural practices that you would like incorporated into your care?"

"Are there any treatments or medications that we have discussed with you that may be hard to continue at home? Yes? In what way?"

How thorough is the planning to assist the client and family as they work through changes?

Is planning comprehensive in identifying problems, issues, and needs that may arise during transition periods? Are key people identified and involved in the process?

"Who takes care of you?"

"Who will make care-related decisions?"

Does planning continue over time based on ongoing assessment and evaluation? Is a timeline developed that shows stages of transition to facilitate an organized approach to planning?

Data from:

Aldersberg, M., & Thorne, S. (1990). Emerging from the chrysalis: Older widows in transition. *Journal of Gerontological Nursing, 16,* 4–8.

Brown, A. M., & Powell-Cope, G. M. (1991). AIDS family caregiving: Transitions through uncertainty. *Nursing Research, 40,* 338–345.

Cantanzaro, M. (1990). Transitions in midlife adults with long-term illness. *Holistic Nursing Practice, 4*(3), 65–73.

Chielens, D., & Herrick, E. (1990). Recipients of bone marrow transplants: Making a smooth transition to an ambulatory setting. *Oncology Nursing Forum, 17,* 857–862.

Johnson, M. A., Morton, M. K., & Knox, S. M. (1992). The transition to a nursing home: Meeting the family's needs. Families face their own transition when a loved one enters a nursing home. *Geriatric Nursing, 13,* 299–302.

Kane, J. J. (1992). Allowing the novice to succeed: Transitional support in critical care. *Critical Care Nursing Quarterly, 15*(3), 17–22.

Kelley, J., & Lehman, L. (1993). Assessment of anxiety, depression, and suspiciousness in the home care setting. *Home Health Care Nurse, 11*(2), 16–19.

Klaich, K. (1990). Transitions in professional identity of nurses enrolled in graduate educational programs. *Holistic Nursing Practice, 4*(3), 17–24.

Loveys, B. (1990). Transitions in chronic illness: The at-risk role. *Holistic Nursing Practice, 4*(3), 56–64.

Robinson, G. M., & Pinckney, A. A. (1992). Transition from the hospital to the community: Small group program. *Journal of Psychosocial Nursing and Mental Health Services, 30*(5), 33–38.

Schumacker, K. L., & Meleis, A. (1994). Transitions: A central concept in nursing. *IMAGE: Journal of Nursing Scholarship, 26*(2), 119–125.

Thurber, F., & DiGiamarino, L. (1992). Development of a model of transitional care for the HIV-positive child and family. *Clinical Nurse Specialist, 6,* 142–146.

Wong, D. L. (1991) Transition from hospital to home for children with complex medical care. *Journal of Pediatric Oncology Nursing, 8,* 3–9.

Consider This Scenario

Mr. Cury, RN, is reviewing the record of Mrs. Blaski, 62, who will be coming in for her first follow-up visit since her hospitalization for a stroke that resulted in permanent right-sided weakness. Her stroke was caused by a small blood clot that occurred as a result of asymptomatic, intermittent heart beat irregularity. Before her discharge, she had been taught to use a cane to assist her with ambulation. Mr. Cury notes in her history that up until this incident she reported herself in good health and was very involved in home and community activities. Her husband is alive and well and employed by a local company. The discharge summary note indicated Mrs. Blaski and her family had voiced no anticipated problems with her care at home.

When Mrs. Blaski arrived, Mr. Cury observed that she seemed uneasy and had little eye contact with those in the waiting room and with him. She was not wearing make-up and her hair was not well combed. With her history of community involvement, this seemed unusual to him. She used her cane appropriately as she walked slowly into the exam room. Her husband seemed attentive to her but appeared very tired. Mr. Cury offered them both a chair and introduced himself as he extended his hand for handshakes. He explained that he would be following Mrs. Blaski's progress and she would see him as well as her physician each time she came to the clinic. He then gave her written information about the clinic and how to contact him or the physician should the need arise.

"This is very helpful," Mr. Blaski stated. "This is all new to us and it sure is nice to have someone to call who knows us."

"You both appear tired. How are each of you coping with all that has happened? Mrs. Blaski?"

"Well, Mr. Cury, this has been so hard. Just look at me, I look like an old lady with this cane and I'm so clumsy having to use my left hand. I'm right handed—no, I *used* to be right handed. I can't even comb my hair right. At home, I can't do my part. John [husband] goes to work and then comes home and has to work some more. I get so down and critical. This is awful. I'm not like I used to be." She starts to cry.

Mr. Blaski holds her and gives her tissues offered by Mr. Cury. He says, "I had no idea how much adjustment this would take. It has left me feeling uneasy, like I'm really not in control of what happens to either of us. It's so unsettling. It's hard to change routines that have been working fine for years. We have both been quite independent, happily so, and the hardest part has been asking each other for help. She has kept our home running smoothly ever since we got married, and I feel so foolish when I even have to ask where things are kept in the kitchen. I know how hard it is for her to see things that need to be done and can't do them. She's always been a 'neatnik' and prided herself in keeping things in good order."

Mr. Cury: "What routines have you been able to keep on track?"

Mrs. Blaski: "Well, John has been able to work, and that is a relief. I guess, even though I need more time, I have been able to at least get up, get dressed, and make my own breakfast, like tea and cereal. It does get messy, though, some days! I just get tired easily and it frustrates me so much."

Mr. Blaski: "I think overall we function OK, but it's at a much slower pace and only the basic things get done, though not as thoroughly as we'd like. We each always seem to look at what is not done, or not done the way we used to do it. We even hesitate to have friends over because things are different. I do miss seeing them and they don't call much right now."

Mr. Cury: "Have you been able to maintain your usual sleep patterns?"

Mrs. Blaski: "It takes me longer to get to sleep because I lie there and think about what I wasn't able to do, what needs to be done. Sometimes I think about how I could possibly have another stroke, and then I feel real anxious. . .talk about not sleeping well!"

Mr. Blaski: "I sleep OK, I guess, but I feel tired all the time. I think it's because, like I said before, I don't feel in control of things like I used to. That has really thrown me. Maybe once we find new comfortable routines, that feeling will decrease."

Mr. Cury: "You both have been able to talk about how you feel, and this is an important part of working through situations and keeping them in perspective. It may prove helpful to establish a time in early evening when you both can identify what needs to be done the next day, make a list and prioritize it. Include on the list time in the day to just relax, to do something you each want to do. As you compare lists on a day-to-day basis, you will begin to realize what you are able to do. That may help alleviate some of the frustration you feel that comes from focusing on what didn't get done and help you feel more in control of your time and home situation. This would allow you to rest better. It could also help you identify those chores important to you that someone else needs to help you with."

"Everyone reacts in his or her own unique way to events that happen and I encourage you to continue sharing your reactions and needs with each other. It is the only way you will be able to understand and help one another. The same is true with us. We are here to help you any way we possibly can. We need to know how we can best help you."

Mrs. Blaski: "I am so glad we can talk like this. It has been so hard to get past the initial shock of all these changes since my stroke. We really do need help to think things through and find new comfortable routines. You just gave us several ideas that I know we wouldn't have had on our own right now, and I think they just might help."

Mr. Cury: "That's good. Try them out and even change them a bit to fit your needs. I'll be interested in hearing what works for you."

"There are a few specific comments you made that I would like to explore a little more. First, the thought of having another stroke made you feel very anxious. Would you like more information and time to talk about what caused your stroke and how your medication works to help prevent that from happening? . . . (*Pause*) Second, you voiced difficulty doing things such as combing your hair and using your left hand. Would you like to talk with the occupational therapist who is trained in assisting people to learn new ways to do tasks that an injury has made difficult to do?"

"Third, about friends: sometimes people really are not sure how to respond when someone is ill or has had a major health problem. They may be waiting for you to make the first move when you feel up to seeing them. If the house isn't in order the way you like, maybe you and Mr. Blaski could meet them at some quiet place for dinner or just for dessert the first time. If you feel self-conscious about the cane, you may consider arriving before they do, and leaving after they do. It's very normal to feel awkward and to lack confidence in managing your right-sided weakness. You are right, your body is different than it was, and it will take a lot of time to integrate those changes into who you are physically. Allow yourself that time, and arrange situations the best you can to minimize the changes. These are thoughts that came to me as you talked. What do you think?"

This scenario is helpful in illustrating how nurses can gain information needed to assess the client-family situation and also incorporate supportive interventions or suggestions for the client and/or caregiver to consider. We will refer back to the scenario as we discuss the following major intervention areas and the role communication plays in each of them:

- Acknowledge and accept where the client and family are emotionally with physical status and treatment needs
- Work with the client and family to identify their understanding of the illness and care involved and their expectations of care providers
- Work to bring client and professional expectations together
- Coordinate care and treatment demands with the client and family's abilities and energy levels

- Support positive coping strategies and tap multidisciplinary resources as needed

Acknowledge and Accept Where the Client and Family Are Emotionally

One of the most important ways for people to deal with emotions of chronic illness is through communication. As you observe and work with the client and family members, there are many opportunities to learn about their feelings and reactions to what is occurring. A key communication intervention to use when these opportunities arise is listening. Several levels of listening can be very therapeutic:

- Acknowledge you heard the other person: Say "uh huh," or nod; these simply let the person know you heard them; just allowing someone the opportunity to talk and put thoughts into words is helpful.
- Acknowledge the content in what was said: Restate what was said, "You've had a very busy day"; this more specific response gives the person an opportunity to clarify any misconceptions on your part or to continue or elaborate further if the person so wishes.
- Acknowledge the emotion in what was said: Reflect back the emotion(s) that were expressed: "This must be extremely painful for you"; responses on an emotional level can bring good results; more expression of feelings usually results (Lorig & Fries, 1992).
- Seek more information: "I don't understand," "Could you tell me more about _____?" This demonstrates you are interested or want to be clear as to what the client is saying or wants or needs.

When you use these supportive listening approaches, you convey to the client and family that their emotions and thoughts are valid and respected. In the scenario, Mr. Cury acknowledged to Mr. and Mrs. Blaski that they appeared tired and asked how they were coping. Then he listened. They shared with him the feelings they were experiencing. As they talked, Mr. Cury noted several comments they made that he wanted to explore further with them. He delayed comment on them while they talked so they could stay focused on their feelings and experiences. Afterward, Mr. Cury then revisited those comments and explored them with Mr. and Mrs. Blaski. It is often difficult to know how to assist family members, regardless of age. When a person has a chronic illness, the unaffected family members may feel isolated, ignored, angry, resentful, or neglected. If they admit their feelings, they may then also feel shame or guilt. Table 8–2 offers a list of questions that would assist health professionals address the concerns and anxieties of the family members that otherwise may stay hidden. If children are quite young and have a limited vocabulary that may make verbal answers difficult, ask them to draw a picture in response to the question. For example, ask the child to draw a picture of:

- What it would be like if your dad was not sick any more
- How you feel about your sister being ill
- How you are different from/same as your friends who do not have a family member who is sick

As you look at the picture with the child, ask the child to tell you about the picture.

Table 8–2   QUESTIONS TO ASSIST FAMILY MEMBERS EXPLORE FEELINGS
RELATED TO A CHRONICALLY ILL SIBLING, PARENT, OR SPOUSE

What questions would you like to ask about your family member's illness?
What feelings do you have because of your family member's illness?
How has the illness affected you? How has it affected your family life?
How would life in your house be different if the illness were not present?
Is more expected of you at home because your family member is ill? If so, how?
Have you ever felt that you are different from your friends because your family member is ill? In what way?
What concerns you most about your family member's illness? How can I help you address this concern?

Work With Client and Family to Identify Their Understanding of the Illness, the Care Involved, and Their Expectations

It is so easy to assume that chronically ill persons and their families understand the disease process and what the necessary treatment is because "they have lived with it so long." What our therapeutic goals for a client are may be totally off base when we find out what the client's goals are. For example, a client with chronic lung disease became very upset when she was put on a progressive ambulation program to increase her strength and endurance, which would allow her to do more things. When the nurse talked with her about this, the client relayed that all she wanted to do was get her arms stronger so she could hold her new little granddaughter; walking had nothing to do with that and was just a waste of her precious energy! When planning care, it is extremely important to talk with the client and family about the activities they want to do or be able to do over time. Ask them how they think the staff can best help them. This discussion with them will give you insight into *their understanding of and ability to accept* the disease process and the impact it has, or will have, on their desired ability to function.

When the client and family are in shock or denial, the approaches focus on supporting them emotionally and sharing and reinforcing basic information about the illness and care routines with them. Repeating information is often necessary. Written information allows them to take in and reinforce information at their own pace. Gradually add more detail and depth to your explanations when they are able to digest more information. Often, they will show their readiness by asking questions or being curious about what is being done. Look for opportunities to help them more fully understand what has happened and the purpose of the interventions being taken. Mr. Cury took advantage of Mrs. Blaski's voiced anxiety about having another stroke to ask her if she wanted information about the cause of the stroke and her medication that is helping to prevent future ones. Her concern about further disability could motivate her to learn about her illness and how she could minimize future risks.

Anger about what has happened may be directed at the staff and how things are done or not done; this should not be taken personally by staff members. Defending yourself is inappropriate; instead, acknowledge the complaints and clarify what is upsetting them. For example: "You seem very upset about his care. I would like to know more about what is concerning you." Avoid nonverbal behavior that is confrontational: stay calm, provide privacy, and sit down if at all possible.

How clients interpret and react to the signs and symptoms they experience can be a clue to their understanding of and reaction to the disease or its progression. For example, pain is not always an inevitable consequence of disease or a sign that the disease is getting worse. But many chronically ill clients may fear pain and worry when it occurs, assuming it may be a bad sign. This is especially true for cancer patients (Cox, Carr, & Lee, 1992). As a result, some may try to deny their discomforts, or seem unusually worried or emotional when discomforts occur. Careful physical assessment and observation that includes the clients' physical responses (pallor, elevated pulse and blood pressure, sweating, guarding, grimacing, sleeping difficulties) and emotional responses (withdrawn or irritable behavior, etc.) must be carried out when pain is suspected or expressed. Explore with clients or their families how they usually express pain. Do they tend to be stoic or private about their pain, or are they emotive or expressive when pain and stress occur? The ways in which persons respond to pain and stress are learned behaviors and often reflect cultural background. (Learning about different cultural groups and their communication patterns can be very helpful as long as stereotyping is avoided. See Chapter 4 for further discussion of culture.) Note responses to medication and comfort interventions.

When medications and care do not bring relief, consider the possibility that pain may be only part of the problem. Talk with them about this. For example: "You seem so anxious, does the pain frighten you? What does the pain mean to you?" When clients experience marked loss of physical function(s) or family roles, their grief may be expressed as pain. In this situation, addressing the grief would play a significant part in addressing the pain (Thiederman, 1989). If pain becomes chronic and is the client's main focus, problems may develop that involve family and social, occupational, pharmacologic, and interpersonal dimensions. Successful treatment requires complete multidisciplinary assessment of each dimension, followed by concurrent, consistent multidisciplinary interventions. This requires clear, consistent, and coordinated communication with the client and family (Wright & Leahey, 1987).

Work to Bring Client and Professional Expectations Together

Once you have identified the client and family's understanding of their situation and what they expect, then you can proceed to find ways to bring their expectations and the health care team's expectations into realistic alignment with each other through a collaborative effort. This requires:

- Sharing information about the disease process and explaining reasons for treatments, therapy, and medications, as well as for any changes that occur
- Establishing appropriate care routines in a way and to the extent that the client can handle
- Encouraging questions and client and family participation in decision making

The more accurate the information the client and family know and the more involved they are in the care, the more organized, manageable, and predictable their world becomes. This does not mean everything that happens from then on will be good. However, their sense of involvement in what is happening increases their sense of being able to cope. The known is much easier to deal with than the unknown (Samuels & Samuels, 1992).

Let clients and families know that changing routines can be hard and frustrating. Ask them how their day is usually structured and establish routines, whenever possible, that can be worked into that structure. If the client is in the acute care setting, establish a routine to the extent possible that can be continued in a similar fashion at home, or maintain the routine that was working well at home. Troubleshoot with them. Give them some suggestions that they can consider, like Mr. Cury did. One idea may lead to another.

Ask them what they need help with or find frustrating and what is working well. So often we tend to only focus on the negatives. Mr. and Mrs. Blaski were having difficulty dealing with not being able to do things the way they had. However, when asked what routines they were able to manage, Mrs. Blaski was able to manage self-care and Mr. Blaski could return to work. Both were very positive. Help them to see their strengths as well as their weaknesses, just as Mr. Cury did with Mr. and Mrs. Blaski.

Coordinate Care and Treatment Demands With Client and Family Abilities and Energy Levels

"I had no idea how much adjustment this would take," Mr. Blaski stated. This is something that is so easy to forget on a busy day, but for clients and families it is a key point for nurses and other caregivers to remember. Chronic illness can decrease clients' energy reserves physically, mentally, and emotionally. For family, the reserves are decreased most often because of emotional and mental stress. For those who also assist with heavy personal care, physical fatigue is common. Financial worries can be a major stressor that can drain mental and emotional energies. When fatigue becomes chronic, it can seriously impact overall health and ability to carry out desired activities. To prevent exhaustion, stressors must be controlled.

Review treatment schedules with them on a regular basis. Explore how it is working for the family group as a whole as well as for the client. Is the household workload shared appropriately by family members? Does the primary caregiver feel comfortable in that role? Is the primary caregiver getting enough rest and personal time? Is the client able to rest? Are treatment demands or energy levels changing? Are expectations too high? Are family communication patterns effective? This can be a very frustrating challenge when aphasia and mental changes are present. Is there a need for supportive services? Asking clients and families questions like these lets them know you are concerned about them on an ongoing basis, and it teaches them to also stop and evaluate their situation periodically. This allows them to see needed changes before overwhelming problems arise.

Support Positive Coping Strategies and Use Multidisciplinary Resources as Needed

One of your key roles in working with chronically ill clients and their families is to assist them in dealing successfully with stress. Strategies focus on preventing or reducing their stress and on improving their ability to deal with it. Often, several strategies are used to address the range of stressors (positive and negative) that are occurring simultaneously. There are many strategies that can be used, and those that are most effective are those that complement a person's lifestyle, belief system, energy level and physical status, personality, family structure, and individual goals (Barton, Magilvy, & Quinn, 1994; Folden, 1994). Strategies to consider are discussed below.

Identify the major stressors, and rank them from easiest to hardest to deal with. Many times when a person is stressed, *everything* seems to be stressful. Feelings of being out of control occur. Help clients and families look at their situation: what are their feelings, what routines have been altered and in what way, what routines are at least somewhat intact. This enables them to see the situation in a more balanced perspective. Mr. Cury did this with Mr. and Mrs. Blaski. They were able to at least begin talking about what had occurred and how they each felt, and they began to sort out the changes and stressors that need to be addressed. Mr. Cury provided some suggestions to help them further clarify and prioritize what they needed to do each day, what they were able to manage, and what they would need more help with.

Address the stressor(s) that are easiest to deal with first. This helps decrease some of the stress fairly quickly and frees up energy to address the bigger stressors. As clients and families experience success in dealing with at least some stress, they begin to feel at least some control over what is happening. Mr. Cury identified specific areas of concern voiced by Mr. and Mrs. Blaski and asked them whether additional information and a referral would be helpful in alleviating their concerns. This demonstrated Mr. Cury's desire to be responsive to their needs and helped to establish a good foundation for addressing more complex concerns and issues.

Help clients and family members, especially the primary caregiver, maintain or regain adequate rest. If sleep and rest patterns are impaired, find out what is interfering with them. Once the cause of the problem is identified, effective interventions can be identified. Fatigue greatly limits a person's ability to cope effectively. Mr. Cury sought this information and discovered both Mr. and Mrs. Blaski were having difficulty in this area, each for different reasons. This provided direction for possible remedies.

Assist the client and family to plan time for relaxation, each in his or her own way. Meditation, imagery, or relaxation exercises; involvement with hobbies; quiet walks; listening to music; and reading are some examples of relaxation activities. Such activities provide positive energy that supports one's coping abilities.

Assist the client and family to identify what makes them feel supported, satisfied, and fulfilled and able to function more effectively. Support can come from positive relationships with family and friends, one's job, activities and hobbies, environment, financial stability, and religious beliefs. People have their own combination of factors and persons that provide them with their support network or system. Once known, assistance can be given to maintain the network as much as possible. Mr. Blaski talked briefly about how he missed seeing his friends. Knowing this, Mr. Cury was able to let him know that sometimes people do not know how to respond when illness occurs and that they often wait for the family to make the first move. He also gave Mr. and Mrs. Blaski a few suggestions that would help them see their friends without putting a lot of additional stress on their situation.

When stress levels are very high and uncontrolled or when further assistance from another member of the health care team is needed, help the family and client seek outside assistance (Crepeau, 1994). Professional counseling and therapy are available from a variety of disciplines that can assist in addressing complex issues on an ongoing basis. Table 8–3 provides a list of organizational resources and referral services available for persons dealing with chronic illnesses or related problem(s). You are often the link clients and families have to information about these services and referral options. In the scenario, Mr. Cury gave Mrs. Blaski the opportunity to talk with the occupational therapist concerning her self-care skills. Often, nurses assume these needs are totally addressed while in an acute care setting. Many times these needs may have been discussed, but the information was not absorbed by the client. Or, the client's needs may not have been evident in the acute care setting and thus were not addressed.

Care Environment Issues

Chronically ill clients are cared for in a variety of settings: the acute care hospital, the long-term care facility, and the home. The unique characteristics of each setting impact how care is given.

For example, in the acute care environment, the chronically ill client may be seen by the same staff members on each visit. This allows the staff members to be more aware of their clients' histories, needs, progress, and treatment plans. However, never assume that what has occurred and has been therapeutic in the past will continue. With the progressive nature of chronic illness, careful assessment of the client and the care plan is warranted with each admission or contact. If a client is completely new to you, frequent interaction with the client will be necessary to establish a client history that truly reflects the situation. If the client is in distress, only the most important questions can be asked initially. Filling in the gaps of the assessment can be done as you interact with the client and family during care. Careful observation of facial expression, body language, and the ability of the client and family to carry out care routines can provide valuable information. The questions you are asked and not asked by the client and family can provide insight into their concerns and possibly fears. As you collect this information, reflect your impressions back to them, just as you reflect verbal comments made, to see if your impressions are correct. Respond to signs of distress. This tells clients you are observant and concerned about responding to their needs correctly.

Because of the chronicity of the client's illness, the client has found ways to cope with activities of daily living. Work closely with the client and family to incorporate these ways into care routines and pace care activities according to physical abilities. If new care routines must be established, work together to establish routines that will carry over into the home routines as much as possible. Let the client know who the caregivers will be and how to inform them if needs arise.

In the long-term care setting, these approaches also work well. The pace of care, however, may be slower. A key area for assessment in this setting must focus on the client's and family's feelings related to long-term care placement. Allow them time to adjust to the new setting. It is not really "home." Provide and respect personal space, no matter how limited. Expect grieving behaviors related to loss of lifestyle, health changes, and family changes. Provide the client and family members opportunities to talk about or express their feelings, in private if at all possible. Include the client and family in planning routines and activities whenever possible.

The major difference when caring for a client in the home setting is that you

Table 8–3 EXAMPLES OF ORGANIZATIONAL RESOURCES AND REFERRAL SERVICES
AVAILABLE FOR PERSONS DEALING WITH CHRONIC ILLNESS OR RELATED
PROBLEMS

Acquired Immune Deficiency Syndrome	National AIDS Hotline	800-342-AIDS
	Minority AIDS Project	213-936-4949
Aging	National Council on Aging	800-424-9046
Alcoholism	National Council on Alcoholism	212-206-6770
Cancer	American Cancer Society	800-227-2345
	National Cancer Information Service	800-4-CANCER
Cerebral Palsy	United Cerebral Palsy	800-872-5827
Chronic Fatigue/Epstein-Barr Virus	Chronic Fatigue & Immune Dysfunction Syndrome Association	704-362-2343
Chronic Pain	National Chronic Pain Outreach Association	301-652-4948
Cystic Fibrosis	Cystic Fibrosis Foundation	800-FIGHT-CF
Deafness and Hearing Impairment	National Association for Hearing & Speech Action Line	800-638-8255
Diabetes	American Diabetes Association	800-232-3472
	Juvenile Diabetes Foundation International	800-223-1138
Disabilities	International Center for the Disabled	212-679-0100
	National Clearinghouse for Disabled Infants	800-922-9234
Down's Syndrome	National Down's Syndrome Congress	312-823-7550
	National Down's Syndrome Society	800-221-4602
Epilepsy	Epilepsy Information Line	800-332-1000
Genetic Diseases	National Maternal & Child Health Clearinghouse	703-821-8955
	National Foundation for Jewish Genetic Diseases	212-682-5550
	National Genetics Foundation	212-586-5800
Headache	National Migraine Foundation	312-878-7715
Hospice	The National Hospice Organization	703-243-5900
Huntington's Disease	Huntington's Disease Society of America	800-245-HDSA*
Ileitis and Colitis	National Foundation for Ileitis and Colitis	212-685-3440
Bladder Control Problems	The Simon Foundation	800-23SIMON
Kidney Disease	National Kidney Foundation	212-889-2210
Liver Disease	American Liver Foundation	800-223-0179
Lung Conditions	The Lung Line Information Service	800-222-LUNG*
	American Lung Association & American Thoracic Society	212-315-8700
Lupus Erythematosus	The Lupus Foundation of America	800-558-0121
Mental Illness	National Alliance for the Mentally Ill	703-524-7600
	National Mental Health Association	703-684-7722
Multiple Sclerosis	National Multiple Sclerosis Society	212-986-3240
Osteoporosis	National Osteoporosis Foundation	202-223-2226
Parkinson's Disease	American Parkinson's Disease Association	800-223-APDA
	National Parkinson's Foundation	800-327-4545
Polio	International Polio Network	314-534-0475
	National Rehabilitation Hospital, Washington, D.C., Dr. Laurel Halstead	202-877-1653
Psoriasis	National Psoriasis Foundation	503-297-1545
Rare Disorders	National Organization for Rare Disorders	203-746-6518
Sickle Cell Disease	National Association for Sickle Cell Disease	800-421-8453
Spinal Cord Injury	Spinal Cord Injury Hotline	800-526-3456
	National Spinal Cord Injury Association	800-962-9629
Stroke/Heart Problems	American Heart Association	214-373-6300

*Cannot be reached in all calling areas.

are providing services in the *client's* environment. Although you have a specific purpose for being there, you are providing care very much within the client's personal home space and you are the one that must adjust to the care setting. However, being in the client's setting provides you with a much more accurate picture of his care situation, including the family interaction and physical environment. What you see may be positive or negative in your eyes. Whichever it is, you must support the client and work collaboratively toward positive care outcomes.

Conclusion

The course of chronic illness is frequently long, complex, and unpredictable. It involves transitions that include changes in identities, roles, relationships, abilities, and patterns of behavior for the client who is ill and the family (Schumacher, 1994). The ability to work through these transitions successfully requires effective planning, collaboration, and support across disciplines to ensure the physical and emotional well-being of those involved. The rewards of caring for chronically ill clients come when you see the client and family work through these transitions in a positive, supported way.

PRACTICAL APPLICATIONS

1. Reflect on transitions you have worked through. Share your thoughts with the group.
   a. What feelings do you remember experiencing during those times?
   b. What was helpful, or could have been helpful, to you during those times?
   c. In what way could this reflection assist you in working more effectively with clients?
2. Call one of the organizational and referral services listed in Table 8–3. Report back to the group on the types of information and referrals each agency offers.
3. Consider a chronically ill client you have cared for. What illness-related losses has the client experienced? How has the client adapted to the losses? To what extent was the collaborative care model used for the client's care?

REFERENCES

Aldersberg, M., & Thorne, S. (1990). Emerging from the chrysalis: Older widows in transition. *Journal of Gerontological Nursing, 16,* 4–8.

Barton, J. A., Magilvy, J. K., & Quinn, A. A. (1994). Maintaining the fighting spirit: Veterans living with multiple sclerosis. *Rehabilitation Nursing Research, 3* (3), 86–96.

Brown, A. M., & Powell-Cope, G. M. (1991). AIDS family caregiving: Transitions through uncertainty. *Nursing Research, 40,* 338–345.

Cantanzaro, M. (1990). Transitions in midlife adults with long-term illness. *Holistic Nursing Practice, 4* (3), 65–73.

Chielens, D., & Herrick, E. (1990). Recipients of bone marrow transplants: Making a smooth transition to an ambulatory setting. *Oncology Nursing Forum, 17,* 857–862.

Cox, B. G., Carr, D. C., & Lee, R. E. (1992). *Living with cancer: A guide for patients and their families* (3rd Ed.) (pp. 110–111). Gainesville, FL: Triad.

Crepeau, E. B. (1994). Three images of interdisciplinary team meetings. *American Journal of Occupational Therapy, 48,* 717–722.

Folden, S. L. (1994). Managing the effects of a stroke: The first months. *Rehabilitation Nursing Research, 3,* (3), 79–85.

Johnson, M. A., Morton, M. K., & Knox, S. M. (1992). The transition to a nursing home: Meeting the family's needs. Families face their own transition when a loved one enters a nursing home. *Geriatric Nursing, 13,* 299–302.

Kane, J. J. (1992). Allowing the novice to succeed:

Transitional support in critical care. *Critical Care Nursing Quarterly, 15* (3), 17–22.

Kelley, J., & Lehman, L. (1993). Assessment of anxiety, depression, and suspiciousness in the home care setting. *Home Health Care Nurse, 11* (2), 16–19.

Lorig, K., & Fries, J. (1992). *The arthritis help book* (p. 173). New York: Addison-Wesley.

Loveys, B. (1990). Transitions in chronic illness: The at-risk role. *Holistic Nursing Practice, 4,* 56–64.

Reimer, J. C., Davies, B., & Martens, N. (1991). Palliative care: The nurse's role in helping families through the transition of "fading away." *Cancer Nursing, 14,* 321–327.

Robinson, G. M., & Pinckney, A. A. (1992). Transition from the hospital to the community: Small group program. *Journal of Psychosocial Nursing and Mental Health Services, 30,* 33–38.

Samuels, M. & Samuels, N. (1992). *Arthritis: How to work with your doctor and take charge of your health* (pp. 63–64). New York, Summit.

Schumacher, K. L. (1994). Transitions: A central concept in nursing. *IMAGE: Journal of Nursing Scholarship, 26,* 119–125.

Siegler, E. L., & Whitney, F. W. (1994). *Nurse-physician collaboration, care of adults and the elderly* (pp. 4–5). New York: Springer.

Thiederman, S. (1989, June). Stoic or shouter, the pain is real. *RN,* 49–51.

Thurber, F., & DiGiamarino, L. (1992). Development of a model of transitional care for the HIV-positive child and family. *Clinical Nurse Specialist, 6,* 146–146.

Weaver, S. K., & Wilson, J. F. (1994). Moving toward patient empowerment. *Nursing and Health Care, 15,* (9), 483.

Wong, D. L. (1991). Transition from hospital to home for children with complex medical care. *Journal of Pediatric Oncology Nursing, 8,* 3–9.

Wright, L. M., & Leahey, M. (1987). *Families and chronic illness* (pp. 38–39). Springhouse, PA: Springhouse.

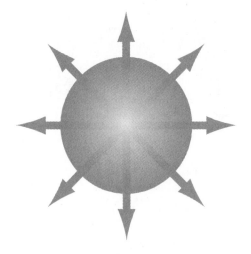

With Clients and Families Experiencing a Loss

In this chapter, we will discuss:

- How to assess the client's understanding of the situation
- Ways to respond therapeutically to common reactions to loss
- Beneficial ways to communicate with grieving families
- The time when death is imminent
- The staff's need to communicate their own feelings and experiences when loss occurs in the clinical setting

How one experiences loss, or grieves, is deeply personal, complex, and unique to each individual. It is a process, a journey of varying length, affected by one's culture, life experiences, age, philosophy and beliefs about life and death, suddenness of the loss, and learned coping strategies. Types of loss can include role or lifestyle change, physical changes and/or altered function, terminal prognosis, and antici-pated or actual loss of a loved one. Such losses precipitate the grieving process, which can be described in various ways. Elisabeth Kübler-Ross is well known for her work in the area of responses to loss. She describes the process as working through five stages: denial, anger, bargaining, depression, and acceptance (Kübler-Ross, 1969). Since her work, other models have emerged that also attempt to describe the process individuals work through in varying ways and to varying degrees when faced with their own or a loved one's mortality. When a person is confronted with a serious illness or loss, either through death or physical injury, fairly common reactions may be seen. These reactions reflect coping strategies used in an attempt to deal with what is happening. Models have been developed that identify certain tasks people face when told of a poor prognosis and as they live with the illness and move toward recovery or death. The family and significant others must also face similar tasks as the process unfolds and when death occurs (Cooligan, Stark, Doka, & Corr, 1994; Corr, 1992; Doka, 1993; Walsh & McGoldrick, 1991; Worden, 1991). Table 9–1 gives an overview of these reactions and when they tend to occur in this grieving process. It also includes the focus of nursing interventions to assist clients as they address tasks common to the stages indicated. Overall, grieving is viewed as a dynamic process involving a variety of reactions and expressions and activity. Many reactions tend to cluster in certain stages. It is important to note that client behaviors often reflect a blending of stages or a fluctuation from one stage to another as the client works through grief.

In caring for clients and families who are grieving, we must be able to identify and accept their reactions and help those involved express their feelings when they feel ready. It is important to provide the client with an emotionally safe grieving environment that allows them to feel supported and accepted, no matter what they say, feel, do, or look like. It is a nonjudgmental environment in which they can be vulnerable without fear or rejection. In this atmosphere, those who are grieving can address their loss and explore their feelings and concerns. Communication plays a key role in establishing this type of environment.

Table 9–1 EMOTIONS IN THE THREE MAJOR STAGES OF GRIEVING AND FOCUS OF INTERVENTIONS*

INITIAL STAGE: FACING THE THREAT OF LOSS

> "I might die of this disease."
> "I know my loved one may die of this disease."

- Emotions, often intense:

Shock	Guilt
Denial	Hope/despair
Disbelief	Bargaining
Anger	Anxiety
Fear	

- Focus nursing interventions to assist client/family to:
  1. Understand the disease.
  2. Maximize health and lifestyle.
  3. Preserve self-concept and relationships with others in the face of disease.
  4. Develop strategies to deal with the issues created by the disease.
  5. Explore the effects of the diagnosis on a sense of self and others.
  6. Ventilate feelings and fears.
  7. Incorporate the present reality of diagnosis into one's sense of past and future.

Table continued on following page

Table 9–1   EMOTIONS IN THE THREE MAJOR STAGES OF
GRIEVING AND FOCUS OF INTERVENTIONS* *(Continued)*

CHRONIC STAGE: DEALING WITH ILLNESS

> "I realize that I will die of this disease but not now."
> "I realize my loved one will die of this disease but not now."

- Acute, initial reactions are gradually resolved.
- Emotions less intense but can resurface at various times, often when physical status fluctuates or treatment regimens change:

Depression (very common)	Denial
Fear	Hope/despair
Anxiety	Bargaining
Anger	Guilt

- Focus nursing interventions to assist client/family to:
  1. Manage symptoms and side effects.
  2. Carry out health/treatment regimens.
  3. Maximize social support and minimize isolation.
  4. Manage stress and examine coping strategies.
  5. Maximize one's coping strengths and limit weaknesses.
  6. Normalize life as much as possible in the face of the disease.
  7. Deal with financial concerns.
  8. Preserve self-concept.
  9. Redefine relationships with others throughout the course of the disease.
  10. Ventilate feelings and fears.
  11. Find meaning in suffering chronicity, uncertainty, and physical decline.

FINAL STAGE: ACCEPTANCE OF LOSS

> "I am dying."
> "He/she is dying."

- At peace with own death; has made "sense" of what has and is occurring, based on belief patterns.
- Emotions: learning and growing from experience; letting go, moving on:
  Acceptance
  Sadness
  Peacefulness
- Focus nursing interventions to assist client/family to:
  1. Deal with disease symptoms, discomfort, pain, and incapacitation.
  2. Manage care procedures and institutional stresses.
  3. Manage stress and examine coping strategies.
  4. Deal effectively with caregivers.
  5. Prepare for death and say good-bye.
  6. Preserve self-concept.
  7. Preserve appropriate relationships with family and friends.
  8. Vent feelings and fears.
  9. Find meaning in life and death.

*Data from Buckman, R. (1992). *How to break bad news*. Baltimore, Johns Hopkins Press, and Cooligan, M., Stark, J., & Corr, C. (1994). Education about death, dying, and bereavement in nursing programs. *Nursing Educator, 19*(6), 38. Used by permission.

How to Assess the Client's Understanding of the Situation

Consider This Scenario

Ms. Cril is assigned to care for Mrs. Karowski, 42, who had her breast removed yesterday because of a malignant tumor. As Ms. Cril prepares for the day, she wonders how Mrs. Karowski is reacting to the loss of her breast and how comfortable she is physically. In report, nothing is said about her emotional status, but it is reported that the physician did see her after surgery and told her and her husband about the tumor. She has not asked any questions or made any comments about this. She has three boys at home, aged 9, 13, and 17. Her pain is being controlled by the ordered medication.

Before seeing Mrs. Karowski, Ms. Cril reviews the medical and nursing progress notes for information that addresses what has been discussed with Mrs. Karowski postoperatively and reactions to such information. The doctor has written that she discussed surgical findings with her and further discussion about treatment would follow. Nurses' notes state she has slept at intervals and that she reports her pain as "much less" after medication. Ms. Cril then checks her other clients to avoid feeling rushed during her time with Mrs. Karowski.

Ms. Cril now knocks on Mrs. Karowski's door and hears a faint, "Yes?" On entering the room, Ms. Cril notes the lights are off and Mrs. Karowski is on her side facing away from the door. "Mrs. Karowski?"

"Yes, it's me," Mrs. Karowski says softly.

Ms. Cril walks up to her bedside on the side she is facing. "I am Linda Cril, a registered nurse. I will be caring for you today." She notes Mrs. Karowski makes very little eye contact and has her sheet pulled up around her tightly. Ms. Cril pulls up a chair next to her bed. "How are you doing with all that has happened to you over the past couple of days?" she asks.

Mrs. Karowski looks at Ms. Cril for a brief moment, and then her eyes tear up. She then covers her face.

Ms. Cril sits quietly, patiently, and allows Mrs. Karowski time with her feelings.

In a few minutes, Mrs. Karowski dries her eyes and looks up. "I feel angry, sad, frightened, numb. One minute I think, oh well, one day at a time, and then a few minutes later, I think, oh, my God, what is happening to me, I could die in a short time! I guess I will just have to stay focused on what I have to do to take care of myself."

Ms. Cril touches Mrs. Karowski's arm: "It must be very hard to have so many feelings about what is happening." She pauses and then continues, "Your doctor was in last evening. What did she say would be the next step?"

Mrs. Karowski: "She said the tumor was found and we'll have to see what the node biopsies show. She is supposed to talk with me more today and that will help me get a better picture of what will be happening. It has surely helped to talk about this. Since I found the lump, everything has been in a fog, kind of suspended. I'm not sure I even hear everything. At home, I've been on automatic pilot. It's so hard to open up; I think it's because inside I'm on an emotional roller coaster."

Ms. Cril: "Let me know of any questions you have or ways I can be of help. I'll be back shortly to do your assessment and give you your medications. Call me if anything comes up before then."

Mrs. Karowski: "Before you leave, let me ask you a question. Do you think I am going to die from this?"

Ms. Cril comes back and takes Mrs. Karowski's hand: "At this point, I really don't know, Mrs. Karowski. I know that doesn't seem like much of an answer, but it is all I can say. I am here for you, though, to help you deal with whatever does happen."

To help clients, you must first understand their needs because their real needs may be very different than what you perceive them to be. How do you go about this? Reflect back on the scenario as we address these questions that will help you assess your client's needs:

- What has occurred?
- What behaviors, verbal and nonverbal, are occurring?
- How can the nurse assist the client to express feelings or concerns so accurate assessment can occur?

What Has Occurred?

Before visiting a client, find out through report and documentation what the client and family have been told thus far, when they were told, and by whom. Also look for cues as to how the client has responded to such information. The acronym "PERSON" can guide you in this psychosocial data collection (Dossey, 1994) (see box on opposite page).

This background information allows you to have a broader perspective of the situation when you interact with your client. For Ms. Cril, this approach provided her with some facts about Mrs. Karowski:

- Mrs. Karowski had been given information on the surgical findings early in the postoperative period.
- She had not outwardly voiced any emotional response to her situation in this initial period.
- Her pain was under control.
- A family support system was available.

Even though the amount of information was limited, it was enough to let Ms. Cril know that because of the newness of the situation, she may need more than a few minutes of uninterrupted time with Mrs. Karowski when she went to see her for the first time. She provided for this by making rounds on her other clients first.

Background information also helps the nurse get a multidimensional view of what is occurring in any given situation. This view helps prevent inaccurate, premature conclusions about what is happening. Knowing what has occurred in a situation thus far can also guide the nurse in deciding what approach would be appropriate and most therapeutic at this particular point in time. There was no way of knowing how Mrs. Karowski felt about her situation, so Ms. Cril provided her with the opportunity to explore her thoughts and feelings about what was happening to her.

What Behaviors, Verbal and Nonverbal, Are Occurring?

Denying a client opportunities to talk about thoughts and concerns can increase feelings of loneliness, sadness, fear, uncertainty, and frustration. But often, clients need assistance in exploring and dealing with their feelings (Spindler, 1991). Signs indicating that clients may wish to express their feelings include (National Cancer Institute, 1990):

- An increased amount of what appears to be idle conversation

The PERSON Method of Psychosocial Data Collection*

P—*personal strengths demonstrated through lifestyle, past activities, or occupation*

Positive examples:	Employed in area of interest; sense of responsibility
	Comfortable with who he or she is as a person
	Balanced activities
Negative examples:	Workaholic
	Voiced disappointment in life experiences
	Lack of commitment to life roles

E—*emotional state/reactions being exhibited by the client*

Positive examples:	Upset but able to focus on situation at hand
	Response is in proportion to seriousness of situation
Negative example:	Lack of any response (total withdrawal) or excessive response to situation (hysteria)

R—*response to stress at present and in past situations*

Positive examples:	Addresses problem directly, seeks information
	Releases feelings in healthy way, e.g., exercise, discussion
Negative example:	Denial of problems
	Abuse, e.g., alcohol, spousal, or child abuse

S—*support systems present*

Positive examples:	Family, significant others
	Uses community resources
Negative example:	Lack of family or significant others network

O—*optimum health goal(s): reasons for getting better; motivation*

Positive examples:	Life goals not yet reached, i.e., parenthood, special projects
	Sees life as a positive experience
Negative examples:	Many negative life experiences, life viewed as string of problems
	Does not view getting better as possible, rather as a debilitating, progressive illness

N—*nexus: mind-body connection; degree of control one feels he or she has over the illness and/or its symptoms; the amount of resignation to being "ill"*

Positive example:	Demonstrates involvement in care and treatments
Negative examples:	Voices being overwhelmed; demonstrates no effort to become involved in care
	Defers decision making to others

*Adapted with permission from "Mrs. Hill needed more than caring . . . and more than a care plan," from the April issue of *Nursing 94,* © Springhouse Corporation.

- An increase in time spent with family members or significant others
- Unusual nervousness

Eye contact and staying with the conversation, as opposed to changing the topic, are also indications of wanting to continue with the discussion that has been initiated.

Behaviors in response to a loss vary. As mentioned before, Table 9–1 presents a wide range of these behaviors. When assessing your clients' understanding of their situations, their verbal and nonverbal communication can assist you in determining how they are perceiving and reacting to their situations. Mrs. Karowski said she had experienced a range of feelings. This is not unusual, but it can be very unsettling and may lead to the client withdrawing from the situation, at least for a while. Mrs. Karowski demonstrated this nonverbally by having her lights off, facing away from the door, having her sheets pulled up around her tightly, speaking in a soft voice, and limiting her eye contact. Seeing only these behaviors, it would be very easy for a nurse to think Mrs. Karowski did not want to talk with anyone at that point. But knowing Mrs. Karowski was facing her first postoperative day and would have to start sorting through some of the information about her condition, the nurse offered her an opportunity to talk about what had been happening to her over the past few days.

How a person reacts to loss can vary greatly and depend on many factors:

- Quality of relationship with significant other(s)
- Circumstances surrounding the loss; was it sudden? unexpected? a gradual process?
- Religious beliefs and ethnic customs; accepted/expected behavioral norms
- Support systems in place (home care, counseling, clergy, etc.)
- Health, physical ability to deal with stressors
- Personality, past established ways of coping

In the next section, discussion will focus on ways to facilitate clients' abilities to express their feelings and concerns.

How Can the Nurse Assist the Client to Express Feelings and Concerns?

A common concern of nurses who encounter clients dealing with loss is fear of not knowing what to say or of saying the wrong thing and upsetting the client (Ufema, 1991a). Several communication techniques are helpful in assisting clients to express their feelings and concerns, including use of open-ended questions and reflective statements, demonstration of caring behaviors, and use of therapeutic touch. They can be used individually or simultaneously.

OPEN-ENDED QUESTIONS AND REFLECTIVE STATEMENTS   Open-ended questions (such as the one Ms. Cril used) and reflective statements can help to initiate communication, especially during first contact. Here are some examples of questions and statements that offer opportunity for the client to share feelings:

> "How are you feeling about what has happened?"
> "What are you feeling about what is happening?"
> "How are you doing emotionally with this?"
> "What can I do to help you through this?"
> "I am not sure what to say, but I am willing to listen."
> "You seem so overwhelmed."
> "It must be difficult to have so much happen so fast."

So many times, clients feel that they must be brave and in control of their feelings. This frequently leads to feelings of isolation. The reality is that clients often experience uncertainty about treatment options and outcomes as well as about the impact of illness outcomes on relationships before the illness. Many clients must

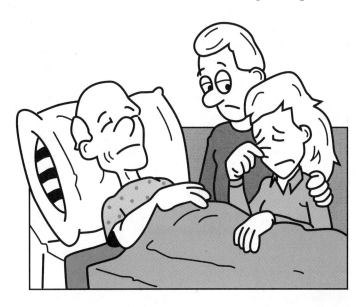

deal not only with the uncertainty of the future but also with physical pain, nausea and vomiting, fatigue, and loss of body function(s). Each of these also takes its emotional toll, especially if there is difficulty controlling such problems. Allowing clients to react honestly to what is happening to them in a nonjudgmental environment validates their individual, unique experiences. Suggest keeping a journal to clients who have voiced difficulty talking about their feelings but feel the need to get in touch with them. Keeping a journal provides them with a way to identify and express how they feel in a private way, which can then be shared if they choose to do so (Chapman, 1994). Table 9–2 contains excerpts from a personal journal that was later published by a woman whose husband had died of cancer. As she worked through her profound sense of loss during the first 6 months after his death, she found that making entries into her journal, rereading them, and sharing them with her children helped her find comfort in releasing her deep feelings of grief.

Also, realize that some clients may choose not to talk about their illness or may do so on one day and not another. Respect their wishes (Stoneberg, 1978). Present the opportunity for clients to share their thoughts, but do not press them to do so unless they indicate a need to talk about them. With length of stays getting shorter in acute care settings, it is not realistic to think clients can discuss and work through complicated, emotional issues within a 3- or 4-day stay in the hospital (Johnson, 1994). The focus of care during this acute time is primarily on comfort measures and assisting the client to deal with care management issues. However, it is very important to be sensitive to the client's complex emotional adjustment that is only just beginning.

DEMONSTRATION OF CARING BEHAVIORS Pay attention to what you do as well as what you say. Your nonverbal communication very often demonstrates caring more than any number of words. Maintain eye contact and a relaxed posture. Sit down in the client's line of vision. Give your undivided attention for whatever time you have with that client (Lillis & Prophit, 1991). In the scenario, Ms. Cril demonstrated

Table 9–2   THE GRIEVING TIME: EXCERPTS FROM
A WOMAN'S PERSONAL JOURNAL*

The first month.—The first few days I feel as though I am sitting in a tree somewhere, watching myself perform. I try to do all the right things—greetings to relatives, the thank-yous, the speech at the service, more thank-yous, more smiles, more greetings. I am outside myself, as if I have switched off my feelings. Except that suddenly right in the middle of a conversation, a wave of reality washes over me and I have to leave, quickly, to hide somewhere. I have to hold on to something when it happens—a pillow, the refrigerator, one of his shirts—because of the terrible pain in my chest. Is it my heart? I think of him, and I have genuine waves of feeling sick as well as the pain.

The second month.—Why can't I dream of him? It is the second month and I can simply not visualize his face or form . . . . I long to see him, but I dare not look at snapshots or home movies. I will be torn apart . . . . I realize that part of my problem is I really cannot share any of my feelings with anyone unless I feel they have recently gone through the same experience. So I bridge social chasms and call up one woman whose husband is dying and another whose husband has just died. I don't even know them, but I stumble through an explanation—maybe I can help them while they help me. We meet, and talk, and it is a help. I feel useful, besides. This is a good move. I'll do it again.

The third month.—I am finally dreaming of him! It is such a comfort, so natural. At first, he was only a shadowy figure, a presence, but now he is there! The practical aspects of life creep up on me. All the business affairs take up time and I prefer them—nothing personal to cope with . . . . The social part of my life is exactly what the books say. Many old friends have disappeared . . . but some friends remain—I appreciate their every gesture.

The sixth month.—One of the children has compared what is happening to me to the unfolding of a butterfly.

*From Brooks, A. (1985). *The grieving time*. Wilmington, DE: Delapeake. Used by permission.

respect for Mrs. Karowski's privacy by knocking before entering her room and softly introduced herself. Ms. Cril observed Mrs. Karowski's behavior and gave her the opportunity to talk about her feelings. She reinforced her interest in Mrs. Karowski's feelings by sitting beside her bed and quietly allowed time for her to respond. The "art of sitting" sends a message of caring and concern. One physician even came up with his own rules for sitting (Morgenstern, 1994):

- Sit.
- Sit close.
- Sit patiently.
- Sit interestedly.
- Look at the patient, not at the chart.
- Do not sit on the bed.
- Sit long enough, but not too long.
- When leaving, offer your hand and some words of warm encouragement and praise. Touch is also therapeutic.

Attention must be paid to small but very important details when working with your clients. Make sure the name and marital status are correct when you address the client. Avoid being too nonchalant in your conversation during procedures. Behaviors such as calling an unmarried woman "Mrs." or allowing conversation during a procedure to *exclude* the client and focus on your weekend social calendar can indicate to the client that she or he is "just another case" and of no particular significance to the staff (Spindler, 1991). Social conversation can be appropriate when the purpose is to lighten, not ignore, the situation or just informally interact with clients. The key to remember is be sure the client is *included* in the exchange. Also, consider what the client might observe during care routines. Clients watch nurses' faces when they care for them and may interpret facial expressions incorrectly. Consider the examples in the box below.

It is very important that you realize what your nonverbal behaviors are and what they communicate to clients. Avoid sending wrong, confusing, or distressing messages. Miscommunication may have occurred if the client suddenly becomes very quiet, changes usual conversing patterns, or disengages from the situation. If you think that there has been miscommunication, talk with the client and clear up any misunderstandings. In the first example in the box, the nurse picks up on the client's not chatting with her when she comes into the room. Then the nurse remembers how worried she had been about her child. She goes in to see the client and says, "I noticed how quiet you have been since this morning when I was in to give you your meds. I had just gotten a call about my child having a fever and was worried. Thinking about how concerned you are about your test results that are due back today, I realized that by looking worried and concerned about that call, I

Examples of Interpretation of Facial Expressions

Nurse's Expression	Client's Interpretation	Reality
Worried, very concerned look	"Oh my, she must know things aren't looking good. I bet my report came back and it's bad. She said it would be back sometime today." The client then becomes very quiet after asking her if the results are back, and she says, "No, not yet."	The nurse has just gotten a call from her babysitter that her 2-year-old child has a fever of 102 degrees.
Distant, angry expression when giving injection	"What did I do to get her so upset. All I asked for was a pain shot!" He doesn't initiate any conversation with the nurse the rest of the day.	The nurse had just been told someone had called in and it was her turn to work a double shift today. She had already made plans for the evening.
Unpleasant look of disgust and an "Oh, my!" when the wound dressing was changed.	"I'm so ashamed and embarassed. Why did this have to happen to me?" the client thought and looked away.	The wound had foul drainage. The nurse thought, "He didn't react to the dressing change; he must be used to it by now." The nurse did not realize she had offended the client and misinterpreted the client's behavior.

Examples of Therapeutic Use of Touch	
Affective Touch	**Task-Oriented Touch**
Holding a client's hand	Turning and repositioning client
Touching a client's arm or shoulder	Range of motion
Backrub	Bathing, skin/wound care
Giving client or family member a hug	Physical assessment

might have given you the wrong impression." When nurses are aware of their own and clients' usual communication patterns and are sensitive to changes in these patterns, miscommunications can often be avoided. If they do occur, this awareness and sensitivity will usually lead to clarification.

THERAPEUTIC USE OF TOUCH   Caring can be communicated very clearly through touch. Touching can be task-oriented (involving nursing procedures or care) or affective (used to convey concern or affection) or a combination of both.

Ms. Cril used touch very effectively when she responded to Mrs. Karowski's question "Do you think I'm going to die from this?" She held her hand as she told Mrs. Karowski she did not know but would be there to help her deal with whatever does happen. Her verbal and nonverbal behaviors both conveyed concern and sincerity. All touch should demonstrate concern and confidence. It should be purposeful and gentle, not sudden, forced, or indiscriminant. Avoid sexual overtones. Before using touch, assess for underlying conditions that may limit the type and amount of touching, such as inflamed, painful joints or easy bruising. Also consider culture, lifestyle, and history of abuse situations that may indicate minimal use of touch. Take cues from use of touch demonstrated by family members (Brady & Nesbitt, 1991).

Clients most in need of touch include (Brady & Nesbitt, 1991):

- Elderly clients in failing health or lacking social contacts
- Clients who are disoriented, disheveled, or foul smelling
- Clients with mental depression, low self-esteem
- Those with multiple tubes or invasive equipment
- Clients in distress: pain, grieving, emotional shock
- Those with diminished level of awareness

Allowing and providing opportunities for physical closeness between family members can be very comforting. Include family members in client care and comfort measures, if they so desire. Arrange tubes and bedside equipment so significant others have "access" to the client and show them ways to touch the client without disturbing invasive equipment. (Often family members are afraid to touch the client for fear of hurting him or interfering with equipment.) Keep personal keepsakes within the client's reach or in line of vision if he or she is unable to handle them. These actions will help sustain comfort and personal relationships (Renz, 1994).

Ways to Respond Therapeutically to Common Reactions to Loss

Let's look at therapeutic ways to respond to expression of grief. Table 9–3 presents common reactions, examples of therapeutic responses, and comments addressing

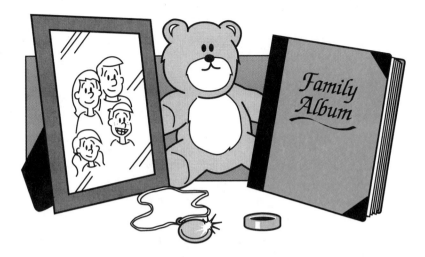

rationale for responses given as well as considerations regarding supportive nursing behaviors.

Beneficial Ways to Communicate With Grieving Families

It is rare that a grieving client is cared for in isolation, without family members present. When family members or significant others are involved in client care, their needs also should be addressed. Assessment of their needs is very similar to that of client needs. However, there are several questions you must answer for yourself when working with family members:

- Who is/are the most involved member(s); who is "in charge" or the main spokesperson?
- What is the family's understanding of the grieving process and where are they in this process?
- Do family members need assistance in finding ways to help the client?
- What must be considered when a child dies?

Who Is the Spokesperson?

When communicating with the family, keep them up-to-date with the client situation, particularly when the client is unable to do this. Often one member of the family will take on the role of family spokesperson. This role may be based on next of kinship, cultural or religious beliefs or roles, or long-term personal relationship with the client. If it is based on religion or culture, seek out a basic familiarity with their belief patterns. This will help you understand family/client dynamics, expressions, and decision-making processes the family follows. It is important that staff and family speak the same language. Social services, clergy, and other outside resources can be tapped for assistance in this communication process. If lines of communication are not kept open, anger and distrust can result, and staff members may avoid the family. This results in more family anger and staff discomfort. If this

Table 9–3 COMMON REACTIONS TO LOSS AND RELATED THERAPEUTIC RESPONSES*

Common Reactions	Verbal/Nonverbal Responses	Nursing Rationale
Shock/numbness.—Difficulty with decision making or functioning related to being overwhelmed with emotion:		
"Oh no, it can't be!"	"This must be overwhelming for you."	Lets person know it is normal to feel overwhelmed and provides an opportunity for response.
"This can't be happening!" Emotional outbursts	"I'm very sorry he died."	Using words such as died or death helps gently reinforce the reality.
	Avoid platitudes such as "Everything will be OK, don't worry," and "It's God's will."	Platitudes belittle the client's feelings or concerns.
Utter silence.—Absence of any attempts to verbalize feelings or reactions to loss.		
	"What are you thinking about right now?"	Lets person know you are willing to listen to whatever he or she has to say.
	Respond with silence.	
	Provide privacy, sit down, avoid unhurried appearance.	Gives opportunity to talk about or express feelings, emotions, concerns; facilitates environment that feels "safe."
	Reinforce, repeat information to help client/family understand situation; write down information for their reference and questions they have for physician and other staff members; write down answers.	Stress level may be so high that information is not processed and decision making is difficult.
Denial.—Inability to acknowledge the loss to limit or control the pain/distress of facing it.		
A client with complete spinal cord injury states, "I can't wait to walk out of here. There's nothing wrong with me."	"It must be hard not being able to move your legs." "I've never taken care of a client with your type of injury who walked again, but I'd never take that hope away from you."	Denying the harsh reality of what has happened decreases anxiety. It is a normal response to an overwhelming loss. Allow client to deny until he or she feels able to deal with it.
		If denial interferes with treatment and/or is prolonged, it can increase distress and requires planned intervention.
Disbelief.—Difficulty taking information in but is attempting to do so.		
"This can't be—I'm so healthy." "How can this be—I've had checkups every year and nothing's been wrong."	"It must be hard to accept this when you feel so well." Avoid confrontation.	Helpful responses reflect effort to understand how difficult it must be to accept what has happened.
Anger.—Resentment toward loss, what has happened; can have many targets against:		
Disease Loss of control, powerlessness: "I hate not being in control of this." Loss of potential: "I'll never be a Mom. It's not fair." Laws of nature/randomness: "Of all the people in the world, why me?" Self: "If only I had not smoked." Friends and family: "It's easy for you to say; you aren't the one who is sick." Medical and other health professionals: "If you had done more tests sooner, this wouldn't have happened." God: "I've been so good. Why is He doing this to me?"	Sit down, your head at lower level than client's; use calm, client-focused response. "You sound angry that _____" "What are you feeling now?" "Your feelings are important; can we talk about them?"	Place emphasis, attention on client and his or her feelings.

Table 9–3 COMMON REACTIONS TO LOSS AND RELATED THERAPEUTIC RESPONSES*
(Continued)

Common Reactions	Verbal/Nonverbal Responses	Nursing Rationale
Guilt.—Self blame with sorrow or regret.		
"I wish I never started to smoke. I brought this cancer on myself."	"Tell me what you are feeling."	Usually maladaptive and rarely useful to client.
	"It must be hard to think it was your fault this happened."	Provides client opportunity to identify feelings and discuss them.
"Why me?"—Often an expression of anger, depair, guilt, or frustration.		
	"Can you tell me what you are feeling right now?"	Need to find out what precipitated the question to be helpful.
	"People can mean different things when they say 'Why me?' May I ask you what you meant?"	This may sound contrived, but it is effective in helping client identify emotion(s) leading up to the "Why me?" Second example may seem more natural to say.
Crying.—Sign of various emotions.		
	If cause unknown:	
	"Are you able to tell me what is making you cry?"	Helps identify cause of tears.
	If cause is known:	
	"I understand."	Supportive; if crying does not taper off, seek assistance for client.
	Move closer to client, or at least do not move away.	Decreases client feelings of vulnerability.
	Offer tissues.	Gives permission to cry, enables client to wipe nose, eyes, face.
		Gives you something to do, brings you into close proximity of client.
	Touch: light touch on arm, shoulder, or a hug.	Communicates concern, support, caring.
Bargaining.—Way of coping with the possible outcomes of illness and reestablishing some degree of control.		
"If I do this, then things will get better . . . ."	Listen.	If it is helping client's adjustment, accept it as one of his coping mechanisms. It is not used by all clients.
Awkward questions		
"Am I going to die?"	"Do you mean from this disease?"	Helps clarify what client is asking.
"Yes."	"I really do not know. It must be very hard not knowing what is going to happen."	Honest response that allows client to talk more about uncertainties.
"What's going to happen to me?"	"Can you tell me what worries you the most?"	Gives client opportunity to identify and/or talk about main fears and concerns.
	"You must be very worried about the future."	More general, last statement is an empathic response encouraging client to talk about what is worrisome.

*Data from: Buckman, R. (1992). *How to break bad news.* Baltimore: Johns Hopkins University Press. Cook, E. A. (1994, April). Understanding your patient's denial. *Nursing '94,* 66–67. Makrevis, C. S. (1994, May). Learning from Ann. *Nursing '94,* 42–44. Milies, A. (1993, December). Caring for the family left behind. *American Journal of Nursing,* 34–35. Taylor, P. B. & Ferszt, G. G. (1994, January). Letting go of a loved one. *Nursing '94,* 55–56.

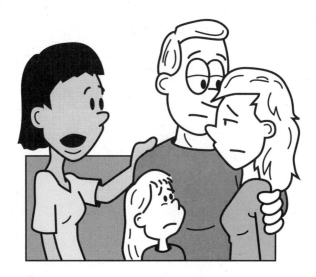

happens, more communication is needed, even though it is difficult. Utilize your resources to prevent or to intervene in this cycle (Edwards, 1994).

As discussed in Chapter 2, it is important that the client identify with whom information can be shared. This should be documented in the record for legal protection as well as for clear paths of communication with appropriate persons designated by the client. This prevents confusion. At times, especially when family members take turns staying around the clock, you may see them keeping written notes about answers to questions, client activities and treatments, and progress reports given to them and by whom. This provides a running account of what has occurred and is a good reference for them. This is helpful when family members are tired and information can be forgotten or misinterpreted over time. If things are not clear or understood by the next reader, questions can be asked and information clarified by the appropriate persons. In an age of liability concerns, this technique may initially be unsettling, but with the intent known, it can facilitate good communication. If there are concerns about such note taking, ask the family member in a nonjudgmental manner, "I find it interesting that you frequently take notes when care is given. Are there any questions or concerns I can help you address?" This gives the family member an opportunity to explain or comment on the note-taking approach and also demonstrates an openness to their questions and concerns.

Client care conferences that include family spokesperson(s), client, social services, clergy, nursing, medical staff, and other therapy representatives involved in the case can be planned at times when all involved can attend. These conferences are very useful in clarifying and sharing information related to clinical decision making as well as assisting in identification and expression of client and family needs. When structured so each person present is given an opportunity to speak and share his or her particular perspective on care issues, the family is assisted in being a positive part of selected approaches to care (Edwards, 1994). It is important to note during such sessions when family members come up with multiple excuses why a plan would not work. Examples include: "I'd love to care for my mom at home, but I don't have any nursing skills" or "I don't have any extra bed linens or pads," or "I don't have a first floor bathroom." Often the task that is proposed to them is overwhelming. Their fears need to be addressed. So provide them the opportunity to explore their fears honestly, in private, away from the client. "What frightens you the most about taking your mother home?" would be one way of opening the conversation. Gentle encouragers, such as "Go on . . ." or "What else?" will facilitate further exploration of feelings and concerns involved. When considering home care, hospice may be discussed as a possible option in selected cases, but it is not for everyone. It is a very supportive, skilled service, but some clients may have their own reasons for refusing this type of care. It may be one of the few decisions they still have control over. It may remind them constantly they will die soon, or they may view it as a sign of weakness that they don't have the courage to tough it out on their own. For these clients, explore other support systems that will meet their care needs and those of their families (Ufema, 1992). Such approaches demonstrate concern for how the clinical situation is impacting both the client and the family.

What Is the Family's Understanding of the Grieving Process?

Knowing the family's beliefs will help you understand to some degree their perceptions about dying and death. As a nurse, you need to go one step further and gain insight into the family's coping skills related to feelings of grief. Just as each client is unique, so is each family member. As each member grieves in his or her own way, for his or her own reasons, at his or her own pace, it is important to remain nonjudgmental about grieving behaviors and be supportive of all family members. This is accomplished through:

- Listening.
- Encouraging expressions of grief: "This must be very painful for you."
- Providing privacy: pull curtain, close door, provide private, quiet area for talks.
- Gently reinforcing the reality of what is occurring: "It must be hard to see your mother so close to death."
- Providing family time with the client.

To learn more about their understanding of grieving, ask if they have had to deal with the death of a loved one before. If they have, ask, "What was the experience like?" or "How did you work through that difficult time?" If they have not, you might ask, "Have you talked about death before?" or "Are there any family traditions related to dying or funerals?" (Brown, 1994). Another question may be, "What has this experience now been like for you?" When family members are showing emotion, such as crying, stay with them. Provide tissues as needed. Placing your hand on their shoulder or arm can be supportive. If they are angry, sit down and let them talk. Do not become defensive. These types of behaviors demonstrate concern and respect for their feelings. Other examples of responses to reactions to loss are discussed in the previous section. As your rapport builds, seek out opportunities for them to talk about their feelings and thoughts.

Explain how the grieving process works, that it is dynamic, that it cannot be rushed, that each person's responses are unique in both how they respond and the length of time it takes to work through the process. Encourage them to share their feelings with other family members and the client. This can help all involved understand their own feelings as well as be more tolerant of other's behavior and feelings. There are times when a person may not be able to express some of his or her thoughts to other family members, for a variety of reasons, but may feel comfortable enough to share them with staff (Lillis & Prophit, 1991):

> Barbara's nurse, Sarah, developed a trusting relationship with Barbara by listening to her cares and concerns. Barbara was terminally ill and also pregnant. As Barbara's condition worsened, she felt comfortable talking with Sarah about her feelings. For example, Barbara told Sarah that she felt guilty because she didn't have strong feelings for her unborn child—something she was embarrassed to bring up with her husband or family.

Assisting the Family To Help the Client

Many times family members do not know how to communicate that they care. Let them know their presence alone says they are concerned. Visits can be short or by phone. Conversation can relate what is happening on a daily basis, the news, or a funny joke that reflects the client's sense of humor can be enjoyed. Just listening to what the client has to say about the day shows concern and interest. Statements that can be helpful are:

> "Tell me about your day."
> "Now that I've told you about my day, tell me about yours."
> "You seem very tired. How about you take a nap and I'll sit here with you for a while and do some reading."

Having something to do can also be helpful. If physical comfort is a problem and family members would like to help, teach them how to reposition the client or give a back rub or a foot massage. Let them know how to participate in care. For example: "If this IV pump beeps before I get back, put the call light on." "This is an incentive spirometer. It measures how deep his breaths are. Remind him to use it every hour or so and encourage deep breaths. We are aiming for 1,200 cc per breath, which is where this marker is right here." If family members are usually there when the physician makes rounds, encourage them to take notes so the client can refer back to them. Family members can also write down questions as they come up and assist the client in addressing them with the physician and other members of the health care team. This is very helpful when the client is on medications that affect his or her level of alertness or is very tired. If listening to music or reading are hobbies, encourage these activities. Family members can bring in new tapes or reading materials at frequent intervals. It is very helpful for them to find a way to keep needed objects within the client's easy reach. Food from home can nourish the spirit as well as the body. Let family members know what types of foods would coincide with dietary orders and would be easily handled if brought in. These are just a few of many ways family members can be helpful to the client. Explore with them what is comfortable for them.

What Must Be Considered When a Child Dies?

It is important to take a special look at the grief that occurs with the death of a child. It is much more intense and things are never the same afterward. The parents often feel they have failed to care for the child responsibly. No matter how the death occurred, the feeling of responsibility for the death persists until the feeling of guilt that occurs with it can be resolved. This shock phase, which usually lasts

What Losses Do Parents Experience With the Child's Death?*

Loss of a piece of themselves
Because of the parents' deep attachment to their child, the child's death is an event that deeply affects their inner and outer worlds; the parent-child relationship is part of who each parent is, and that part has been taken away. ·

Loss of comforting illusions
The belief that parents can protect and provide security for their children too often is an illusion; this loss totally rocks one's self-esteem, and the feeling of failure as a protector and as a parent takes over. Even after these feelings are dealt with, life is much harder without this once-comforting illusion.

Loss of order in their universe
It is natural for parents to raise their children, grow old, and their children bury them; this is the way things are supposed to be. When a child dies, no matter how old, this order is violated. "You're not supposed to bury your children."

Loss of the future
Parents' hopes and design of the future is changed forever because their child had been part of that design; no longer can the parents see their child grow and mature. Birthdays and holidays become painful reminders of the child's absence. As years pass, parents often think about the child growing up and what the child would be like.

*From *The worst loss: How families heal from the death of a child* by Barbara D. Rosof. Copyright © 1994 Barbara D. Rosof. Reprinted by arrangement with Henry Holt and Co.

up to 2 weeks or so in most types of loss, can last up to a year or longer after a child's death (Sanders, 1992).

Parents deal with these losses in their own unique ways. A number of factors impact on how each parent grieves: gender, families they grew up in, losses they have already experienced, and what is going on in their lives now. Each of these contribute to how they have learned to approach life experiences and deal with their feelings. Many men have learned to "get the job done" and focus on the tasks more than on the feelings or relationships involved. They have not been encouraged to practice and develop skills in identifying what they are feeling and putting it into words, and thus when they grieve they find it very difficult to express themselves. In contrast, many women have been encouraged to build and nurture relationships, which requires being in touch with their own feelings and the feelings and needs of those around them. It is no wonder that when a couple faces the same deep loss at the same time, their differences in how they react, their needs, and the expectations each may have for the other to meet those needs often lead to unexpressed feelings of isolation, hurt, not being understood, and anger. This comes just when they need each other the most (Rosof, 1994; Knapp, 1986). As they work through their grief, the relationship between them either weakens or becomes stronger. It will never be the same.

When you care for grieving parents who are having difficulty, these approaches may be helpful to them (Rosof, 1994):

1. Assist them with the tasks and decisions that must be addressed quickly: help them contact someone they trust and know well to be with them, and then use the 4-D system (following page) to sort out what needs to be done, when, and by whom. For each task or decision that needs to be addressed, ask if it is one they can:

- Delegate: Can this be delegated to someone I/we trust? If so, to whom? Allow friends to help.
- Defer: Is it something that can wait? Many things can and should wait, such as what to do with the child's possessions.
- Decline: Is it something I'd rather not do and is not necessary to do now? There are few things that must be done immediately.
- Decide: Is it something I/we must or want to decide now? Sometimes the answer will or must be "yes." These are the questions/decisions that must be focused on now.

This method is a concrete way of sorting through the decisions, tasks, and demands that the family will be faced with and can be used in any crisis situation.

2. Encourage them to let their partner know how they feel, even if it is just a short statement, i.e., "I wish I could stop crying, but the tears just come up like unpredictable waves. How are you doing with all of this?" This helps each one look at and express his or her feelings and helps establish some communication that focuses on the partner, too.
3. Encourage them to help each other when they can, but to also give their partner some space; often, time alone and apart is necessary when grieving styles, moods, and energy levels vary.
4. Assist them to seek sources of help other than each other. Even though both may want to help the other, they are so drained they cannot give what the other needs. And that is OK. Social services and chaplaincy services can assist you in helping them connect with appropriate support services and groups.
5. Encourage them to let each other know what each needs. The risk that the other may not be able to meet the need is present, but at least it makes each one look at the relationship, presents opportunities to talk as a couple, and allows both to know what their partner's wants and needs are. Not to speak up will most certainly guarantee the needs will not be met.
6. Remind them to take it slow. Grieving is a bad time to make decisions. Allow the relationship to evolve.
7. Demonstrate caring of where they are in their grieving process.
8. Discuss with them and assist them to seek out a mental health professional if one or more behaviors of unresolved grief (see Table 9–4) persist for more than 6 months past the acute grief phase with no sign of improvement.

In some families, children are kept isolated or protected from what is occurring, or it is thought that children do not grieve. This can lead to feelings of abandonment, first by the sibling who has died and then by the parents and relatives. Ways to help children as they grieve that can be shared with the parents or the children's temporary caregiver(s) include (Sanders, 1992):

- Be honest about what has and is happening, detailed in a way the children can absorb.
- Have family time set aside at least weekly to give children a chance to talk and reinforce the family as a unit.
- Give the children opportunities to plan meaningful rituals that include remembering the child who has died and support grieving.
- Do not be afraid to let the children see you cry—this gives them permission to cry, too.

Table 9–4   BEHAVIORS THAT MAY INDICATE UNRESOLVED GRIEF*

Formal behavior that masks intense feelings of anger.

Development of physical symptoms your child experienced in illness.

Furious hostility toward specific persons connected with your child's death.

Chronic guilt and lowered self-esteem.

A feeling that the loss took place yesterday, even though it occurred months or years ago.

Loss of patterns of social interaction, interruption of friendships and formerly valued social activities.

Searching that continues over time, with a great deal of apparently purposeless behavior, restlessness, moving around.

Panic attacks, physical expressions of fear, such as shortness of breath and choking sensations.

Avoidance of customary mourning rituals (funerals, visits to the grave, etc.)

A relatively minor event triggering a major grief reaction.

Self-destructive and self-punishing behavior.

Radical changes in lifestyle.

*From *The worst loss: How families heal from the death of a child* by Barbara D. Rosof. Copyright © 1994 Barbara D. Rosof. Reprinted by arrangement with Henry Holt and Co.

And when children voice ideas or perceptions concerning guilt or their causing the death, ask them to tell you more about these feelings and listen respectfully. Your serious appreciation for how badly they feel gives them room to rethink things. They will then talk about it again at a later time when they feel the need to do so. For example (Rosof, 1992):

> "Jessie wasn't even there when Will drowned," her Dad remembers. "She and Allie were way down the beach, looking in tide pools. When Allie and I found out she thought her not saying her prayers was what caused it to happen, we were dumbfounded. I charged in with a whole bunch of explanations, but Allie had the good sense to shut me up. She just let Jessie talk about how much she missed Will and how important it was to say your prayers and that you let God down if you didn't."
>
> Allie: "I didn't say much, because I didn't know what to say. After that time she clammed up for weeks. Then one day we were driving to gymnastics, and out of the blue she said, 'Maybe Will would have drowned no matter how much I prayed.' I said, 'I'm afraid you're right, honey. We don't know why God took him, but I don't think it

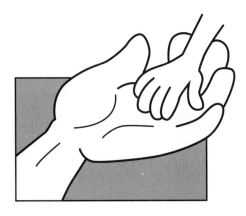

What Losses Do Siblings Experience When a Child Dies?

Loss of family as they have known it
   When they lose their brother or sister, they lose their parents at least temporarily, because parents are so disabled by their own grief. Their places in the family are forever changed and so is the family itself. And they have fewer tools to handle it than do adults.

Loss of an unspoken, yet strong, constant presence of each other that has been an ever-present, important part of their lives

Loss of playmate, confidant, competitor
   Siblings learn to know each other very well, and they share thoughts and feelings even parents may never know about; to lose a person who knows you that well is losing a piece of yourself.

Loss of someone who shares "the inside view" of what life is like in the family
   Very personal information and experiences that no one else could possibly understand.

Loss of illusions
   "I'm safe. My family is safe. My parents will always take care of me. Nothing bad will happen to any of us. Nobody I love is going to die." When illusions are lost too early and too harshly, significant damage is done to their capacity to feel safe. "I know I'll always see things differently. It's more fragile than people know. You can't count on things lasting."

Loss of ability to enjoy life again, to put death in perspective
   Children often believe their thoughts or actions caused the death, even children who were not directly involved in the death. This creates a great feeling of guilt, one they often will not reveal. It is reflected, however, in changes in mood and behavior.

Loss of someone to talk to
   Even though friends can comfort children and provide some diversion from their grief, they usually cannot talk to them about what they are going through and cannot help them grieve. The younger the child, the more this is true. This loss is magnified when the child's parents are unable to comfort them or help them grieve.
      Example: A mother sees herself alone on a tiny life raft. She can see her husband and her children each in their own rafts, battered by the storm. But she is so close to sinking herself that she must focus all her energy on staying afloat; she has none left to help them. Children often sense this in a parent and they will suppress their feelings.

*From *The worst loss: How families heal from the death of a child* by Barbara D. Rosof. Copyright © 1994 Barbara D. Rosof. Reprinted by arrangement with Henry Holt and Co.

was a punishment for you.' I wanted to make a whole speech, but I bit my tongue. I think what helped her was the chance to think it through herself and talk to me when she needed to."

It is consistently recommended that we listen to what the children have to tell us. A group of fourteen students, ages 11 to 14, came together to write a book on death and dying when the father of one of the class members became ill with a life-threatening disease. Over the period of a year, the students engaged in learning about their own and others' views and feelings about what dying is like, what is death, and what happens when death occurs. They shared their personal experiences with death and their reactions through discussions, drawing, and writing.

They talked with other children of all ages and adults, including their parents, about the topic. They talked with those who had different experiences and perspectives than they had and with professionals who worked with and supported those who were dying. They watched a variety of multimedia presentations on the subject. As they completed their work, they offered some advice that could prove very helpful in our work with grieving children and their families (Rofes & the Unit at Fayerweather Street School, 1985):

> We found it helpful to talk about death. It seemed easier to talk about being afraid of dying with other kids than to talk about it with adults. Lots of times adults get nervous, change the subject, and tell us that we shouldn't think of things like that.
>
> Drawing pictures about what we thought death was like and talking about the pictures with each other made it less scary to talk about.
>
> It was helpful to find out how other kids looked at death.
>
> It is difficult for anyone to tell a person that he or she is dying, but it is important for people to be told this information directly and honestly, rather than to learn about it through an unfortunate slip. The doctor (or the friend or family member) should say something like, "You have/your family member has a serious illness for which there is no cure. This disease usually causes death." Then the doctor should answer any questions, telling the truth to the best of his or her ability. He or she should be honest but leave some room for hope.
>
> It is also important for adults to become more comfortable with the subject of death and dying . . . we look forward to the time when all people will better understand and accept the cycle of life and death, so that they will be able to live richer and more satisfying lives."

A Special Look at When Death Is Imminent

"I don't think most people are aware of the extent of the trauma. It's mental, it's emotional, it's physical, and it takes your whole being." "You can know intellectually that someone you love is going to die, but when it actually happens, it's still a shock." Even though an illness may have been long, when death is occurring and after death occurs, many feelings emerge. An individual may feel like he or she is beginning to grieve all over again. Sometimes feelings of guilt over what should have been said or done take over, or the "what ifs" keep coming. Grief can affect one physically as well as emotionally. Exhaustion, loss of appetite, headaches, shakiness, insomnia, indigestion, and palpitations are often experienced (Fraser, 1991).

Communicate that you are available to them. If the family is visibly upset or appears anxious, ask if they would prefer you stay with them for a while, if this is possible. If this is not possible or if they prefer time alone with the loved one, let them know you will be close by and to call if they need anything. If religious faith is important to the client or family, ask if they would like their clergyman called or would it be comforting to have a favorite passage read to them (if you feel comfortable doing this). Ask if there are any religious practices or rites they would like to carry out. If at all possible, make arrangements for them to do so. Provide privacy and check on them frequently. This nonverbally demonstrates sincerity in your concern for them. This can be reinforced by a squeeze of the hand, a hug, a hand laid on the shoulder. Words are often not necessary. Let them know how the client is doing physically and focus on comfort measures.

It is important to listen carefully to what the dying client says. Research is

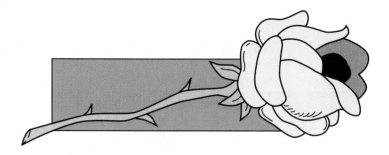

being done in the area of "nearing death awareness" that develops gradually in clients who are dying slowly (Callanan, 1994). Many such clients express special knowledge of what dying will be like for them and may communicate needs that must be met or deeds that have to be done for them to die peacefully. Symbolic language may be used and may reflect the client's lifestyle or events. For example, a client enjoyed traveling in her lifetime, which required frequently standing in line for tickets, boarding, and so forth. While dying, she called out, "It's time to get in line!"

These expressions are often accompanied by a change in mood or behavior. Many times such responses and behavioral changes are considered confusion or hallucinations, changes caused by physical status or medications. These assumptions can leave a client with unmet psychological or spiritual needs. If the staff and family listen, these statements may give insight into what the client is experiencing and trying to communicate. In the above example, when the client was asked if anyone was in line with her, she said her daughter was. Her daughter had died a year before from cancer. Another client had made a comment in August that Christmas can be sad. He died on Christmas Day. These forecasts or glimpses can be comforting for the family. If a client dies alone, often the family feels guilty. But the client may have chosen to do this to minimize stress on the family. Sometimes, clients may need permission to die and appear restless, picking at the sheets as they try to decide whether to "stay" or "go." Often, the family can help by letting the client know it is OK to "go" even though they will miss him.

After a client dies, assist the family as they begin to work through the loss (Ufema, 1991b). Ask the family if they would like to spend some quiet time with the body before it is prepared for the morgue. If so, allow privacy and stay close by the room. If there are family members not wishing to be in the room, accompany them to a quiet, private area. You may begin their closure by sharing your thoughts about the deceased client. For example, "Sam was special to me. His sense of humor was priceless and helped me through some difficult moments." Allow time for family members to share their thoughts. Ask if any family members would care to assist in preparing the body. This can be very helpful closure for some, but others may not want to do this. Be sure that the family does not feel obliged to assist. It is very much a personal decision. Avoid rushing the family through the decisions that need to be made, such as funeral home selection, and be sure questions are understood. Provide tissues. Let them know it is all right to cry.

Staff's Need to Discuss Feelings and Experiences

"As an emergency department nurse in a metropolitan hospital, I deal with death almost daily. But every patient who dies still leaves a scar on my heart." After taking care of a

Strategies That Will Assist the Client to Share What Is Being Experienced and Help Family and Staff Understand Messages the Client Attempts to Communicate*

Pay close attention to everything the dying person says. Any communication, no matter how obscure, may have meaning. Keep a pen and pad at the bedside so notes can be jotted down about any unusual comments or gestures made by the patient.

Watch for signs in the patient's behavior that may indicate nearing death awareness: a glassy-eyed look, distractedness, strange gestures (such as pointing at or waving to someone you cannot see), efforts to get out of bed for no apparent reason.

Respond to patient's statements with gentle, open-ended questions that will encourage him or her to explain. When a patient whose mother died long ago says, "My mother's waiting for me," say, "I'm so glad she's close to you. Tell me about it."

Accept what the patient says, and don't argue with it. Don't say, "But your mother died 10 years ago."

When a patient speaks in metaphors, respond in kind. If the patient says, "I've got to catch a train," you might say, "When does the train leave? Do you know anyone on board? Do you want to get on?"

If you don't understand what the patient is saying, admit it. You might explain, "I think you are telling me something important, but I'm not getting it. Don't give up trying—I won't."

*From Callanan, M. (1994, May). Farewell messages. *American Journal of Nursing*, 19–20. Used by permission.

man for an hour in an effort to get him to surgery and working with another nurse to provide him time for a brief visit with his son, this nurse wondered "Could I have done more?" The man had told her, "I'm not ready to die. Please, not yet." She had responded, "We'll do everything we can and you'll never be alone." "It was all I could promise." Her patient died in surgery. She may never know the answer to her question, but she did hope she did as much as she could with the time she had with him (Dubiel, 1992).

Such reflection on an incident is not unusual. Often nurses ask searching questions, such as: could something more have been done? or done differently? or

A Special Word About AIDS Patients and Their Loved Ones*

When a gay man dies of AIDS in the Midwest—or wherever the gay community is still largely in the closet—his lover, friends, and family may have few people to comfort them. They may be unable or unwilling to help each other, and the outside world may not offer solace. Grieving, always painful and difficult, becomes harder when there's no support system to ease the ache of loss. In conducting grief groups for the lovers and families of AIDS patients. . .we've learned just how difficult it is for these survivors to accomplish the tasks of mourning—to accept their loss, adjust to it, and carry on with life. . . .Whatever your own feelings about homosexuality, your acceptance, understanding, and intervention can be enormously helpful as they begin to deal with bereavement.

*From Lamendola F., & Wells, M. (1991, May). Letting grief out of the closet. *RN*, 23–25. Used by permission.

more quickly? This is true even when everything humanly possible was done. It is important to realize that as we support clients and families in their grief, we may also need to be supported as we experience feelings of loss, frustration, conflict, fear, and sadness. When situations elicit strong feelings, consider "Where did these feelings come from?" "How do they affect my behavior?" "Did my values conflict with those of my client?" "What makes me angry?" "What makes me so burned-out?" The more critical the incident, the more important it is to explore and share feelings with colleagues. Not taking time to "debrief" can lead to being over-whelmed emotionally and sometimes physically (Laing, 1994). Sharing of personal feelings is not always easy, however. For example, there are times when the fine line between compassion and emotional overinvolvement is crossed. Fear of seeming unprofessional or unable to handle work stress may prevent one from seeking assistance from colleagues. Today, nurses are encouraged to get to know clients and their families well, but how well is not defined. Many nurses have had experiences with clients who become very special to them even when the nurses try to keep a professional distance. It is part of being human. The sharing of experiences can foster understanding and assistance in dealing appropriately when overinvolvement occurs (Heinrich, 1992).

Staff helping staff prevents too much self-criticism and cynicism and helps increase the value of caring for each other as well as clients and families (Wahba & Dodaro-Surrusco, 1994). The chaplain, social services, psychiatric clinical nurse specialists, and grief support group facilitators may prove helpful in assisting staff to address their needs. It is only in staying healthy, physically and emotionally, that we as caregivers can be therapeutic when caring for others.

PRACTICAL APPLICATIONS

1. Take some time to answer these questions:
   What do you think death is like?
   Do you believe in life after death? Why? If you do feel there is life after death, describe what you think it will be like.
2. Choose a way of describing your thoughts to the above questions. (Examples: drawing, poem, narrative description, music/song, etc.) Share your work with others in your group.
3. Think about how you felt when a person or a pet you deeply loved died.
   How old were you?
   What comforted you?
   What upset you?
   Did you have to go to a funeral service? What was it like? How did it make you feel?
   Discuss your experiences with group members.
4. Read and report on one book or article that addresses grief.
   Consider: How did the information broaden your personal views of the grieving process?
   Did you find the information comforting? Discomforting?
   How can you use the information gained in nursing practice?
5. Have each group member select a different religious faith. Explore its beliefs and practices related to death and dying. As a group, devise a chart that shows the similarities and differences between the religious faiths. Discuss how this information would help you in providing client care.

REFERENCES

Brady, B., & Nesbitt, S. (1991, May). Using the right touch. *Nursing '91,* 46–47.

Brooks, A. (1985). *The grieving time* (pp. 10, 14, 15, 18, 32). Wilmington, DE: Delapeake.

Brown, M. (1994, September). Lifting the burden of silence. *American Journal of Nursing,* 62–63.

Buckman, R. (1992). *How to break bad news.* Baltimore: Johns Hopkins University Press.

Callanan, M. (1994, May). Farewell messages. *American Journal of Nursing,* 19–20.

Chapman, K. (1994, July). When the prognosis isn't as good. *RN,* 55–57.

Cook, E. A. (1994, April). Understanding your patient's denial. *Nursing '94,* 66–67.

Cooligan, M., Stark, J., Doka, K., & Corr, C. (1994). Education about death, dying, and bereavement in nursing programs. *Nurse Educator, 19*(6), 37–39.

Corr, C. A. (1992). A task-based approach to coping with dying. *Omega, 24,* 81–94.

Doka, K. J. (1993). *Living with life-threatening illness.* Lexington, MA: Lexington.

Dossey, B. (1994, April). Mrs. Hill needed more than caring . . . and more than a care plan. *Nursing '94,* 68–70.

Dubiel, D. (1992). Finding the right words. *Nursing '92,* 74.

Edwards, B. (1994, January). When the family can't let go. *American Journal of Nursing,* 56.

Fraser, L. (1991, September/October). Getting through grief. *In Health,* 88–89.

Heinrich, K. (1992, November). What to do when a patient becomes too special. *Nursing '92,* 63–64.

Johnson, J. R. (1994, May). Caring for the woman who has had a mastectomy. *American Journal of Nursing,* 25–31.

Knapp, R. (1986). *Beyond endurance: When a child dies* (pp. 50–51) New York: Schocken.

Kubler-Ross, E. (1969). *On death and dying.* New York: Free Press.

Laing, M. (1994, August). Letting the healing begin. *American Journal of Nursing,* 49–50.

Lamendola, F., & Wells, M. (1991, May). Letting grief out of the closet. *RN,* 23–25.

Lillis, P., & Prophit, P. (1991, December). Keeping hope alive. *Nursing '91,* 65–66.

Makrevis, C. S. (1994, August). Learning from Ann. *Nursing '94,* 42–44.

Milies, A. (1993, December). Caring for the family left behind. *American Journal of Nursing,* 34–35.

Morgenstern, L. (1994). The art of sitting. *Western Journal of Medicine, 161,* 93.

National Institutes of Health, National Cancer Institute. *Taking time: Support for people with cancer and the people who care about them.* No. 93-2059. Revised 1990, reprinted April 1993.

Renz, M. (1994, November). Healing touch. *Nursing '94,* 46–47.

Rofes, E. & The Unit at Fayerweather Street School. (1985). *The kids' book about death and dying* (pp. 94, 110–114). Boston: Little, Brown.

Rosof, B. (1994). *The worst loss: How families heal from the death of a child,* (pp. 8–39, 35–36, 71, 90–106, 116, 124, 145). New York: Henry Holt.

Sanders, C. (1992). *How to survive the loss of a child* (pp. 2, 22, 24, 97–99). Rocklin, CA: Prima.

Spindler, J. (1991, May). Seeing through the mask of cancer. *Nursing '91,* 37–40.

Stoneberg, M. (1978). *Listen with your heart.* American Cancer Society.

Taylor, P. B., & Ferszt, G. G. (1994, January). Letting go of a loved one. *Nursing '94,* 55–56.

Ufema, J. (1991a, February). Meeting the challenge of a dying patient. *Nursing '91,* 42–46.

Ufema, J. (1991b, October). Helping loved ones say good-bye. *Nursing '91,* 42–43.

Ufema, J. (1992, September). Insights on death and dying. *Nursing '92,* 26–28.

Wahba, A., & Dodaro-Surrusco, D. (1994). Caring and . . . curing, comforting. *RN,* 39–40.

Walsh, F., & McGoldrick, M. (1991). Loss and the family: A systemic perspective. In F. Walsh, & M. McGoldrick (Eds.), *Living beyond loss: Death in the family* (pp. 1–29). New York: Norton.

Worden, J. W. (1991). *Grief counselling and grief therapy: A handbook for the mental health practitioner* (2nd Ed.). New York: Springer.

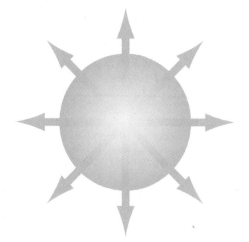

10

With Other Nurses

In this chapter, we will discuss:

- Situational assessment
  - Deciding with whom to speak
  - Deciding what information you need
  - Timing of business communication
- Sharing information
  - Verbally
  - In writing

An important nursing function is the ability to communicate effectively with other health care personnel. On a typical day, in addition to clients, nurses may interact with physicians, respiratory therapists, dietitians, student nurses, and many other types of health care providers. As a nurse, you need to think about what types of information you have to share with these people and how you will contact them to provide it.

What are some important communication skills for nurses? Although this can vary depending on the situation, nurses need to be able to provide information to others in a fashion that is easily understood by the receiving person. Nurses need to vary their styles of providing data depending on the perceived abilities of the listener. The nurse would speak very differently to a confused elderly client than he or she would to a physician.

Another communication skill that nurses need to be able to use is the ability to receive and process data. The nurse needs to be able to seek out information, process it, decide what it means, and express it to others.

Communicating with other health care professionals is usually not difficult for an experienced nurse, but it can be very challenging for a student or graduate nurse because this type of communication is a learned skill that a newcomer may not have had time to practice.

How Do Nurses Communicate?

Because nursing is a professional endeavor, how you communicate reflects on your ability as a nurse. Sometimes nurses give and receive information on a formal basis, such as during shift-change report or when telephoning a physician. At other times, nursing communication can be very informal, such as during a coffee break.

It is important to be able to know when formal communication is needed and when it is all right to be informal. To judge the formality of a situation, look around you. How are other people interacting? What communication style do you see? If others are talking and laughing, then the style is probably informal. If people are quietly talking to each other, the communication style is probably of a formal nature. When considering which style is appropriate, keep in mind that as a newcomer, it is always better to be more formal than the occasion calls for than to be too informal in a formal environment.

In this chapter, we will examine how nurses communicate with each other. First we will discuss how to decide to whom you need to talk and when to do it.

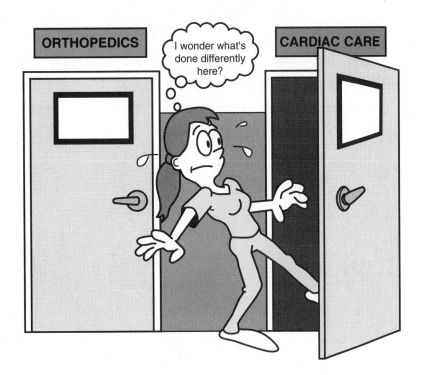

Then we will examine verbal communication methods that nurses use. The latter part of the chapter is devoted to written communication methods.

Many hospitalized clients have complex illnesses, requiring complex nursing care. Even the most experienced nurses have questions regarding care for their clients. But whom do you ask for help if you are unfamiliar with the care your client needs? Should you ask the nurse manager, the team leader, the primary nurse, the LPN, the unit aide, the unit secretary, or maybe even the candy-striper? To whom should you go with your questions and what is a good time for you to ask?

To help you with this, you need to assess your situation. When you need to talk to another person, consider using the old adage of "what, who, and when" to guide you. First, you need to decide what information you need. Once you have figured out what you need to know, you can use this information to give you clues about who is capable of answering your question. Knowing whom to talk to will provide information about the time frame for which you need your answers.

Consider This Scenario

Ernestine Rubin, RN, arrives on the step-down cardiac unit at GetWell Medical Center at the beginning of her shift. She sees a note telling her to report to the medical-surgical unit, 6 Main. Ernie immediately becomes concerned because this is the first time she has been "pulled" (this means that she is going to work today on another nursing unit because her regular unit is overstaffed and the other unit is understaffed) in the 6 months she has worked at GetWell. Ernie gathers her things together and gets on the elevator. The thought keeps running through her head: "I wonder what they do differently on 6 Main."

As the morning passed, Ernie had multiple questions that were answered quickly because she knew whom to ask: She asked the other RNs about the nursing management system used on 6 Main. They told her that the unit uses a modular approach to client care. As Ernie was introduced to the LPNs and the nurse assistant on the team, each person told her that he or she was familiar with the clients assigned to the team. This was very helpful, because they were a good source of information about the clients. A visitor asked about the location of the outpatient surgery unit. Because Ernie didn't know the answer to this, she asked the unit clerk for directions to the unit.

In this scenario, a nurse arrived to work at an unfamiliar nursing unit. She had to determine:

- What information was needed
- Whom to ask
- When to ask

What Types of Information Do You Need to Know?

The type of information you need can help direct you to the appropriate person to ask, because asking the appropriate person will certainly increase your chances of getting the correct answer. The majority of questions relate to the client, unit policy, or the institution.

Does your question deal with the client's physical condition, such as what to do about a temperature elevation? If it does, you probably need to speak with the primary nurse or the nurse providing care for the client.

Does your problem relate to unit policy or procedure, such as "What type of dressing does this nursing unit use on a tracheostomy stoma?" If so, any nurse on the unit can answer your question—you would not need to specifically ask your client's nurse. The best reference for unit policy questions is the hospital standards or procedure manual.

Does your question relate to the hospital environment, such as "When is the cafeteria open?" or "Where is the laboratory located?" If so, nearly anyone employed by the hospital can answer a question of this type. The unit secretary is usually knowledgeable about many hospital environment issues and is a good person to ask.

To Whom Do You Need to Speak?

After you have decided *what* information you need to know, you need to think about *who* can answer your questions. You will need to consider:

- Client care management style for the nursing unit
- The type of information you need as discussed above

What type of care management is being practiced on your unit? Knowing this information can help you decide to which person you need to talk, because it is usually best to direct your questions about the client to the LPN or RN who is providing his or her care. Are the nurses using a primary care type of arrangement, in which one nurse is providing most or all of the care for the client? Are they using the management style of team leading or modular nursing? In this type of client management, an RN directs the nursing group, usually made up of LPNs and aides, in providing care. Or perhaps the unit uses a combination of several management styles. When assigned to a nursing unit, ask the nurses about the method of care delivery for the unit.

When Do You Need to Speak With Them?

Another thing to consider about communication is appropriate timing. When do you need the information? Appropriate timing will help to ensure that both parties have the time to communicate accurately. Do you need to talk to the nurse immediately, or can it wait 5 or 10 minutes? You should set priorities for the information you need, and act or plan accordingly. If you need to tell the nurse that your client is not breathing, you must do so immediately. But if you want to ask a question about a procedure that you will do in several hours, you probably can wait until the nurse is finished with the current activity.

It might be helpful to use an organizational table to help you decide priorities. When faced with an unknown situation, think about these questions:

1. Is this a crisis or an emergency? (Will someone be injured if I don't act right now?)
2. Is this important to the ongoing care of the client? (Will interventions for the client be disrupted if I don't act right away?)
3. Is this important to the management of the hospital? (Will operations on the unit or the hospital be disrupted if I don't act right away?)
4. Is this a housekeeping or clerical issue? (Can action be delayed until more time is available?)

After you have decided with whom you need to speak and you recognize that the period for your conversation is not immediate, determine when the person with whom you need to speak will be available. Remember that nurses are busy people, and you may not get their undivided attention for very long periods of time. This doesn't mean that they don't want to help you; it means that they have a lot to do. You might find a nurse finishing the charting at the end of the shift, saying good morning to several people, and gathering paperwork for report all at the same time. Keep in mind that even though people are capable of doing several things at once, it doesn't mean that this is conducive to good communication. When possible, you should avoid disturbing others when:

- They are counting narcotics
- They are speaking on the phone
- Several people are speaking to each other
- The nurse is talking to a physician, client, or a client's family
- The nurse is in the middle of a timed activity, such as preparing a preoperative injection that is due in a few minutes

When the person with whom you need to speak is currently busy, you could say, "I see that you are busy. Is there a good time for me to ask you a question?"

Table 10–1 presents some situations you may encounter. Keeping in mind what

Table 10–1   LET'S PRACTICE THIS INFORMATION

Situation	Whom Should You Ask for Help?	When Should You Ask for Help?
The client tells you he can't breathe.		
An IV pump is beeping and you don't know how to fix it.		
The client wants you to use nonallergic soap on him.		
You overhear a client talking about a gun in his bedside stand.		
You need help to ambulate a client.		
A visitor asks you for directions to the cafeteria. You don't know where it is.		
A physician asks you to help him do a procedure. You don't know how to do it.		
A new procedure is added to your client's interventions and you don't know how to do it.		
A client asks you about his medication and you don't know the answer.		

has been discussed so far, try to fill in the two right-hand columns. Answers appear at the end of the chapter.

How Do You Communicate With Other Nurses Verbally?

Giving and Receiving Report

The word *report* has many meanings. In the profession of nursing, its general meaning is the act of providing pertinent client information to other nurses who may be unfamiliar with the client. With this information, the on-coming nursing staff can provide safe, purposeful nursing care. There are several occasions in which report is used. It usually is done at the beginning of the shift, with the off-going nursing staff providing information to the on-coming nurses, as will be depicted in the scenario following. Report is used when a client is being transferred from one nursing unit to another. This type of report can be either written or verbal. Often, the nurse will call the report to the nursing unit that is receiving the client. For example, if a client is being admitted to the cardiac unit from the emergency department, the nurse in the emergency department will call the nurse in the cardiac unit.

First, let us examine the idea of a beginning-of-shift report. Although there are several report formats, there are elements common to each:

1. Report commonly takes several minutes per client. So for a unit with 49 clients, report can be lengthy.
2. It is common to use abbreviations during report as Ms. Rodriguez did when she gave report in the scenario. These abbreviations can make it difficult for a nursing student to understand everything that is being said. If you don't understand a term used in report, write it down, and ask someone later to define it.
3. Most nurses use a report sheet to write down the information obtained during report.

What Does a Good Beginning-of-Shift Client Report Consist of?

Client's name, room number, admitting physician
Problems encountered during the shift
Alterations in physical/mental condition resulting from interventions
Problems/orders to be clarified
Things that should have been accomplished during the shift but weren't
    IV levels
Abnormal laboratory values
Special precautions such as masks, hourly I & O's, etc.

What Usually Doesn't Need to Be Stated in Report?

Results from interventions that are as anticipated
Routine events, such as "a.m. care done," unless this has been a problem for the client
Vital signs, unless abnormal
Medication given, unless there was an unusual occurrence

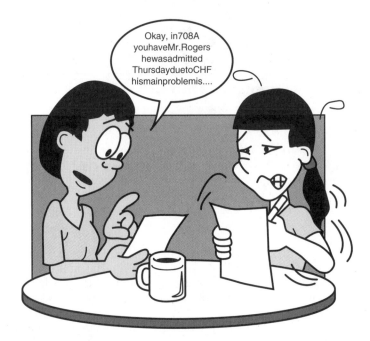

4. Learning how to give report takes practice. First, you need to know the style for the unit you are on. Is it done in person, taped, or written? Are there any specific guidelines to tell you what is included in report? If so, you need to use them. It is helpful to make notes of what you want to say during report. Use the Kardex, your charting, and your observations about the client to guide the report. Try practicing giving report on a tape recorder at home or at school until you are comfortable with the technique.

The Scenario Continues

The report system used on 6 Main is one information provider using a tape recorder to give report to multiple information receivers. The *left-hand column* is a transcription of the report Ernie received this morning from the off-going nurse. The nurse on the recording used many abbreviations and talked fast. The *right-hand column* explains some of the abbreviations and jargon.

"This is Claudia Rodriguez giving report on the clients in rooms 212, 213, and 214. Mrs. Franklin is in 212A. She was admitted on Thursday due to CHF. Her main problem continues to be activity intolerance. She was in a chair for one half hour, but became short of breath. She was OK when we put her back to bed. She has D5 1/3 up, going at 125. 500 up."

CHF = congestive heart failure
was OK when we put her back to bed = condition became better when placed back into bed
D5 1/3 = the IV solution is 5% dextrose and 1/3 normal saline
going at 125 = the IV is running at 125 cc per hour
500 up = the IV has 500 cc remaining in the bag

"Carron Sponte is in Room 212B. She came in 2 days ago for an infected mastectomy site. She had the mastectomy several months ago in an out-of-state hospital. She says that the wound hasn't healed right since the surgery. She was admitted after a debridement of the wound. Now it's wide open and draining. You need to irrigate it, pack it with gauze, and then put a pad on top. Her temp is 101° and her antibiotics were changed today because of the wound cultures. If her temp goes above 103°, you need blood cultures and you have to notify Dr. Selden."

"Jerome Bell is in 213. He was admitted today with a diagnosis of R/O TB. Respiratory isolation was instituted. His main problem is airway clearance because the sputum is very thick. I taught him about increasing his fluid intake and have included this in the care plan. Could you reinforce this? I have a call out to Dr. Reddy's service to clarify his streptomycin. He's allergic to the mycin drugs."

"Soo Bakta is in 214. He had an exploratory lap yesterday for a bowel obstruction. He appears to be in a lot of pain, but he says the PCA is taking care of it. His lungs had crackles bilaterally when I came on, and I called Dr. Kim. He ordered 40 of Lasix IV as a one time. Since the Lasix, he has put out 600 and the crackles are significantly better. He knows how to use the incentive spirometer, but I found that I needed to encourage him to use it. He has D5 LR up at 125. Just hung a new bag a minute ago. N/G to low intermittent with 400 out. His K was 3.1 at 8 a.m. He had a bolus, and we added 40 of K to each liter. He has a repeat K at 4 p.m."

debridement of the wound = surgical procedure in which nonhealing tissue is removed from a wound

wide open and draining = after surgery, the surgeon left the wound open to heal. The most common usage for this is to heal an infected wound.

blood cultures if she goes above 103° = if the client's temperature goes above 103°, the nurse will call the laboratory to draw blood cultures

notify Dr. Selden = call the physician and give a status report on the client

R/O TB = rule out tuberculosis (decide if the client has tuberculosis or not)

have a call out = the nurse has placed a call to Dr. Reddy's answering service to ask him to call the nursing unit

clarify streptomycin = the physician has written an order that cannot be carried out because the client is allergic to the ordered medication. The nurse needs to tell the physician about the allergy and ask what should be prescribed instead.

exploratory lap = exploratory laparotomy

PCA = patient-controlled analgesia

had crackles bilaterally = both lungs had increased fluid in the alveolar space

when I came on = at the beginning of my shift

40 of Lasix IV as a one time = received 40 mg of Lasix IV push on a one-time basis, not as an on-going medication order

put out 600 = had a urine output of 600 cc

just hung a new bag = added a full IV bag (this could hold 1,000 cc, 500 cc, or 250 cc. The nurse should have stated which amount was in the IV bag.)

N/G to low intermittent = the nasogastric tube was placed to low intermittent suction

K was 3.1 = his serum potassium was 3.1

had a bolus and added 40 to each liter = because his potassium was low, they put potassium in a small amount of IV fluid, and gave it to the client. Also, they placed 40 mEq of KCl into each liter of IV fluid he will receive.

Repeat K at 4 p.m. = Mr. Bakta will have a potassium level drawn at 4 p.m.

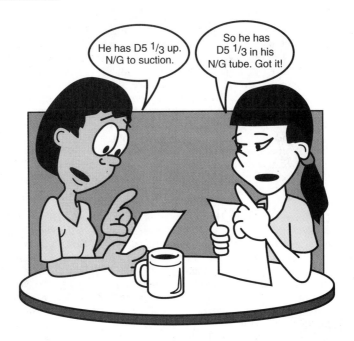

There are several methods of giving report to the on-coming nursing staff. Each unit may use a different style, or the style could be consistent throughout the institution. Some factors that may vary are:

- Who gives the report (Table 10–2)? In the scenario, the primary care nurse, Ms. Rodriguez, provided the report.
- Who receives the report (Table 10–3)? In the scenario, the on-coming primary nurse will listen to the report.
- Is it done in person, on tape, or in a written format? In the scenario, the report was taped.
- Do the on-coming nurses listen to report on all the clients or just the clients for whom they will provide care? This can vary from unit to unit and from shift to shift.
- Is it a bedside report or is it done in the conference room?

The Scenario Continues

During the day, you are told that you are getting a new client who is being admitted from the emergency department. Soon, the unit clerk tells you that a nurse from the emergency department is on the telephone and wants to give report on your new client. You pick up the phone and he says, "This is Aaron Cornwall, RN, and I want to give you report. I am bringing you a 67-year-old man named Joshua Green. He came into the ED with complaints of abdominal pain. I put down an N/G and got coffee-ground returns. His admission diagnosis is R/O GI bleed. His vitals are 130/68–99.2–96–24. He has an IV with 600 cc of NS. His wife is with him. Dr. Bunch is called on consult but hasn't seen him yet. I'll be up with him in 10 minutes."

Table 10–2   WHO GIVES AND RECEIVES THE REPORT?

Method	Advantages	Disadvantages
One Information Provider, One Receiver		
The off-going charge nurse gives report to the on-coming charge nurse, who then provides each nurse with information about the clients.	Time effective.	If the off-going charge nurse does not collect adequate data, he or she is unable to provide enough data to the on-coming nurses.
One Information Provider, Multiple Information Receivers		
The off-going charge nurse gives report to the on-coming charge nurse and staff nurses.	All listeners able to receive information and able to question information provider if necessary.	Time consuming. Report can easily take 20 minutes. If there are 10 nurses in report for 20 minutes each, 200 minutes of the shift is used just for report.
Each Care Provider Giving Report to the Client's Care Provider		
Each off-going nurse can give report to the on-coming nurse who will provide care for the client.	Able to get in-depth report. This is a good system for units that require large amounts of client data, such as critical care units.	The nurses are not familiar with clients other than the ones for whom they are caring. May take a lot of time to find each nurse to whom to give report.

Table 10–3   IS THE REPORT DONE IN PERSON, ON TAPE, OR IN A WRITTEN FORMAT?

Method	Advantages	Disadvantages
In-Person Report		
At the end of the shift, the off-going nurses provide information to the on-coming nurses.	Able to get in-depth information. Able to ask questions of the information provider.	Time consuming. Who's watching the clients if everyone is in report?
Taped Report		
The off-going nurses dictate report into a tape recorder for the on-coming nurses to listen to later.	Good use of time. Can tape report at a slow moment. Able to be out with the clients while the next shift is listening to report. Able to replay tape if listener did not understand information.	Able to obtain only information that is on the tape. Can't ask questions of the tape recorder.
Written Report		
The off-going nurse writes the report on paper for the on-coming nurse to use at a later time.	Good use of time. However, may take longer than oral report.	Only able to obtain the information that is written on the paper. Poor handwriting can be a concern.
Walking Report		
The off-going and on-coming nurses have report at the client bedside.	Able to include client in the discussion. Able to show the on-coming nurse specific aspects of the client's care.	May breach confidentiality when discussing each client in a two-bed room.

Transfer Report

When a client is transferred from one nursing unit to another, a transfer report is usually telephoned to the nurses on the receiving unit. Many institutions have also made interunit transfer forms to help ensure that the receiving nurse receives enough information about the client who will be transferred. The receiving nurse should have paper and pencil handy to record pertinent information. What is typically included in this type of report?

- Client name
- Admission medical diagnosis
- General statement describing the client's health progress while on the nursing unit
- Patient orders (medical and nursing)
- What has been done for the client and what still needs to be accomplished

On the Telephone

Many people are hesitant to answer the telephone if they believe that they cannot easily answer questions the caller may have. This may be true for anyone who is not familiar with a specific nursing unit, such as nursing students or nurses "pulled" to an area. The assumption they make is: "I don't know a lot about this unit or its clients. I probably can't answer the questions people may ask, and then I'll feel dumb. So, I'll let someone else answer it." So the phone rings and rings. People might be surprised to find that many questions callers ask are really very simple, such as "What are visiting hours?" or "Is Dr. Fillip on the unit?"

The Scenario Continues

The phone at the nurse's desk rings and you answer it like this: "6 Main. Charlotte Homestead, RN, speaking. May I help you?" The caller says that she has just been discharged and that she has left her bathrobe in the closet of her room. You tell her that you will go look, and you place her call on hold. You find the robe and bring it back to the nursing station. You pick up the phone and tell the caller that you have found the robe and she can pick it up at the nursing station.

You overhear the phone conversation of another nurse in the nursing station. When the phone rings, the nurse picks it up and says, "What do you want?" Although you can't hear what the caller is asking, you can hear your co-worker's response. "Hey, I don't know who that person even is, much less where she is. Call the operator and ask where this Sandra Dupp works." With that, the nurse hangs up the telephone and walks away. You wonder if the caller is angry about how he or she has been treated, because you know that if you had been treated this rudely, you'd consider it a reflection on the nursing care of that nurse and perhaps of the nursing unit.

Try to answer the phone within the first three rings. Pick up the phone and state the name of the unit, your name and title, and ask, "May I help you?"

It is important to listen closely to what the caller is saying. If you can't understand the caller, say, "Excuse me, but I was not able to understand you. Could you say it again, but more slowly?" To help ensure the caller can understand you, do not eat, drink, or chew gum while on the phone.

If you cannot answer a question the caller asks, simply say, "Let me put you on hold and I'll find the answer to your question." To put a caller on hold, push the hold button on the telephone. Then find someone who can answer the question and come back to the phone as quickly as possible. In the scenario, the nurse overheard made no attempt to help the caller find the information that was needed.

Delegating to Others

In many nursing settings, nurses are delegating portions of the client care routine to LPNs, nursing assistants, or aides. It is important to understand what delegation is. It can be defined as assigning tasks to someone who has the appropriate proficiency for the task. The power and the responsibility to delegate tasks appropriately come from your state nurse practice act (Barter & Furmidge, 1994).

There are several factors that must be considered to delegate appropriately. The task must be within a person's job description, a person must have the education to perform the task, and a person must have the ability to do the task (Herrick, Hansten, O'Neil, Hayes, & Washburn, 1994).

Delegation of activities is a very important task, with a high potential for problems if the task is not performed correctly. If you delegate tasks inappropriately or your staff assumes tasks inappropriately and you do not intervene, you could be held accountable.

Consider This Scenario

In this scenario, the nurse delegates a task to a nursing assistant. In the first part of the scenario, the nursing assistant *thinks* she understands what the RN said. The RN also *thinks* the aide understands. In reality, neither understands what the other is doing.

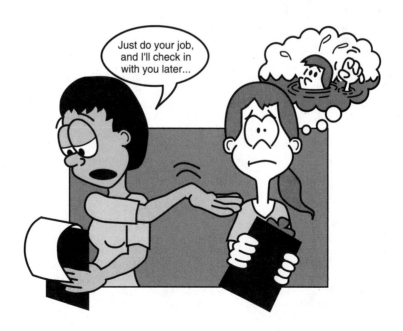

In the second part of the scenario, the RN correctly communicates with the nursing assistant so that *both* of them know what they need to do.

The INCORRECT Way to Delegate

Harriet Trumbell, RN, notes that Mr. Gilbert needs to be encouraged to ambulate and he also needs his dressing changed today. She sees on the assignment sheet that Ms. Hamilton is assigned to be Mr. Gilbert's aide.

Harriet usually works on a nursing unit that doesn't have nursing assistants, and so she isn't very sure of herself in delegating activities to the aides.

She asks who Ms. Hamilton is and approaches her. "Ms. Hamilton, I am Harriet Trumbell, the RN who is going to be working with you today. I see that Mr. Gilbert needs to have a dressing change and he also needs to be ambulated. OK with you?" Ms. Hamilton nods her head to suggest that it is OK and Harriet goes to check on her other clients.

Later that morning, Harriet sees Ms. Hamilton. "How are you doing with Mr. Gilbert?"

"Oh, we are fine," says Ms. Hamilton.

A few hours later, Harriet notices that she hasn't seen Mr. Gilbert walking in the hallway, so she goes into his room to check on him. She finds Ms. Hamilton irrigating a wound on Mr. Gilbert's coccyx.

Harriet asks to speak to Ms. Hamilton in the hallway. "What are you doing? I didn't tell you to do this dressing! I wanted you to change the dressing on his arm! And how come he hasn't ambulated yet?"

"Oh, I didn't know that you wanted his arm dressing changed. All I saw in the Kardex were the instructions for his coccyx dressing, so that's what I did. And you didn't tell me when to ambulate him, so I was going to do it now."

The CORRECT Way to Delegate

Harriet Trumbell, RN, a nurse on a medical-surgical unit, receives her assignment for the day. Among her clients is Mr. Gilbert. As Harriet looks over his Kardex, she notes that he needs to be encouraged to ambulate and he also needs his dressing changed today. Because she is not familiar with Mr. Gilbert, she goes into his room and quickly assesses the situation. She finds that Mr. Gilbert is alert and oriented and requires a moderate amount of assistance to ambulate. She notes that he has a dressing on his arm and also one on his coccyx.

Harriet usually works on a nursing unit that doesn't have nursing assistants, and so she isn't very sure of herself in delegating activities to the aides. Because of this, she talks with the nurse manager about what the aides are allowed to do and what they cannot do. To be sure that she understands the nurse manager, Harriet lists the activities that she wants to delegate to the nursing assistant. She is told that simple dressing changes and helping clients to ambulate are within the nursing assistant's job description.

Harriet looks on the assignment sheet and finds that Ms. Hamilton is assigned to be Mr. Gilbert's aide. She asks who Ms. Hamilton is and approaches her. "Ms. Hamilton, I am Harriet Trumbell and I am the RN who is going to be working with you today. I see that you are assigned to Mr. Gilbert in 596-B. I have written out what you need to do for him. Let's go into the conference room and go over it."

They move into the conference room and Harriet continues, "Mr. Gilbert needs to have a dressing change done on his right arm dressing. It currently has a 4×4 on it. You just take the old one off and put a new sterile one back on it. Tell me if it is red or has any drainage coming from it. I also want to know if his temperature is elevated. He also has a dressing on his coccyx. You don't need to change that dressing. I will do it later."

"I also see that he needs to be ambulated. I would like to see him ambulate once before lunch and once after lunch. We will have to check with another nurse to find out how far he can ambulate. OK with you?"

Ms. Hamilton nods her head to indicate that it is OK.

"Now, to make sure that we have everything straight, tell me what you need to do for Mr. Gilbert."

Ms. Hamilton repeats the information back to Harriet in her own words, except that she forgets to say that Mr. Gilbert needs to be ambulated twice. This is clarified by Harriet, and both set off to do their tasks.

An hour later, Ms. Hamilton says to Harriet, "Mr. Gilbert's temperature is 99.5. His arm wound is healing. No redness or drainage. I am going to walk him now."

Harriet walks away, thinking, "I believe I might like working on this nursing unit."

The task of delegation is best broken down into three sections:

- Assessment of the situation
- The delegation itself
- Evaluation of the activity that was delegated

Assessment of the Situation

Some things to consider before you delegate a task to someone:

1. Of what does the task consist?
2. Is it a straightforward task or is it a complicated one? For example, is the task a simple 4 × 4 dressing or perhaps a dressing that requires irrigation and packing with gauze?
3. What does the client need? What are the client's abilities?
4. Who is available to do the task? You will need to consider if the person has the time available to be able to perform the task.
5. Does the task fall within the person's job description? You can usually find this information in the institution policy manual. All job positions have job descriptions that list the activities and skills needed for a specific job. But remember this caution: You will find that there are always people who want to do more than their job description or official training allows. Monitor this closely. You cannot let people perform activities for which they are not trained. Tell them that these actions cannot be allowed. If this continues to be a problem, you will have to discuss this with your supervisor.
6. What is the proficiency level of the person you want to do the task? In addition to considering if the task falls within the job description, you need to think about whether the person actually knows how to do the task. This information can be obtained only by asking the person or observing his or her work. If the person does not have the skills to perform a task, it cannot be delegated to that person.
7. Is the person doing any other activities at the time? Before you delegate, you need to know what else the person has to do. For example, if the person has two incontinent clients who need to have their beds changed, you cannot ask that person immediately to ambulate a different client.

Delegation

1. Tell what you want delegated to the person to whom you are delegating. Be very clear in your descriptions. Use lay-person English, not hospital jargon. Remember that the person to whom you are delegating may not

have an extensive medical background; you cannot assume that he or she will understand what you are saying (Huber, Blegin, & McCloskey, 1994).

2. Do not abbreviate anything. You cannot assume that everyone knows what the abbreviations mean.

3. State when the task should be done. Does it need to be done immediately or simply during the day? You might need to help the person organize priorities to fit the new task into the proper order.

4. Tell the person if there are any specific parameters for which to watch. Examples of this would be vital signs that are out of the client's normal range or whether a wound is healing.

5. Tell the person what parameters to report and to whom to report them. There are times that you want to know specifics about a client. For example, you ask a nursing assistant to take a client's oral temperature. You could add to this, "I want to know if the temperature is above 100.5°."

6. If the task is complex or lengthy, write it down and go over it. If you are giving more than one task at a time, write it down. Always give both the client name and room number in addition to a description of the tasks needed. The person can use this task list to help keep track of what needs to be done. During the day, you could go over the task list to see what has been done and what still needs to be accomplished. At the end of the day, the task list serves as a reminder for you to use when you give report to the on-coming nurses.

7. When you are finished describing the task, have the person restate the task in his or her own words. This is vital to do because it will show whether the person understands what you want done. You can clarify any misconceptions before they turn into problems.

8. Tell the person if you want to be told when the task has been completed. This could be useful for several reasons. You might need to do an activity after completion of a delegated task. Or you might want to evaluate the client's response after the task is completed.

9. Encourage the person to come and ask you if there are any questions or concerns. Make sure that you are available and nonjudgmental. Remember the old adage: The only stupid question is the one that you are afraid to ask.

10. It is often a good idea to pop in and check on the person doing the delegated activity. This is helpful to ensure that the task is being completed correctly. It also gives you the opportunity to observe the client's response to the treatment.

Evaluation of the Activity

1. Did the person tell you when the activity was finished (if you asked to be notified)?

2. Did the person report the appropriate parameters?

3. Did the person do the activity you requested?

4. Did the person document the activity correctly? Does the documentation match what the person told you and what you observed?

In conclusion, nurses will be delegating many more activities than they used to delegate in prior years. The delegation must be done appropriately, with correct supervision.

How Do You Communicate With Other Nurses: In Writing?

The Chart

The information collected during a client's hospitalization is usually compiled into the client chart. The client chart could be as simple as a collection of papers placed into a loose-leaf notebook or it can be as extensive as a 3-foot pile of papers. The usage of the term *client chart* varies. In some institutions, the information could be contained in one client chart, whereas in other institutions, the information could be divided into several charts. They might have a main chart, a computer chart, a bedside chart, and a medication chart, all located in different places.

All these charts contain client information, and some charts may overlap information contained in other charts. You will need to spend time in your institution determining what types of client charts are used and what information will be found in each type of chart.

Although the primary purpose of keeping a written record of the client's condition is to provide direction for the client's health care, there are several other reasons to ensure that a client's chart is a useful document. The chart is a legal document that reflects the health care standards of the institution and describes the health care the client receives. It serves as a communication tool describing the client's ongoing status and the response to treatment.

The chart is used as a data collection tool for research and educational purposes. It also is used by insurance and regulatory bodies such as JCAHO to decide if the institution is delivering safe, appropriate care.

Because there are many types of health care providers who provide care during a client's hospital stay, documentation within a client's chart can take many forms. Physicians, nurses, physical therapists, nutritionists, and social workers are some of the health care providers whose contributions may be included in a client chart (Table 10–4). Each type of health professional may have his or her own documentation methods and forms. In this section, we will discuss nursing's role within client documentation.

The profession of nursing has a variety of documentation functions within its arena of record keeping. The most common nursing documentation methods relate to care planning and other written communication methods such as the Kardex, nurses' notes, transfer forms, discharge teaching forms, and incident reports, which are discussed in the following sections. The time spent in documenting nursing activities can be quite extensive; some report that as much as 15% of nursing time is spent in documentation (Gwozdz, 1992).

Let's define some common terms. *Charting* is a term usually used to denote the actual act by the nursing staff of writing or typing in the client's record about a client's condition. *Nurses' notes* is a term that describes the pages or computer files where nurses record information in a client chart.

Kardex

If you quickly need information about a client's care, where can you find it? There are several places you could look. One place is the client's chart, but the chart can

Table 10–4 WHAT IS FOUND IN A CLIENT'S CHART?

	Who Fills Out the Original?	Who Adds to It During the Client's Stay?	Where Is This Document Located?	Where Does It Go at the End of the Client's Stay?	Comments
Nursing Notes	The nurse who is providing care for the client fills out the nursing charting.	Any nurse can add information to the nursing notes, but usually the majority of the information comes from the nurse providing care for the client.	It can be found in the client's chart or at the client's bedside.	It is placed into the client's chart as evidence of the nursing care received.	If the nursing notes are kept at the bedside, they should be placed in an inconspicuous place. This helps prevent unauthorized people from reading them.
Client Orders (Physician Orders)	The physician or physician designee writes the original client order. After it is written, the unit clerk provides this information to the appropriate nurse or department. Usually an RN must check over the unit clerk's work for accuracy. (This is called noting the order.)	Each physician or physician designee can write client orders as needed.	It is usually found in the client's chart toward the front of the chart.	It is placed into the client's chart to document the medical treatment plan.	It is a good idea to check the client's chart periodically to see if new orders have been written.
Graphic Sheets	Typically, the nurse, nursing assistant, or unit clerk fills in the appropriate information (I&O, vital signs, blood sugar).	Any nursing personnel can add information to the graphic sheet.	It can be found either in the client's chart or at the client's bedside.	It is placed in the client's chart at the end of the client's stay.	Sometimes graphic information must be written in several locations. Have you filled in all the right areas?
Kardex	The unit clerk fills out the Kardex when the client is admitted.	When the client's orders change, the unit clerk or the nurse updates the Kardex.	It is usually found in a looseleaf notebook or a flip chart at the nursing station.	In most institutions, the Kardex is not a part of the permanent record, and thus is disposed of on discharge.	The Kardex is useful only when it is updated whenever the client's condition changes.
Laboratory Reports	These are usually computerized reports and come from the laboratory.	As new laboratory tests for the client are completed, a new report comes from the laboratory and is placed in the chart in front of the previous results.	These reports are usually found in the client's chart.	This information is kept in the client chart on discharge.	Many lab report sheets put an "H" or "L" next to lab results that are high or low to alert you to possible complications.

History and Physical (H&P)	There are two types of history and physical reports. One primarily has a medical focus; the other comes from nursing. The physician doing the H&P usually dictates it, and the nurse fills out the nursing H&P forms on admission.	These are usually not altered once they are completed.	The medical H&P is usually found in a different section of the chart separate from the nursing H&P.	Both types of information are kept in the client chart on discharge.	These forms can provide a wealth of information. Plus, the medical H&P is usually typed, which can make it very easy to read!
Discharge Instructions	The nurse who is providing care for the client fills out the discharge information.	The physician can add information to the discharge instruction sheet.	Many times, on admission, the discharge instruction sheet is placed at the client bedside, or it may be in the client's chart.	One copy goes to the client, one copy goes to the physician, and the original goes into the client's chart.	Start filling out this form as soon as you know the client is going home.
Transfer Summary	This form is filled out by the charge nurse or the nurse who is providing care for the client.	Any nurse, physician, or physician designee can add information to the transfer summary.	It is usually kept in a filing cabinet until it is known that the client will be transferred.	When it is filled out, the form will go with the client to the new institution.	To fill out this form requires a lot of time. Start filling it out as soon as you know the client will be transferred.
X-ray Reports	After the radiologist reads the x-ray and dictates the report, the report is typed and sent to the client's nursing unit.	When the client has further x-rays or x-ray procedures, new reports will come to the unit.	These reports are usually found in the client's chart.	This information is kept in the client's chart on discharge.	These reports can be quite lengthy. You may want to just read the radiologist's findings or impressions.
Consents	Some consent forms are filled out before the client is admitted to the hospital (this is usually filled out by admitting department personnel). A consent form is also needed for any invasive procedure (such as surgery).	Policies vary among institutions as to who is allowed to witness consent forms. In some institutions, a witness is simply stating that the correct person is signing the form. In other institutions, the witness is responsible for determining if the client is adequately informed about the surgery/procedure.	The hospital consent for treatment is usually kept in the client's chart. The blank consent forms are kept in a filing cabinet until needed.	Because these are legal forms, they are kept in the client's chart on discharge.	Policy varies from institution to institution about which type of procedures require a consent form. Typically, any procedure that is invasive or has significant risk requires informed consent. Nursing students may not be allowed to witness a consent form being signed. Check the institution's and your school of nursing's policy.

Table continued on following page

Table 10–4 WHAT IS FOUND IN A CLIENT'S CHART? *Continued*

	Who Fills Out the Original?	Who Adds to It During the Client's Stay?	Where Is This Document Located?	Where Does It Go at the End of the Client's Stay?	Comments
Operative Reports	After the surgery or procedure, the physician or physician designee dictates a description of the procedure and how the client tolerated it. This is typed, and the report is sent to the nursing unit.	Only the person who dictated the report can add to or alter the report.	This report is kept in the client's chart.	These are kept in the client's chart on discharge.	These reports can be very informative. For example, you could read the report to note the vital signs during the procedure or about the client's positioning in surgery.
Physician Progress Notes	The physician or physician designee uses these forms to describe the response or lack of response to treatment.	Any physician or physician designee assigned to the client's case can add to the progress notes.	The physician progress notes are kept in the client's chart.	These are kept in the client's chart on discharge.	Although many handwritten progress notes are difficult to read, they can provide a tremendous amount of information to the nurse.
Consultations	Any person that provides consultation to the client case fills out these forms. These consultants could be physicians or nurses.	Only the consultant who filled out the consultation form can alter it.	Consultation reports are kept in the client's chart.	These are kept in the client's chart on discharge.	Although these can also be difficult to read, they can provide very specialized information about the client's care.
Face Sheet	These forms are usually filled out before the client is admitted to the hospital (this is usually done by the admitting department). These forms contain demographic information such as the client's home address, insurance information, employer, whom to call in an emergency, and client's religious affiliation.	These forms are not usually altered during the client's stay.	They are usually kept at either the front or back of the client's chart.	These are kept in the client's chart on discharge.	The face sheet can provide a lot of information about the client.

be an extensive document several inches thick, and if you need to find something within the chart, it could take you a long time. A better place to look would be the client's Kardex. The Kardex is a nursing form that is usually kept in a notebook or a flip-rack near the nursing station. Pertinent data are written on the Kardex to allow the nursing staff to have a quick reference for the information needed to plan a client's care. The Kardex usually provides the following data:

1. Admitting medical diagnosis
2. Surgical intervention and date
3. Attending physicians
4. Consulting physicians
5. Consulting nurse practitioners
6. Client allergies
7. Current nursing interventions and assessments
8. Diet
9. Physical activity
10. Laboratory specimens to be obtained
11. Other pertinent data, such as client nickname or family telephone numbers

The Scenario Continues

During the clinical day, you removed a Foley catheter from a client at 2 p.m. By hospital policy, the client must void in sufficient amounts by 8 hours later or the catheter must be reinserted. Along with noting this information in the nurses' notes, writing the catheter removal time on the Kardex will be very helpful to monitor the client's condition.

At shift change, the on-coming nursing staff saw the notation in the Kardex about the catheter removal and made a note to check on the client's ability to void.

The scenario demonstrated that putting information in the correct place is vital. When a client is admitted, information is written in the Kardex and updated as needed. Because typically it isn't an official or legal part of the chart, the information is usually written in pencil.

Remember that the Kardex information is only as accurate as the person who wrote it in the Kardex. A major limitation for Kardex usage is the fact that it may not be updated as the client's condition changes. For example, a client who had been ambulatory had a stroke and became comatose. On the Kardex, the activity order still read: "Bathroom privileges." The client order wasn't still pertinent; it just hadn't been updated as the client's condition changed. If the Kardex information seems incorrect to you, check the client orders in the chart or ask the nursing staff or the physician. If the client orders change, the Kardex must be changed also. If the client order is still pertinent but the information in the Kardex is incorrect, erase the incorrect information on the Kardex and write in the correct data. You should tell the primary nurse that you have altered the Kardex.

The Kardex may also include notes that will be helpful for client care that may not have been included in the care plan. For example, some clients don't wish to have ice in their bedside water pitcher. This probably wouldn't be important enough to be a care plan item, but it is easy to handle by placing this information in the dietary section of the Kardex. Before you provide care for a client, look over the Kardex for pertinent information. Typically, nurses do this while they are listening to report for that client.

Care Planning

A care plan is a description of the nursing plan for a client. The nursing process was developed to help nurses provide client care in a systematic format. One of the strongest reasons to develop a care plan is that the care plan serves as a communication tool. Although a client's plan of care is usually developed by only two or three nurses, the plan is written so that the entire nursing staff is aware of the client's goals and thus can work toward these goals. Without a care plan, each nurse might be working independently on a set of goals different from those of the previous nurse. This would certainly lead to fragmentation of care.

The nursing process is well documented elsewhere. Basically, the goal is to deliver nursing care to clients, assess them to learn their strengths and limitations, analyze these data to formulate nursing diagnoses, decide appropriate goals, and apply nursing interventions to achieve the goals. During and after the nursing interventions, nurses reassess clients to decide if goals have been met.

When does your client need a care plan? The answer to this is easy: a care plan is needed every time a client is in the health care system. A better question would be: What *type* of care plan does the client need? Should you use a standardized care plan, a completely handwritten plan, a hybrid of the two, or a standardized plan that allows for individualization?

Does the Profession of Nursing Need Care Plans?

Care planning for professional nursing really came into power in the 1970s. Although the idea was embraced enthusiastically by JCAHO* and many nurses, it wasn't universally accepted. In fact, many experienced nurses questioned why they needed to write out a plan of care when "everyone knew what needed to be done" to deliver safe, competent care.

Because of this initial care planning mandate, many institutions developed standardized care plans. This type of care plan described the generic nursing care that would be required for a person with a certain condition. In time, however, most institutions have changed to handwritten care plans.

What was wrong with standardized nursing care plans? The answer to this question was easy. JCAHO didn't believe that they directed individualized nursing care, therefore, they did not like them. If institutions wanted to be accredited by JCAHO, they needed to use handwritten, individualized nursing care plans.

But times have changed. Now JCAHO accepts and even encourages standardized nursing care plans that allow for individualization to the client. These take less time to write and actually may allow for more individualized care because the nurse concentrates only on how the standard care plan must be altered to fit the client's condition.

Does this mean that the nursing process is also dead? Of course not! The new JCAHO mandates have altered the format of the care plan, but they have not abandoned the idea of the nursing process. It still is the method nurses use to provide client care.

*Joint Commission on Accreditation of Healthcare Organizations.

Although in nursing school the nursing care plan is usually quite extensive, those used in actual client care are much more succinct. To keep the institutional document practical, it is common for clients to have only two or three priority nursing diagnoses listed in the care plan.

The method for care planning is different in each institution. Some organizations are now using standardized care plans, others are using handwritten plans, and some are using the computer to help generate a care plan (see box). To design a care plan for a client, you'll need to know the care planning policy in your institution.

To find out which type of plan to use, you'll need to assess your client and consider all the applicable nursing diagnoses and determine the priorities. Then look at the standardized care plans. If your institution does not have standardized care plans already written out, there are many good care plan books available for purchase. Do your client's problems fit within the scope of the standard plan? If they do, then a standardized plan may work well for you. If the client's problems are unique and you think the nursing staff will need more direction than that given in a standard plan, then you must either alter the standard plan or write a completely new plan.

Whatever the system for making a care plan, the most important thing is that it really must reflect the client's needs. Put information in the care plan that will help others provide appropriate care for the client.

The Scenario Continues

A care plan can be a very useful tool. In this scenario, the lack of a useful care plan meant that the nurse wasted a great amount of time simply learning how to provide care for a client.

During report, you were told that one of your clients, Ms. Sponte, had a very extensive wound that required irrigation, packing, and application of several types of dressing materials. The Kardex and physician order read "dressing change q.s." (q.s. means each shift). Hoping for more guidance, you checked the nursing care plan, which addressed the issues of "Alteration in Comfort, Acute Pain and Alteration in Coping," but there wasn't anything mentioned about the dressing change. The nursing notes for the prior shifts described the wound but not the method for the dressing change. Knowing you needed more information, you asked the other nurses if they had ever done this dressing. One of the nurses said that she had done it yesterday and that the following materials were needed:

- Three large dressing pads
- Sterile field
- Sterile saline
- Iodine-soaked packing gauze
- 60 cc syringe
- Two boxes of gauze pads

You decide to talk to the client about the dressing change. Ms. Sponte tells you that the dressing change is very painful for her, but she doesn't really know what the nurses have been doing with the dressing. You check to see that she can have some pain medication 30 minutes before the dressing change.

You give Ms. Sponte the pain medication, and 30 minutes later, you start the dressing change. After you remove the old dressing, you discover that you will need more gauze pads than you brought into the room. You ask the client to put on the call light, and when

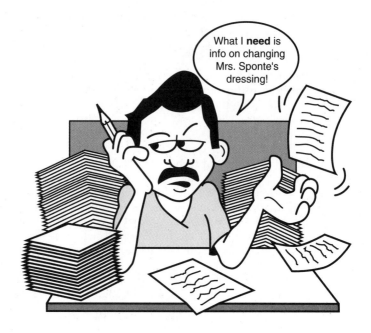

it is answered, you tell the nurse to bring you two more boxes of gauze pads. With them, you could complete the dressing change.

This procedure required 25 minutes of your time, not including the time waiting for the pain medication to take effect. If you had known how to do the dressing change, this time could have been decreased by half.

After the dressing change, it occurs to you that it would be a lot easier to write up a "recipe" for this dressing. This way, the next nurse will know exactly what is needed and how to do the dressing change easier and yet with correct technique.

Nursing Charting

Nurses place a multitude of information into client records and they do it many different ways. Nursing charting must reflect everything the nurse does for a client. This is a far-ranging goal, because this must include an assessment of the client's condition, interventions received, the client's response to those treatments, and communications to other health care personnel about the client. These activities fall basically within four major groups: initial assessment, intervention, teach, and consult (Table 10–5). With all the information that needs to be included, most nursing charting systems will be quite complex. What does a good charting system look like? A good system:

- Will be legally sound
- Will reflect the nursing process
- Will provide a complete description of the client's status
- Will record all nursing interventions

Table 10–5 CATEGORIES FOR INCLUSION INTO NURSING CHARTING

Initial Assessment	Physical condition Emotional condition Actual problems Potential problems

Intervention	Prevention of harm
	Interventions
	   Physician ordered
	   Nursing ordered
	Response to treatment or interventions
	Unexpected response to treatment

Teach	Physical condition Prevention of harm Home care Medications Nutrition Response to teaching Activity level
Consult	Reason for consult Nurse experts Physician Family Ancillary staff Nutritionist Discharge planner

- Will provide useful communication among disciplines
- Will provide useful information for research and chart audits (Lampe 1985).

There are two types of charts: paper and computer (Table 10–6). To document events correctly, you need to know your institution's charting policy. Correct charting procedure in one institution may be totally incorrect in another. You can usually find the details of the charting policy in the policy manual. If you need more help with following the institution policies, talk to one of the institution's nursing educators.

No matter what type of charting system your institution uses, there are some charting interventions you should always use. These interventions, discussed below, relate to correct timing, legal issues, correct format, and accuracy (Bergerson, 1988).

Timing

1. Chart after you deliver the care, not before. If you chart a bed bath as given before it really is done, what would you do if the client dies before you really give the bed bath? Never chart medications as given until the client has actually received them.
2. Chart events immediately after they occur. Although this may not always be possible, at least make it a point to stop and chart every hour. During an emergency it may be impossible to take the time to chart. Instead, note the

Table 10–6   WHAT IS THE CHART FORMAT?

Method	Positives	Negatives
Paper Chart Documentation about the client's condition is done using standardized paper charting forms.	Easier to learn to use than a computer charting method. Much less start-up cost.	Can easily lose parts of the chart. Only one person can use the chart at a time. May spend much time in simply locating the chart. Labor intensive. Client orders must be noted and the order sent to the appropriate department. Long-term storage of chart can be a problem. Poor handwriting can make reading the chart difficult.
Computerized Documentation Systems Documentation about the client's condition through the use of a personal computer with charting documentation software.	Less redundant information. Easy to search for specific information. Easy long-term storage of client records. Poor handwriting not a concern. Multiple people can use the chart at the same time. Rapid interdepartmental communication. Physician can type an order into the computer and it goes directly to the appropriate department.	Extensive start-up costs. Much education needed to learn to use system (what to do with agency nurses, student nurses, etc.). Many people have an aversion to computers. Confidentiality of chart can be a concern. How do you chart when the computer is down? Difficult to remember how to use if on an intermittent basis.

time as events occur. For example, if you are working quickly to stabilize a client until the client can be moved to the intensive care unit and don't want to stop to chart events until after the client's condition is stable, note the time you gave medications, the client's vital signs, etc. on your report sheet.

Legalities

1. Chart in permanent ink. No erasable ink or pencil allowed!
2. Close your charting with your legible signature, including your official title.
3. Don't alter your charting after you have written it. If you make an error, draw a single line through it, write "mistaken entry," and initial it. Don't draw multiple lines through it, completely obscuring the entry, or use "white-out." This looks as if you are trying to hide something (Iyer 1991).
4. Chart only what you have observed or done. Don't chart for others.
5. Don't leave any spaces after your entries. Draw a line through unused space. Doing this will make it so others cannot add to your charting.

Correct Format

1. Use only institutionally approved abbreviations. A list of these can usually be found in the policy manual.
2. Use correct spelling. Incorrect spelling makes the reader wonder about your level of education and perhaps your professional competency. If you are a poor speller, consider investing in an electronic spelling aid or a pocket dictionary.
3. Write neatly and make sure it is legible. Many people hold the misconception that they will not be held accountable for something if it can't be read. This is not true. You are still accountable for your actions despite poor documentation. In fact, a real problem with illegible writing is that it may be so illegible that it cannot be used to defend your actions, even though these actions may have been appropriate. Another problem is that poor writing casts you in a poor light as a professional nurse. How can you be a good communicator if others are unable to read your writing? Poor handwriting may also give the appearance that the writer is trying to hide something or that poor-quality care was delivered.
4. Don't use words like "rude," "obnoxious," "nasty," "fat," or other derogatory terms. These are personal descriptors, not professional ones. Instead of using these types of words, describe the client's behavior. For example, instead of writing "client is uncooperative," it would be better to describe it as "client yelling for the nurse instead of using call light. States, 'I will do whatever I want to and you can't stop me.' "
5. Don't use the chart to settle disagreements with other staff members. Consider what you would think if you found the following charting statement

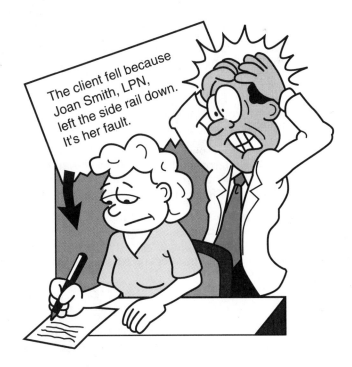

in your mother's chart: "Found client with much dried feces on her buttocks. Obviously not cleansed well by previous nurse." How would this reflect upon the nursing care provided?

6. Don't document a problem without documenting your intervention. Consider the brief notation "Client temperature 103°." Well, what did you do about it? It would be much better to write, "Client temperature 103°, Tylenol given, blood cultures drawn. Call placed to Dr. Seller's service about temp."

7. Don't chart items in more than one place. For example, if your documentation system uses a graphic sheet for recording the vital signs, you needn't chart these also in the nurses' notes unless they are abnormal, thus requiring a nursing intervention.

Accuracy

1. Fill in all areas of the charting form. Leave no area blank. If it isn't applicable to your client, write N/A instead of leaving it blank.

2. Review your charting before the end of your shift. Have you included everything you needed to say? Some common things to include in charting are:
   - Assessment data (physical and emotional)
   - Client response to nursing interventions and required medications
   - Reason for omission or alteration of treatments
   - Notification (or attempted notification) of physician regarding client status
   - Client/family teaching and response to teaching

3. Use client quotes whenever possible. This helps to show what the client is really feeling and may avoid misinterpretation.

4. Document client behavior accurately. Instead of writing "client is agitated," write "client pacing back and forth in his room, yelling loudly."

5. Chart completely, accurately. Write what you saw, not what you assumed happened. For example, if you find a client on the floor, you must chart it as such. You cannot say "client fell" unless you saw it. However, you could chart the fall as "client states that he fell."

6. Make your intention clear. Consider the statement "Dr. Jansen called." This could be interpreted as "call *received* from Dr. Jansen" or "call *placed* to Dr. Jansen." It would be much better to write "0800 Call placed to Dr. Jansen's service" or "08:30 Call received from Dr. Jansen."

7. Chart client response to treatment. With increasing attention being given to client outcomes, it is important to document the client's progress or lack of progress toward attainment of his or her goals. Although this may be done daily or per shift, compare the client's progress against the goals on the nursing care plan.

Transfer Forms

Many institutions have created transfer forms to help with continuity of care. The forms may be used when a client is transferred from one type of nursing unit to another or from one institution to another. They are also used for transfers between nursing units. For example, a client may be transferred from the intensive care unit to a general medical floor. The transfer form would be helpful to ensure that all members of the nursing staff understand the client's care.

The transfer form is especially useful for client transfers between institutions, because only portions of the chart are photocopied and sent with the client. The transfer form can provide a data base to help the receiving institution plan the client's care.

Before you can fill out the forms, you first need to obtain some basic information from the client and the chart. When is the client leaving the unit? Where is the client going? What types of information will be especially pertinent to the receiving nurses?

Because the forms can be quite extensive, start filling them out as soon as you know that the client is to be transferred. Some topic areas to be included on the transfer form are (Fig. 10–1):

- Latest physical assessment data
- Activities of daily living capabilities
- List of ordered medications and the times they were last given
- Nursing care plan with a list of unresolved nursing goals
- A summary of the hospital stay

Depending on the length of the hospitalization, the summary could range from only a few sentences to a page of information. The summary usually includes reason for admission, surgical procedures, response to treatment interventions, and any major problem during the hospitalization. Also to accompany transfer forms are copies of the following:

- Current physician orders
- Nursing care plan
- Client history and summary of the hospital stay

Discharge Forms

A hospitalization can be a mind-boggling event, just from the viewpoint of information overload. A client and family enter the institution, encounter people who appear to be speaking a language other than English, and have a multiplicity of details thrust upon them. Yet, when they go home, the client and family are expected to assume responsibility for the client's care. Discharge instruction sheets were developed to help clients understand their posthospitalization care. Giving clients a copy of the discharge instructions in addition to verbal explanations really helps reinforce discharge teaching. It also serves as a written description of the discharge teaching, if clients later say that they did not receive discharge teaching (Fig. 10–2).

The forms are usually multiple-copy, carbonless paper. A copy of the form is usually given to the client and the physician. The signed original of the form is placed in the chart.

Before you can fill out the forms, there are some things you need to consider. When is the client to be discharged? What is the client's educational level? Can the client read English? Will the client be able to read the small print on the forms? What is the client's current level of understanding of his or her illness and its posthospitalization care?

PATIENT TRANSFER FORM
SAGINAW GENERAL HOSPITAL
Saginaw, Michigan

NAME Sundwick	First Mary	Middle K	Sex ☐ Male ☒ Female	Marital Status ☐Single ☐ M ☐ D ☒ W ☐ Sep.

Address 1156 Hazelton, Clio, MI | Birthdate 4-8-01 | Religion Catholic

Date of Transfer 7-22-95 | Facility Transferred to: Rest-More | Physician in charge at time of transfer - Physician Signature

Facility Transferred from: Get Well Medical Center | Dates of Stay at Facility Transferred from: Admitted 7/03/95 Discharged 7/22/95

Relative or Guardian Claire Sundwick | Relative Notified Yes ☒ No ☐ | Address 1156 Hazelton, Clio | Phone Number 555-2130

DIAGNOSIS:
(a) Primary (active) Diabetes

(b) Secondary (inactive)

Allergies: Penicillin

Surgical Procedure 7/06 Open reduction Right hip

Current Meds | Time of Last Dose

Humulin NPH 44 U am | 8am
Humulin NPH 12 U 5pm | 5pm 7/21
Lasix 40 mg qd | 8am
Tylenol #3 c q4° prn | 11am 7/18

Diet 1800 ADA, low salt

Rehabilitation Program

O.T. 1/2 hour daily

P.T. 1 hour daily

Speech none

ACTIVITIES OF DAILY LIVING INFORMATION

Speech:	☒ Normal	☐ Impaired	☐ Absent
Hearing:	☐ Normal	☒ Impaired	☐ Deaf
Sight:	☐ Normal	☒ Impaired	☐ Blind
Mental Status:	☒ Alert	☐ Forgetful	☐ Confused
Feeding:	☒ Independent	☐ Needs Help	☐ Dependent
Dressing:	☐ Independent	☒ Needs Help	☐ Dependent

ELIMINATION
Bowel: ☐ Independent ☒ Needs Assistance ☐ Bed Pan ☐ Incontinent
Bladder: ☐ Independent ☒ Needs Assistance ☐ Urinal ☐ Incontinent
Last B.M. or Enema: Date _7/21_

Bathing:	☐ Independent	☒ Needs Help	☐ Bed Bath
Ambulatory Status:	☐ Independent ☐ Bed Bound	☒ Needs Help	☐ Transfer Only

Indwelling Tubings: (Include insertion date and size)
none.

Appliances - Supports - Equipment:
☐ Hearing Aid ☒ Dentures (Upper, Lower, Partial)
☐ Contacts ☒ Glasses ☐ Other

Nursing Assessment and Recommendations and Treatments:
(include body marks and size, seizures, attitude, vital signs, etc.)
132/70 - 99' - 88 - 20.
Lungs clear, good peripheral pulses, incision right hip - clean + dry, no drainage. Blood sugar range 69 - 136. Insulin usage unchanged during hospitalization. Gives own insulin

Nurses Signature April Suh Rn | Date 7/22/95 10an

THE FOLLOWING MEDICAL RECORD FORMS MUST MUST ACCOMPANY THIS FORM:
1. CHEST X-RAY   2. HISTORY & PHYSICAL   3. DISCHARGE SUMMARY   4. CARE PLAN(S)   5. LABS

A

Figure 10–1 Examples of transfer summaries. **A,** patient transfer form.

NURSING TRANSFER SUMMARY
Cardiac Care
Saginaw General Hospital

Form #41753
Rev. 4/92 D-12
Side 2 of 2

Transferred from CCU to ____7 - Main____.

Stamper

ADDRESSOGRAPH

Date Admitted: __6/14/95__   Today's date: __6/20/95__

Date Transferred to CCU: __6/14/95__

Primary Diagnosis: __Acute CHF__

Secondary Diagnosis: __diabetes__

Code Status: __no-code__   Mask Precautions: __no__

Cardiac Work-Up: EKG __Sinus tach__   X-ray __CHF__

Pertinent Lab Results: _____

Stress test (date) __∅__   Results: _____

Cardiac cath (date): __∅__   Results: _____

Arrhythmias / treatment: __none__

Treatments/Care required: __needs help when ambulating, unsteady,__

Culture results: _____

Activity level: __up with help to bath room__ Knowledge level: __Understands he is very ill__

Last Epidose of chest pain: __none__

Family Support: __no family in area__

Glasses: Y____ N____ NA __✓__ Prosthesis? Y __ N __ NA __✓__ Describe _____

PCA Pump Value Transferred: __∅__   Dentures? Y __✓__ N __ NA __ Describe __upper + lower__

Physical Assessment at time of transfer: __Rhonchi bilateral, alert + oriented, Skin warm + dry, decreased pulses bilateral legs. edema bilateral legs to knees, IV in ℝ forearm, infuses well. D5W @ KVO__

Kardex updated and reviewed: Y __✓__ N ____
Medication orders updated and reviewed: Y __✓__ N ____
Plan of Care updated and reviewed: Y __✓__ N ____
Family Notified of transfer: Y __✓__ N ____

Transferred via __W/C__ with belongings, medications, chart, and stamper at __11 am__.

*Signature of Nurses: __G. Stevens Rn__

Transferring Unit   Receiving Unit

B   *Signature denotes agreement with and understanding of the above.

Figure 10–1 *Continued* **B,** Nursing transfer summary. (Courtesy of Saginaw General Hospital, Saginaw, Michigan.)

DISCHARGE ORDER/INSTRUCTION SHEET

Saginaw General Hospital
Saginaw, Michigan

Form #F41919
Rev. 4/94 D-43

Stamper

ADDRESSOGRAPH

PHYSICIAN ORDER SECTION

☑ Discharge - __9__ / __21__ / __95__

☑ Office Follow-up with Dr. __Achu__ in __2__ days/weeks (make appointment) # __732 - 1556__

Dr. __Peddi reddi__ in __1__ days/weeks (make appointment) # __757 - 1040__

Dr._____ in ____ days/weeks, make appointment # _____

Diet: ☐ Regular ☐ Cardiac (Low Salt, Low Fat) ☒ ADA (Diabetic) __1800__ Calories ☐ Other: _____

Activity: ☒ No Restrictions ☐ Light/easy gradual return to normal over next_____ weeks.

☐ Restrictions _____

Special Testing: Lab work in __1__ days/weeks __Saginaw General Outpatient Lab__

X-rays in ____ days/weeks at _____ Phone # _____

Other _____

Special Procedures (dressings, drains, equipment) ☐ NA ☐ Follow doctor's specific instruction sheet.

Medication	Dose/Frequency
Capoten	25 mg, three times a day
Lasix	40 mg each morning
Prednisone	5 mg each morning
Tagamet	300 mg three times a day

☐ Contact your family physician for instructions regarding all other medications.

Physician Signature: __Dr. Achu__ Date: __9/21/95__ Time: __09⁵__

NURSING

Other Instructions/Post Discharge Needs: ☐ Not Applicable

Written Materials: __Taking Medications Safely__

Nurse's Signature: __April Suh Rn__ Date: __9/21/95__ Time: __1325__

ALLIED

Social Service/Discharge Planning

Nutritional Services

R.T./O.T./P.T./Speech/Other

I have received and understand the above instructions.

Patient/Family Signature _____ Date: _____

WHITE COPY: MEDICAL RECORD   YELLOW COPY: PATIENT   PINK COPY: PHYSICIAN

Figure 10–2 An example of a discharge summary. (Courtesy of Saginaw General Hospital, Saginaw, Michigan.)

Try to fill out the form *during* the hospitalization so that you won't have to do it all at the time of discharge. Print in large letters while completing the form. Press hard—you are making several copies. Use only plain English—no hospital jargon. You must pay attention to this, because jargon can become quite ingrained in a person's writing style. One of the authors wrote a note to her child's teacher, using several nursing abbreviations. The teacher wrote a note back, asking for a translation.

Typically included on a discharge instruction sheet are:

- Posthospitalization diet, activity level, and activity restrictions
- Special equipment needed
- Wound care or treatments
- Medications (times to take them, reason to take them, and any special instructions for their use)
- Follow-up visits and when
- Complications—what to watch for after discharge

After you fill out the form, review the information with the client. If someone other than the client is responsible for posthospitalization care, wait and review the discharge teaching with that person. After you have explained the discharge plan, ask the client or caregiver if there are any questions. Tell the client or caregiver whom to call with questions after being discharged.

Incident Reports

The American public has the general belief that the delivery of health care is perfect and that mistakes cannot happen. But simple logic will tell you that this isn't true because health care is provided by human beings who are not perfect. Even so, we must provide the most incident-free health care possible. Incident reports are a method for reporting any circumstance out of the ordinary (Fig. 10–3). These reports are not meant as punishment, but as a means to document unusual events. Health care providers need to document incidents for a variety of reasons:

1. JCAHO and other accrediting bodies mandate such reporting.
2. With such reporting, an agency could make changes based on the reasons for the incident.
3. Reporting provides the opportunity for quick follow-up on situations. This would help make sure that the client receives appropriate care after an incident or that something broken would be fixed quickly.
4. If a pattern of incidents occurs, policy may need to be changed or staff may need to be educated.

To make tracking of incidents easier for the risk management team, many institutions use two types of incident reports: one for incidents that concern clients and families and one for staff injuries, accidents, etc. What are some common occurrences that require the use of an incident report?

1. Client fall
2. Medication error: wrong client, wrong medications, wrong time, wrong route, medication given to client with a medication allergy, missed doses
3. Adverse effect from medication (severe allergic reaction)
4. Incident with client, family, or visitor
5. A potential accident (loose stairs, handrails, etc.)

INCIDENT NO. _____

① MEDICAL RECORD NO. 35259-1

Hurley Medical Center
VARIANCE/INCIDENT REPORT

MONTH _____ INDICATES REVIEW _____

② White   Marilu   K
LAST NAME   FIRST   M.I.

DEFINITION:
AN INCIDENT IS DEFINED AS ANY HAPPENING WHICH IS NOT CONSISTENT WITH THE ACCEPTED ROUTINE OPERATION OF THE HOSPITAL OR THE ROUTINE CARE OF A PARTICULAR PATIENT. IT MAY BE AN ACCIDENT OR A SITUATION WHICH MAY OR MAY NOT RESULT IN AN INJURY. **THIS IS A HOSPITAL RECORD. IT IS NOT PART OF THE PATIENT'S RECORD**

1577   Caring Road, Clio
HOME ADDRESS

Whenever an incident or accident occurs involving a patient or visitor, the person in charge of the area or patient must complete this report. Obtain all pertinent and accurate facts through interviews with other staff members, patients or visitors.

③ DIAGNOSIS R/O Sepsis

Submit the pink copy to Quality Assessment and the remaining copies to the Department Head, Supervisor, or Designate for evaluation to determine the cause and if additional action is necessary to prevent recurrence. He/she will then keep one copy for their records and **immediately** forward one copy to the Risk Manager.

④ DATE 2/1/95   ⑤ 1 ☐ VISITOR   3 ☐ OUTPATIENT   ⑥ AGE 77   ⑦ SEX 1 ☐ M 2 ☒ F
TIME (7-3) 3-11 11-7   2 ☒ INPATIENT

⑧ DAY OF THE WEEK
1 ☐ SUN   3 ☒ TUES   5 ☐ THUR
2 ☐ MON   4 ☐ WED   6 ☐ FRI
                          7 ☐ SAT

PRIOR TO INCIDENT

⑨ SERVICE
1 ☒ MEDICAL   4 ☐ OB/GYN   8 ☐ ER
2 ☐ SURGICAL 5 ☐ PSYCHIATRY 9 ☐ CLINIC
3 ☐ PED   6 ☐ SPECIAL CARE 10 ☐ SUB ABUSE
              7 ☐ HEMO   11 ☐ OTHER

⑩ LOCATION OF INCIDENT
1 ☒ PATIENT'S ROOM   5 ☐ RADIOLOGY
2 ☐ HALLWAY   6 ☐ OPERATING ROOM
3 ☐ BATHROOM   7 ☐ EMERGENCY ROOM
4 ☐ SHOWER   8 ☐ OTHER _____

⑪ ROOM NUMBER
103-B

⑫ ABILITY TO FOLLOW INSTRUCTIONS
1 ☐ NO PROBLEM   4 ☒ DISABILITY IN
2 ☐ CHILD   COMPREHENSION
3 ☐ LANGUAGE   5 ☐ NOT
   BARRIER   APPLICABLE

INFORMATION ABOUT INCIDENT

⑬ **ACTIVITY LEVEL**
1 ☐ UNLIMITED
2 ☐ COMPLETE BED REST
3 ☒ LIMITED WITH ASSISTANCE
4 ☐ LIMITED WITHOUT ASSISTNACE (SPECIFY IF LIMITED)
5 ☐ SUPERVISED BY ADULT (FAMILY/STAFF)
6 ☐ RESTRAINED

⑭ **SEDATION WITHIN PAST 8 HOURS**
1 ☐ YES
2 ☒ NO
TYPE AND AMOUNT

⑮ **OTHER PERTINENT MEDICATIONS WITHIN PAST 8 HOURS**
1 ☐ YES
2 ☒ NO
TYPE AND AMOUNT

⑯ **BED RAILS   UP   DOWN**
RIGHT UPPER   1 ☒   2 ☐
RIGHT LOWER   3 ☒   4 ☐
LEFT UPPER   5 ☒   6 ☐
LEFT LOWER   7 ☒   8 ☐

FULL   UP   DOWN
RIGHT 9 ☐ 10 ☐
LEFT   11 ☐ 12 ☐

⑰ **TYPE OF INJURY**
1 ☐ LACERATION
2 ☐ HEMATOMA
3 ☒ ABRASION
4 ☐ SPRAIN OR STRAIN
5 ☐ FRACTURE
6 ☐ INTERNAL
7 ☐ BURNS
8 ☐ PUNCTURE WOUND
9 ☐ NO APPARENT INJURY

⑱ **OTHER SAFETY DEVICES**
1 ☐ SAFETY JACKET
2 ☐ SAFETY BELT
3 ☐ SAFETY STRAPS
4 ☐ COVERED CRIB
5 ☐ LOCKED LEATHER
6 ☐ RESTRAINTS
7 ☐ OTHER – SPECIFY

⑲ **POSITION OF BED**
1 ☐ HIGH
2 ☐ LOW
3 ☐ NOT ADJUSTED

⑳ **MENTAL CONDITION**
1 ☒ ORIENTED
2 ☐ DISORIENTED
3 ☐ OTHER

㉑ **HOSPITAL PERSONNEL WITH PATIENT**
1 ☒ YES   2 ☐ NO

㉒ **X-RAY TAKEN**
1 ☒ YES   2 ☐ NO

㉓ **SEEN BY**
1 ☒ PHYSICIAN
2 ☒ SUPERVISOR
3 ☐ OTHER

㉔ **WHO WAS NOTIFIED**
1 ☒ PHYSICIAN Dr Reddi   2pm
2 ☒ SUPERVISOR Mrs Walski 2pm
3 ☐ OTHER _____
☐ AM ☐ PM

TYPE OF OCCURRENCE

㉕ A **MEDICATION ERROR**
1 ☐ WRONG PATIENT
2 ☐ WRONG MEDICATION
3 ☐ WRONG DOSE
4 ☐ WRONG ROUTE
5 ☐ WRONG TIME
6 ☐ MED. NOT GIVEN
7 ☐ MED. ERROR TRANSCRIBE
8 ☐ MED. ERROR – NO ORDER

㉕ B
9 ☐ IV INFILTRATION
10 ☐ IV – WRONG RATE
11 ☐ MEDICATION ALLERGY
12 ☐ WRONG MED. DISPENSED
13 ☐ WRONG DOSE DISPENSED
14 ☐ NOT DELIVERED IN TIMELY MANNER
15 ☐ OTHER

㉗ **CONTROLLED SUBSTANCE**
1 ☐ INCORRECT SHIFT COUNT
2 ☐ MISSING DOSE
3 ☐ OTHER

㉖ **TREATMENT ERROR**
1 ☐ ORDERS NOT DONE
2 ☐ TEST/PROCEDURE NOT DONE
3 ☐ PREP NOT DONE
4 ☐ WRONG DIET
5 ☐ WRONG BLOOD
6 ☐ STAT-ORDER NOT DONE
7 ☐ TREATMENT NOT GIVEN
8 ☐ ORDERS NOT NOTED
9 ☐ WRONG PROCEDURE/TEST
10 ☐ WRONG RESULTS REPORTED
11 ☐ WRONG PATIENT
12 ☐ TREATMENT DELAYS
13 ☐ STERILE TECHNIQUE BROKEN
14 ☐ OTHER

㉘ **FALLS**
1 ☐ FROM BED
2 ☐ FROM CHAIR, STRETCHER, ETC.
3 ☐ GETTING IN/OUT OF BED
4 ☒ WHILE ABULATING
5 ☐ UNAUTH. – OUT OF BED
6 ☐ GETTING ON/OFF TOILET
7 ☐ WHILE RESTRAINED
8 ☐ OTHER

㉙ **OTHER OCCURRENCE**
1 ☐ SURGICAL PERMIT NOT SIGNED
2 ☐ INSTRUMENT COUNT-INCORRECT
3 ☐ EQUIPMENT FAILURE
4 ☐ ELECTRICAL INJURY
5 ☐ PROPERTY DAMAGE
6 ☐ SPECIMENS LOST
7 ☐ EXPOSURE TO TOXIC
8 ☐ FIRE
9 ☐ CONTRABAND SEARCH
10 ☐ SELF INFLICTED INJURY
11 ☐ SUICIDE ATTEMPT
12 ☐ PATIENT ALTERCATION/ASSAULT
13 ☐ ELOPEMENT/AMA
14 ☐ OTHER

WRITTEN DESCRIPTION OF INCIDENT (FACTS ONLY)

While ambulating with help to the bathroom, client slipped and hit her head on the bathroom door. No change in level of consciousness. Client helped back to bed with 2 assists.

DATE 2/1/95   SIGNATURE S. Coleman Rn

CORRECTIVE ACTION/FOLLOW-UP

_____

DATE _____   SIGNATURE _____
STATEMENT OF PHYSICIAN

DATE _____   SIGNATURE _____

USE BACK FOR FURTHER INFORMATION
WHITE COPY TO RISK MANAGER – YELLOW COPY: DEPT. COPY – PINK COPY TO QA (AS SOON AS WRITTEN)

FORM 32965 (Rev. 4/90)

Figure 10–3   An example of a variance/incident report. (Courtesy of Hurley Medical Center, Flint, Michigan.)

6. Loss of property (client or institution)
7. Injury to staff, client, family, or visitor

What to Write on the Incident Report

The priority after an incident occurs is to ensure that the client, family member, visitor, or staff member doesn't sustain further harm. After the incident and when the resulting treatment is over, you must complete an incident report. To fill out the incident form correctly, you absolutely must know your institution's policy for correctly filling out the form. Does your institution have separate forms for clients and staff?

It may be helpful to have each person who witnessed the incident fill out a separate form, giving their view of the incident. Fill out the form using objective terms. Write what you saw, not what you think might have happened. However, you could include the client's statement of what happened. Describe the injuries (if any) and the immediate care the victim received. For example, "Client said that her leg hurt but that she felt that she could walk on it. Helped by two staff members back to bed. Client did not put full weight bearing on the leg." Note the time you notified the physician and any orders received.

A completed incident report should be given to the nurse manager, who will go over the report with the institution's risk manager (usually a lawyer).

What Not to Write on the Incident Report

Even if you think that someone is to blame for the incident, don't suggest this on the form. When filling out an incident report, it is not appropriate to include your opinion of the competence of the other health care providers involved in the incident.

What to Write in the Nurses' Notes About the Incident

Chart objectively and accurately. Write what you saw happen. For example, you are walking in the hallway and hear a thump. You go into the client room and find the client on the floor. Instead of charting "The client fell out of bed," it would be more appropriate to write "Nurse walked into room, found client on the floor beside bed. Client stated, 'I fell down when I was trying to go to the bathroom. You told me not to get out of bed but I did it anyway.' "

Describe the client's condition and any immediate care you provided. State the time that the physician was notified and if any orders were received. Document throughout the day about the condition of the injured area (if any). For example, if the client injured a hip, you should assess for pain, leg movement, pulses, and other neurovascular symptoms. If the client's condition alters, you need to notify the physician.

What Not to Write in the Nurses' Notes About the Incident

Although you need to write a careful description of the incident, you must *not* write that you have filled out an incident report. The incident report is an institutional worksheet; it's not a part of the client's chart. If you write in the nursing notes that you filled out an incident report, it can tell anyone reading the chart that an incident has occurred. It also can now be obtained by the client's attorney and be used in a court of law. If you do not mention the incident report in your nursing notes, the client's attorney will not be able to obtain a copy of the incident report as part of the client's chart (Iyer & Camp, 1991).

PRACTICAL APPLICATIONS

Nursing communication is a complex act. Let's look at an example of nursing communication and how it can go wrong.

Duramorph

You were told that you have a client coming back from the postanesthesia care unit (recovery room). You look up to see that the client is being pushed on a stretcher into the room. You go into the room to help and the nurse starts to give you report on the client. The nurse giving the report is speaking fast and is in a big rush. In fact, she says, "Hurry, I've got to get back to my other clients." During report, she goes over the client's vital signs, condition of the client's dressing, and the client's level of consciousness. Because of the speed in which you receive the report, you feel rather overwhelmed.

As she leaves the unit, the nurse says, "Oh, I almost forgot, she's a Duramorph." You don't know what this means and want to ask the postanesthesia care unit nurse, but she is already gone. When you ask another nurse what Duramorph means, she doesn't know either. Undaunted, you ask a second and third nurse what this term means. "Oh, that's a new drug that they're putting in the epidural space for pain relief. It lasts for about 2 or 3 days. It usually works really well."

Now that you know a small amount about Duramorph, you assess the client for immediate postoperative needs. After you have found that the client is resting comfortably, you know that you need to obtain more information about this method of pain relief. Because you know it is a pain medication, you know where to go for more information: the pharmacy. A pharmacy staff member brings you some information about Duramorph to the nursing unit. The information states that the client shouldn't receive any other pain medication simultaneously.

Later, you have time to look at the physician orders and are very surprised to see that the surgical resident has ordered the client to receive pain shots every 4 hours. Either the resident doesn't know what Duramorph is or he doesn't know that the client has received it.

If you had not questioned the meaning of information that had been told to you, the client could have been seriously overdosed on pain medication, which could have resulted in client injury.

1. What could you have done to ensure that you received the correct information from the recovery room nurse?
2. What could you do to prevent this type of event from occurring in the future?
   (Answers to these questions are found at the end of the chapter.)

REFERENCES

Barter, M., & Furmidge, M. (1994). Unlicensed assistive personnel: Issues relating to delegation and supervision. *Journal of Nursing Administration, 24*(4), 36–39.

Bergerson, S. (1988, April). Charting with a jury in mind. *Nursing '88,* 51–56.

Brider, P. (1991, May). Who killed the nursing care plan? *American Journal of Nursing,* 35–39.

Carpenito, L. (1991). Has JCAHO eliminated care plans? *American Nurse, 23*(6), 6.

Eggland, E., & Heinemann, D. (1994). *Nursing documentation: Charting recording and reporting.* Philadelphia: J.B. Lippincott.

Fondiller, S. (1991, September). The new look in nursing documentation. *American Journal of Nursing,* 65–76.

Gwozdz, D. (1992). Streamlining patient care documentation. *Journal of Nursing Administration, 22*(5), 35–39.

Herrick, K., Hansten, R., O'Neil, L., Hayes, P., & Washburn, M. (1994). My license is not on the line: The art of delegation. *Nursing Management, 25*(2), 48–51.

Hildman, T. (1992). Registered nurses' attitudes toward the nursing process and written/printed nursing care plans. *Journal of Nursing Administration, 22*(5), 5.

Huber, K., Blegin, M., & McCloskey, J. (1994). Use of nursing assistants: Staff nursing opinions. *Nursing Management, 25*(5), 64–68.

Iyer, P. (1991, January). New trends in charting. *Nursing '91,* 48–50.

Iyer, P., & Camp, N. (1991). *Nursing documentation.* St. Louis: Mosby.

Kerr, S. (1992, January/February). A comparison of four nursing documentation systems. *Journal of Nursing Staff Development,* 26–31.

Lampe, S. (1985). Focus charting: Streamlining documentation. *Nursing Management,* 43–45.

Mantel, D. (1992, January). How to protect yourself when the patient gets hurt. *RN,* 69–72.

Murphy, J., Beglinger, J., & Johnson, B. (1988, February). Charting by exception: Meeting the challenge of cost containment. *Nursing Management,* 56–72.

Reiley, P., & Stengrevics, S. (1989). Change-of-shift report: Put it in writing. *Nursing Management, 20*(9), 54–56.

Rosalinda, S., Albardo, V., & Thrane, J. (1989, June). Computerized nursing documentation. *Nursing Management,* 72A–72H.

ANSWERS TO THE PRACTICAL APPLICATIONS

1. What could you have done to ensure that you received the correct information from the recovery room nurse?

   You could ask her to slow down when talking to you. If the nurse has already left the nursing unit, and you have questions for her, call her.

2. What could you do to prevent this type of event from occurring in the future?
   It would be helpful to repeat the information you received back to the nurse. This would allow time to clarify misconceptions.

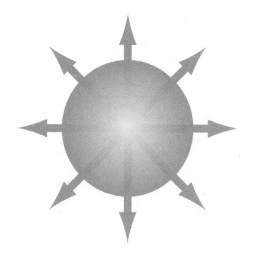

11

With Physicians and Ancillary Health Care Personnel

In this chapter, we will discuss:

- Nurse/physician relationships
- How to determine with which physician or health care provider you need to speak
- Typical methods of communication: verbal and written
- How to write a client order
- Communicating with personnel in ancillary departments

Because nurses are managers and providers of the client's care, there is a lot of client information that needs to be passed from the client to other health care providers. Nurses serve as a central repository for much of this information, passing it out as needed to the appropriate people. Every day of their working lives, nurses talk with physicians and other ancillary health care staff members. In this chapter, we will examine how to communicate with physicians and other members of the health care team.

Relationships Between Nurses and Physicians

The goal of health care workers is to provide excellent client care. To do this, they must be able to communicate effectively. For many aspects of communication, the relationships between the persons doing the communicating can affect the quality of that communication. This is true of the relationship between physicians and nurses.

A study conducted by *Nursing '91* examined the physician/nurse relationship. In this study, 1,000 registered nurses in the United States were asked to comment on their relationships with physicians. More than half reported dissatisfaction with these relationships, and only one third reported that they had a collegial relationship with physicians. Fifty-seven percent reported that nurses are treated as physicians' subordinates. Three fourths of the nurses believed that physicians do not treat nurses as partners within the health care field, although the majority of nurses saw themselves as equal partners with physicians. This survey clearly shows that physician/nurse relationships have a great deal of room for improvement (*Nursing '91* Editorial Staff, 1991).

Physicians report many frustrations with the current health care system, with the greatest number of complaints directed at the nursing staff (Burns, Andersen & Shortell, 1993). Because older physicians have had to contend with the majority of changes in the health care system, it was anticipated that they would have the most complaints. Yet younger physicians were found to have the most complaints of all groups.

Studies have shown that physicians and nurses report little communication difficulties within their respective professional groups, but they report major difficulties when trying to talk with members of another professional group. It was also noted that interns reported greater difficulty communicating with nurses than did

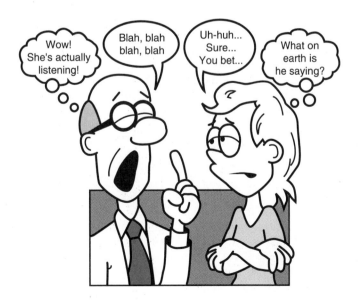

more experienced physicians (MacKay, 1991). Maybe this happens because communication skills are a learned behavior, and interns simply haven't learned it yet.

Thirty to 40 years ago, the health care industry was certainly different from what it is today. It revolved around the medical field. The physician was absolutely in charge, and the nurse was expected to follow orders without question. The typical nurse behavior pattern was focused primarily on carrying out the medical plan of care, rather than acting as a client advocate. If a nurse needed to give the physician information, it was done in a deferential manner. Nurses were nonintimidating to physicians, and they were expected to be very helpful to them in many small ways. They carried the charts when physicians made client rounds. They obtained coffee and ran errands. When a physician entered the room, the nurse stood up and offered him the chair.

During this era, the vast majority of physicians were white males and the nurses were mainly white females. Although it was common to hear physicians call the nurses collectively "the girls," a physician was always referred to by his professional title. To call a physician by his first name or call him "one of the boys" was unthinkable. This is still quite prevalent today in many settings.

Physicians and nurses were socialized into this pattern of behavior by a multitude of events. Medical education, nurses' training (as it was called in the 1950s through the 1970s), the gender roles of the day, and perhaps even expectations of society shaped these behaviors and attitudes.

Fifteen to 20 years ago, events in health care began to change. Women were becoming more assertive, and the profession of nursing began to define its professional boundaries. The educational level of nurses increased, both through formal education such as college classes and through specialization of practice, such as critical care nursing or pediatric nursing. More men and members of minorities entered the field of nursing. The legal system began to render decisions regarding nontolerance of harassment in the work place. These events contributed to the profession of nursing becoming more autonomous and expecting respect from medical practitioners.

What is the state of physician/nurse relations today? It is improved from what it was in the World War II era, but a power struggle is still going on. One of the largest problems has to do with autonomy of practice. The absence of a clearly defined distinct domain of nursing is related to the lack of collaboration between physicians and nurses (Prescott & Bowen, 1985). Is the physician in charge of the client and therefore in charge of the nursing staff? Or is each profession autonomous and in collaboration with the other? Although nursing is an independent profession, the reality is that many physicians believe that they "own" the client and therefore the nurses work for them.

Another element of the power struggle relates to the ability to admit clients to the hospital, bringing business (clients) to the institution. Historically, only physicians have been allowed to admit clients. Because physicians were bringing business and money to the institution, the hospital administration was cautious not to offend them. Nurses did not have the same power. They were viewed by hospitals as costing money, not making money. Events are changing, however, and several states have granted nurse practitioners the independent ability to prescribe medications. In many other states, nurse practitioners can prescribe medications under the authority of a physician. With this ability to prescribe medications, many institutions are allowing nurse practitioners to admit clients to the hospital. The increasing trend toward outpatient services and home care has altered the balance of power between physicians and nurses and will continue to do so in the future.

During the early 2000s, the trend toward primary care usage is expected to increase, and it is anticipated that nurse practitioners will be delivering much of this primary care. If so, nurse practitioners will be co-gatekeepers to the health care system, along with physicians. This will dramatically enhance the balance of power for nurses. Factors that will increase nurse empowerment include (Havens & Mills, 1992):

1. A stronger voice in the management of nursing units, including being involved with the budget process.
2. Participation in the hiring of new staff members.
3. Unit-based quality assurance programs.

Consider This Scenario

In this scenario, we will show how miscommunication can occur when male and female health care workers talk to each other. Both *think* they know what the other person has said. But neither actually knew what the other was saying.

As Angelica Rowland, RN, performs a physical assessment on her client, she notices that his lungs sound congested and his ankle edema is more pronounced than it was yesterday. The client tells her that he took Lasix at home, but his physician had not ordered it in the hospital. A few minutes later, Maurice Campbell, MD, comes into the room. Ms. Rowland has worked with Dr. Campbell several times before. She doesn't think that Dr. Campbell likes her because he doesn't seem to respect her as a nurse. He does not appear to listen when nurses contact him about clients. Instead, it seems that he just wants everyone to work together. He especially wants the staff nurses to be available when he wants information about the clients. Dr. Campbell thinks, "I wish Ms. Rowland was more of a team player."

"Dr. Campbell, I notice that Mr. Mott's lungs are more congested and his ankle edema is increased. He tells me that he used to be on Lasix, but he isn't now." She is very careful *not* to say that Dr. Campbell should put him back on Lasix, but simply provides all of the information to lead him to that conclusion.

Dr. Campbell asks Ms. Rowland several questions. While Dr. Campbell is speaking, Ms. Rowland nods her head and says "yeah," indicating that she is listening to him. Later, she looks at the client orders and notes that Dr. Campbell has ordered several laboratory tests for the client. This is puzzling, because these tests had already been performed earlier that day. When she calls him to tell him this, he asks her why she nodded her head when he suggested having the tests run. Ms. Rowland replies that she didn't realize that she had nodded her head. "I was just listening to you. I didn't say that I agreed with you."

Gender roles have certainly changed or blurred. Although the medical student population in the 1990s is 50% female, the majority of physicians in practice are male. And even though nursing schools have approximately 15% male students, the majority of nurses in practice are female. Thus, gender roles still play a major factor in physician/nurse relationships. Research shows that females value mutual respect and trust, and males value competence and people working together as a team (Tannen, 1990). This was also shown in a study by Prescott and Bowen (1985) in which nurses stated that they valued the attributes of mutual respect and trust above

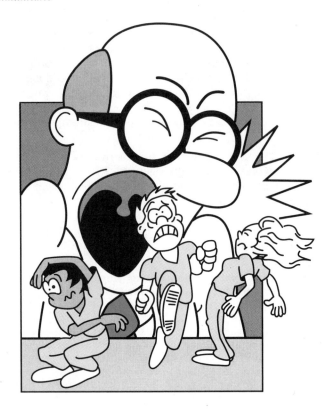

all others. Physicians, however, valued competence in nurses and the willingness to provide help to the physicians when needed.

The female nurses in Prescott and Bowen's study reported difficulty in using a straight open communication style with male physicians. When a female nurse needed something from a male physician, the general method was to state her needs in a way that didn't seem overbearing or threatening. This is a common problem when women are talking with men. In the scenario, Ms. Rowland communicated in such a way as to not seem that she was telling the physician what to do. This "beating around the bush" approach can be very frustrating for both sender and receiver.

Another interesting gender difference is the use of signals to suggest listening behaviors. Women use the word "yeah" to suggest that they are listening, whereas men say "yeah" only when they agree with the conversation. So when Ms. Rowland nodded her head and said "yeah" during the conversation with Dr. Campbell, he may have incorrectly assumed that she agreed with him, when she was really only saying that she was listening. These differences can certainly be the basis for misunderstandings (Tannen, 1990).

Suggestions: How Should You Act Toward Physicians?

Although nurses should act in an assertive manner, they should not treat physicians rudely. Physicians and all members of the health care team should treat each other with respect, as one professional to another. You should act the same toward physicians as you would toward any other health professional. If you are able to help them, do so.

For example, you are sitting near the coffee pot in the conference room and a physician asks you for a cup of coffee. Hand it to him!

If you are unable to help a physician, explain why. For example, if you are busy doing a dressing change and a physician asks you to help him find a client chart, estimate how much longer you will be, and tell him that you will be available then.

Communicating With Physicians About Clients

As a nurse, you will be communicating with physicians and health care providers about clients on a regular basis. One of the most difficult aspects of this is determining with which physician or health care provider you need to speak and when. To get the correct answers to your questions, you need to consider:

- Who is responsible for what aspect of the client's medical care?
- Which health care providers are included in the client's case?
- What information do you need to tell them?

Consider This Scenario

Kathy Rogers was shot and stabbed during a fight. She was taken to the nearest trauma center and underwent surgery for internal abdominal bleeding and a collapsed right lung. She is HIV positive. After the surgery, she will remain in the intensive care unit for 5 days. Because she is so malnourished, she develops a reddened area on her coccyx during her stay in ICU. You need to inform her care providers of this reddened area. You look at the chart and discover that the following physicians and nurse practitioners are on Ms. Rogers's case:

1. Dr. Martin Canto, trauma surgeon
2. Dr. Marybeth Penski, pulmonologist
3. Dr. Jose Rodriguez, pulmonologist
4. Dr. Jeffery Shaven, infectious disease
5. Tonya Swarthier, nurse practitioner, skin management
6. Fay-Anne Mantel, nurse practitioner, women's substance abuse
7. Dr. Seij Ramadan, pulmonology fellow
8. Dr. Raj Moody, third-year internal medicine resident
9. Dr. Seth Johnson, first-year internal medicine resident
10. Dr. Randolph Pierce, first-year surgery resident

After you consider the role of each health care provider, you decide to call the nurse practitioner who specializes in skin management to come see Ms. Rogers for this problem.

The second day after surgery, Dr. Penski and Dr. Rodriguez come to see Ms. Rogers. They ask you, "How is she doing?" The translation for this is, "How is she doing from a pulmonology point of view?" You tell them about her lung sounds, the drainage from the chest tubes, her lab reports, and her vital signs.

Ms. Mantel comes to see Ms. Rogers later that day. She asks, "How is she doing?" The translation for this is, "Is she alert enough to talk about what happened?"

Dr. Shaven visits that day also. He asks, "How is she doing?" The translation for this is, "How is she doing from an infectious disease point of view?" You tell him about her lab values and the open sores on her arms and legs.

Ms. Rogers slowly improves and is discharged several weeks later.

This scenario looked at the complexity of health care providers caring for a critically ill person. In this situation, you will need to learn:

- Which physician or nurse to talk to
- Who is who and what they do
- How you find out who is on the case
- How you find the physician or nurse

With Which Physician or Nurse Practitioner Do You Need to Speak?

To learn this, you will need to consider several factors. For example, you need to know if your institution is a teaching hospital or a private institution. In a teaching hospital, much of the client's medical care is delivered by interns and resident physicians, and so the majority of questions concerning medical care will be directed to them. In non–teaching hospitals, attending physicians will be delivering the client's medical care, and so you will be directing questions to them. In Ms. Rogers' case, the nurse was able to decide which health care provider to call by analyzing the problem and deciding whose scope of practice would be able to fix the problem.

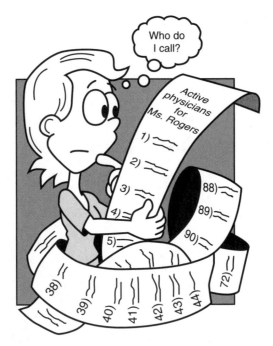

Who's Who and What Do They Do?

In Ms. Rogers' scenario, she had several different types of health care providers. The following is a brief description of the different health care team members and their scope of practice.

MEDICAL STUDENT   During the second, third, and fourth years of their medical education, medical students make visits and check on clients in a manner very similar to nursing students. This gives them exposure to clients in a way that cannot be done via textbook education. In most states, medical students cannot write client orders independently until after they graduate from their medical program. It is usually acceptable for them to write client orders under the direct supervision of a physician, who will countersign the order.

INTERN   Physicians spend the first year after medical school in an internship at a hospital. This gives them in-depth practical application of the information they learned in medical school. Many interns work long hours, such as being on-call for 24 hours straight. After an internship, a physician may practice as a general practitioner. Some states do not use the term *intern*; instead, the first year of postgraduate physician education is residency. You will need to find out what is practiced in your state.

RESIDENT   After completion of an internship, a physician may want to specialize in an area of medicine such as surgery or internal medicine. This residency usually takes three or four additional years. During this time, the physician will see clients who are within the specialty area. To help distinguish the various levels of education, many institutions use the terms *first-year resident, second-year resident, third-year resident,* etc.

FELLOW   Some medical specialties have subspecialties, such as pulmonary medicine, which is a subspecialty of internal medicine. A fellowship requires one to five additional years after residency. Fellows see only clients who are within the scope of their practice.

HOUSE STAFF   This is a term that includes all the medical staff members employed by the hospital in a learning capacity, such as interns, residents, and fellows. A similar term from the military is *house officer*.

NURSE PRACTITIONER   A nurse practitioner is a registered nurse who has completed a practitioner course and usually has a master's degree in nursing. Their practice level varies from state to state and institution to institution. In some institutions, nurse practitioners can admit clients to the hospital and manage their care. In other institutions, they must work in a collaborative practice with physicians. Some nurse practitioners specialize in areas such as nurse-midwifery or diabetic management. You can see that the definition of "nurse work" and "physician work" is blurring. As a matter of fact, many of the references to physicians in this chapter also could include nurse practitioners. As the health care system evolves, the practice of nurses and nurse practitioners will continue to change.

PHYSICIAN ASSISTANT   A physician assistant practices under direct supervision of a physician, as a subgroup of the medical profession. Because of this, physician assistants cannot be independent practitioners. They are usually employed by hospitals, clinics, or private physicians. Their level of practice can vary from state to state. Their educational level starts with an associate or bachelor's degree followed by two years of physician assistant training. Physician assistants (commonly called PAs) usually specialize in a field such as surgery or internal medicine.

ATTENDING/PRIMARY PHYSICIAN OR ATTENDING/PRIMARY CARE GROUP   This is the client's private physician or nurse practitioner or, in a group practice, the name of the group practice to which they belong. The attending is considered to be in charge of the client's medical care. The name of the attending is usually listed on the face sheet of the chart and on the client name band. In many teaching institutions, most clients are seen by interns and residents, in addition to the attending physician or nurse practitioner.

STAFF PHYSICIAN   If a client does not have a private physician, he or she is assigned to a staff physician. The staff physician or practitioner is in charge of the client's medical care. This is most common at teaching hospitals. In non-teaching hospitals, the client may be assigned to the emergency room physician or a private physician who is accepting new clients.

How Do You Find Out Who Is on the Case?

There are a variety of strategies that you can use to help you figure out which health care providers are included in the client's health care regimen. You could look at the face sheet of the chart to find out who is the client's attending or staff physician. Another method is to read the progress notes, because a progress note is usually written each time the health care provider sees the client. You could also look to see who is writing client orders. If you can't read the writing or the signature, ask the unit clerk (also known as a unit secretary or health unit coordinator) to help interpret this information.

If the health care provider is a member of the house staff or is in a group practice, you'll have to decide which member of the staff or group practice to call. There are usually posted on-call schedules for house staff and group practices. For the house staff, you could call the hospital operator and ask who is on call. For group practices, you could call the answering service to learn who is on call.

To Which of the Client's Care Providers Should You Speak?

Simply knowing which health care providers are included in the client's health care is only part of the information you need before you can talk with them. You also have to decide which person will need to know the information—in other words, who is capable of handling the problem?

To decide who needs to know the information, assess your situation. Does this client have multiple physicians and nurse practitioners or simply an attending physician or nurse practitioner? Are there specialists on the case? If so, it's usually best to direct questions about a body system to the appropriate specialist, e.g., if you need to tell a physician about the client's blood gases, call the pulmonary physician.

One of the complicating issues can be the number of physicians or nurse practitioners on a client's case. Sometimes critically ill clients have 15 or 20 physicians or nurse practitioners directing their care. (Ms. Rogers has 10 physicians and nurse practitioners.) Sometimes it can get difficult to figure out which specialist to call for a problem, because the client's problem either overlaps several body systems or perhaps doesn't exactly fit into any of them. For example, suppose Ms. Rogers develops a fever. Should you call the pulmonologist (thinking the client may have pneumonia), the surgeon (thinking the client may have an infected wound), or the infectious disease specialist (thinking the client may have complications resulting from her HIV-positive status)? If she had an attending physician, you would call that physician about the fever, and he or she would decide if one of the specialists would need this information. However, not all clients have an attending or primary physician. This is a very complicated issue. If the client does not have an attending or primary care provider, you may need to call each of these physicians and discuss the client's fever. It would be helpful to consult the staff nurses about which specialist to call.

Do you need to relate a rather simple problem, such as getting an order for medication to relieve constipation, or is the problem very complex, such as reevaluating the pain medication for a dying client? If it is a relatively simple problem, the resident can probably take care of the problem. If it is very complex, it may need to come to the attention of the attending or one of the specialists. However, the resident could contact them; you wouldn't have to do this. It can be very hard for a nursing student to figure out if a client problem is simple or complex. Ask the nursing staff or nursing instructor for help in deciding whom to call for a problem.

In most cases, a nursing student will not call a physician because the student cannot take verbal orders. However, calling a physician is a skill that needs to be practiced. The student nurse could call the physician and have an RN listen in on an extension phone. (Make sure that the physician understands that someone else is on the line.) In this manner, the RN is able to hear the conversation, add any necessary information, and write any verbal orders received.

Ways to Find the Physician or Nurse Practitioner

Once you have figured out which nurse practitioner or physician you need to contact, the next step is to actually talk to them! The first thing to do is to determine whether they are on the nursing unit. If they are not on the nursing unit, determine whether they are in the facility. If so, you could page them.

What do you do if they aren't currently on the nursing unit or in the institution? You call them! Although this may seem difficult, it really isn't. With the vast number of electronic communication devices available, no one is out of communication range for very long. Some of the most common ways to reach physicians and nurse practitioners include *overhead page, personal pagers, answering service*, a *call to their office*, and a *call to their home or car*.

Most physicians and nurse practitioners have personal pagers, answering services, and phones in their homes, cars, briefcases, and offices. Which of these methods or locations is the best? Of course, it depends on the situation.

Some of the most important questions to answer have to do with timing. What time of day is it? Is it a weekday, weekend, or holiday? Knowing this will be helpful because many practitioners follow a set schedule: they have office hours at certain times and see clients in the hospital at certain times. So, trying to predict where they may be will help you find them faster. It makes sense to call the place where you think they will be.

Does the physician have instructions that all calls go to his or her answering service or home after a certain time? This type of information can usually be found in a physician directory or Rolodex. Ask other nurses where to call first.

If you don't know where to find the physician, try the answering service first. Usually the service can tell you where to find the physician.

OVERHEAD PAGE   The overhead page system is one of the most common communication devices in many hospitals. It is used the most during daytime hours, because it can be very noisy to use at night while people are trying to sleep. The hospital telephone operator usually operates the overhead page system. To page someone, simply dial the telephone to get the operator and tell the operator whom you want paged and the phone number to call. You need to know what type of paging system your institution uses.

PERSONAL PAGERS Personal pagers are primarily of two types: voice or digital. The voice pager is used for voice messages and the digital pager displays telephone numbers. Some paging systems have online messages that guide you through the process of using the pager. You dial the telephone number for the pager and then follow instructions. A typical message would be, "Leave a message after the tone," or, if it is a digital pager, it might instruct you to, "Insert phone number to be called now." Other types of pagers do not give verbal instructions; after you dial the telephone number, you hear a beep, which is your indication to start speaking.

For voice pagers, keep the message short and repeat it twice. Include the person's name and the telephone number you want the person to call. Speak slowly and clearly. A sample message would be, "Dr. Tucker, please call 8577, please call 8577." It is much better to have the physician call the nursing unit than it is to provide information over a pager system.

For digital pagers, leave the telephone number of a multiline phone system. This way, the line will not be busy when the call is returned. If you cannot wait by the phone, leave a note stating where you can be found.

Consider This Scenario

The nurses have just called the Leibowitz family to come to the hospital because their mother's condition is deteriorating. When the family comes to the hospital, they get into the elevator with several other people. While they are in the elevator, they hear a physician's personal pager deliver the following message: "Dr. Columbine, Mrs. Leibowitz has died. Please come to 6 North to pronounce Mrs. Leibowitz, please come to 6 North to pronounce Mrs. Leibowitz."

In this situation, misuse of a physician's pager could have a devastating effect. Think how the family members felt when they heard the message. It would have been much more tactful and kinder to simply say, "Dr. Columbine, please call 6 North 4555, please call 6 North 4555."

ANSWERING SERVICE Many professionals have an answering service to take their calls when they are not available. After calling a physician's office telephone number, if no one is available to answer your call, the answering service would pick it up. They usually need to know the client's name, room number, hospital, name of the caller, nature of the problem (just a general description), and whether the call is an emergency.

OFFICE During business hours, there's a good chance that you will find physicians and nurse practitioners in their offices, seeing clients. You would call the office and ask to speak to them. If they are unavailable, you will probably be asked to leave the client's name, room number, hospital, name of the caller, and the nature of the problem (just a general description).

HOME Most institutions have policies that nurses call a physician's answering service to find a physician. However, some physicians would prefer to be called at home. You would know to call the physician at home by a physician statement of such. However, it is more common to call the answering service and the physician would later return your call.

Consider This Scenario

A group of resident physicians and nurses are making client rounds. (This means that as a group, they are seeing each of their clients on the nursing unit. This is commonly done as a teaching method.) You need to tell one of the physicians of your client's problem with constipation. You could make rounds with them and, as they come to your client, provide them with the information about the client's condition, including the problem of constipation. This method really simplifies nurse-physician-client communication. If you are unable to make rounds with them, another method is to wait until rounds are finished to speak with the physician. If it seems that it will be a long time until they finish, you could talk to the physician after the client currently being seen.

When you need to speak with a physician or a nurse practitioner who is present on the nursing unit, it is really important to use an appropriate location for the discussion. It is always better to try to have your discussion in a quiet place, rather than in the middle of a bustling nurses' station. But, the reality is that often this is where the conversation takes place, either in person or on the telephone.

Remember, too, that client confidentiality must be considered, so you do not want to have a discussion in an elevator, a visitor's lounge, the cafeteria, or a hallway with other persons nearby. If you must talk about work-related issues in these places, keep your voice low and ensure that you never violate client confidentiality.

Appropriate timing of a conversation is also important. Unless it is an emergency, you should wait until the physician is finished with the current activity before you talk to him or her.

Consider This Scenario

You are taking care of Cheryl Cathews, who had surgery 3 days ago. While you are doing her a.m. care, Cheryl pulls out the N/G tube by accident. You know that usually the client has an N/G tube for 3 to 4 days after this type of surgery. The client asks you to leave the tube out. You assess her bowel sounds and ask her if she is passing gas. You find that her bowel sounds are active in all quandrants and she says that she is passing gas.

In her chart, you see that Dr. Minaret, a surgical resident, has been writing client orders and progress notes. You see by the resident on-call schedule that she is on call, so you page her. After you dial the telephone number, you state, "Dr. Minaret, please call 9175, please call 9175."

A few minutes later, Dr. Minaret calls the nursing unit and you say, "Dr. Minaret, this is Merlin Williams, RN. I'm taking care of Cheryl Cathews. You assisted Dr. Highland to do a colostomy revision on her 3 days ago. Ms. Cathews inadvertently pulled out her N/G tube. She has active bowel sounds in all quadrants and is passing gas. Can the N/G tube be left out?" Dr. Minaret agrees to this and states that she will come to the nursing unit in a few minutes to write the order.

"Oh, while I've got you on the phone, would you please tell me what Ms. Cathews' hemoglobin was today?" says Dr. Minaret. Because you knew that you might be asked for additional information, you had brought the chart to the telephone with you. You look up the lab reports and respond, "Her hemoglobin is 9.9 this morning."

This scenario illustrated several important items to consider when talking to a physician.

- When to call
- What to relate
- How to prepare for the discussion

What Information Do You Need to Relate?

One of the most important reasons to call a physician or nurse practitioner is to report changes in the client's condition. You should call the physician if the client's condition becomes worse, if laboratory values are significantly different from normal, if the vital signs are unstable, or if you have questions about the client orders (Table 11–1). Document in the nurses' notes the time that you called the physician, the information that you gave, and the response. If you received client orders because of the conversation, simply write "orders received," and the reader can refer to the client order sheet for further information (Tammelleo, 1992).

What Do You Need to Know Before You Speak With a Physician?

Before you approach the physician, make sure that you have all the necessary information available. Typically, this would be any data that supports the information you are presenting. It is common for the physician to ask for other information about the client's condition than just the problem you have brought up, so it is a good idea to bring the client's chart to the conversation, as Mrs. Williams did in the scenario. Having the chart nearby will be helpful if you expect to receive client orders as a result of this verbal interchange.

Because many physicians have such large practices, it is always good to begin the conversation with the client's name and a short description of why the client is hospitalized. Then state what you wanted to tell the physician and provide the supporting data.

Because everyone, including health care providers, takes vacations and days off, a physician or nurse practitioner may be on-call for another physician or nurse practitioner. This is commonly referred to as "Dr. So-and-So is covering my practice

Table 11–1 WHAT SHOULD BE BROUGHT TO A PHYSICIAN'S ATTENTION?

Situation	What Needs to Be Said?	Sample Conversation

Altered physiologic state
  Temperature
  Lung sounds
  Blood pressure
  Pulse
  Respirations
  Abnormal lab results
	Person's name you are calling
	Your name, title, and location
	Client's name and reason for admission
	What is the problem?
	What have you already done for the problem?
	Pertinent vital signs, physical assessment parameters
	Your suggested treatment of the problem (if you know one)
		"Dr. Smith, this is Mr. Brace, RN, calling from 2 Main at GetWell Medical Center. You admitted Mrs. Fissile yesterday for high blood pressure. I gave her 10 mg of Procardia sublingual 1 hour ago for a blood pressure of 210/110. Her current blood pressure is 188/104. She is alert and oriented and says she has a headache. What would you like us to do for the current blood pressure?"

Question about client orders	Person's name you are calling Your name, title, and location Client's name and reason for admission What is the problem?	"Dr. Lily, this is Ms. Hollally, RN, calling from 3 North at GetWell Medical Center. I am taking care of Ms. Carpenter. You admitted her today for low back pain. You ordered Tylenol #3 for her for pain. She is allergic to codeine. What should we give her for pain medication?"

Altered mental state
  Anxiety
  Depression
  Anger
  Confusion
	Person's name you are calling
	Your name, title, and location
	Client's name and reason for admission
	What is the problem?
	What have you already done for the problem?
	Pertinent vital signs, physical assessment parameters
		"Dr. Flushing, this is Ms. Yak, RN, calling from 9-C at GetWell Medical Center. I am taking care of Mr. Farmer. You admitted him 2 days ago for sickle cell crisis. He is becoming extremely anxious and unable to sit still. There is no change in his vital signs or physical assessment as compared to yesterday. He is asking for a sedative. None is ordered. What would you like us to do?"

Failure to respond to therapy
  Pain medication
  Blood pressure medication
	Person's name you are calling
	Your name, title, and location
	Client's name and reason for admission
	What is the problem?
	What have you already done for the problem?
	Pertinent vital signs, physical assessment parameters
		"Dr. Malady, this is Mrs. Chishom, RN, calling from 3 Main at GetWell Medical Center. I am taking care of Ms. Crim. She had a hysterectomy performed this morning. She is in a lot of pain despite the 75 mg of Demerol I gave her 3 hours ago. Her dressing is dry and her vital signs are within normal limits. Can we shorten the time between Demerol injections?"

Table continued on following page

Table 11–1 WHAT SHOULD BE BROUGHT TO A PHYSICIAN'S ATTENTION? (*Continued*)

Situation	What Needs to Be Said?	Sample Conversation
Consultation	Person's name you are calling Your name, title, and location Name of person asking for the consult Client's name, location, and reason for admission Reason for consultation Speed in which the consultation needs to be done (urgent means as soon as possible, routine means within the day or the next day)	"Dr. Green, this is Mr. Auker, RN, calling from 5 South at GetWell Medical Center. Dr. Zito has asked you to consult on Mrs. Von Drak. She is in room 511A. She had a colostomy revision 4 days ago and has spiked a temperature of 104°. Dr. Zito says that the consult is routine, so he would like you to see her today."
Family considerations	Person's name you are calling Your name, title, and location Client's name and reason for admission Problem Suggested solution	"Dr. Raj, this is Mrs. Skarsten, RN, calling from 4 Main at GetWell Medical Center. I am taking care of Mr. Kennedy. You admitted him last week for his abdominal pain. His wife is here and wants to talk to you before she will sign the permit for his surgery. Do you want to talk to her now or do you want to call her?" When he says that he wants to talk to her now, Mrs. Skarsten says, "Here is Mrs. Kennedy." (Hands phone to Mrs. Kennedy.)
Unusual incidents	Person's name you are calling Your name, title, and location Client's name and reason for admission What is the problem? What have you already done for the problem? Pertinent vital signs, physical assessment parameters What does the physician need to do?	"Dr. Al-Medina, this is Ms. Patmore, RN, calling from 4 North at GetWell Medical Center. I am taking care of Mrs. Pontiewski. You admitted her yesterday for vertigo. While going to the bathroom, she fell. We got her back to bed and had the medical PA (physician assistant) come to see her. Her hip was x-rayed and it's not fractured. She says her right hip is sore but she can walk on it. I filled out an incident report."

248

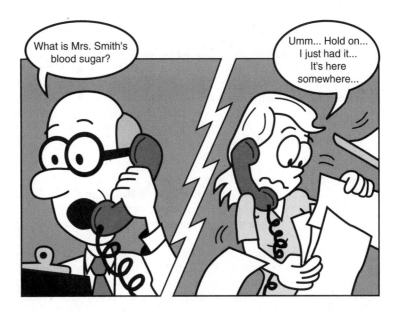

for me." If this is the case, you will need to provide more background data on the client, because the on-call physician may be totally unfamiliar with the client.

Communicating Verbally and in Writing

Via Telephone

The telephone can be an extremely valuable tool for health care providers. On many units, the phone rings day and night.

Many physicians and nurse practitioners are called on a regular basis. It is a good idea to try to consolidate information to decrease the number of calls. For example, on a surgical unit, a surgeon may have ordered a.m. blood work for many clients. He told the nurse manager to call him when the results of the ordered laboratory tests come back. Because they will probably be finished at different times, the physician could be called several times during the day with lab results. Because it would be more efficient for you and the physician, wouldn't it be better to wait until all the lab reports are back and call them all at once to the physician? (Remember, though, that you wouldn't wait if any results were abnormal. You would call these to the physician right away.)

Here's another method to consolidate information on phone calls: Before you call a physician, ask other nursing staff members if they need to speak with that physician as well.

If the physician or nurse practitioners are not available when you call, provide the number of a multiline phone so that the phone will not be busy when they try to call you back.

If you can't wait by the phone, put a note near the phone indicating from whom you are expecting a call and where you can be found.

Progress Notes

Whenever a physician makes a visit to a client, he or she writes a *progress note* that describes the client's condition, response to treatment, and any changes in the medical regimen. Much valuable information is available in the progress notes. Sometimes, though, they are difficult to read because they are handwritten.

Physician Orders (Client Orders)

Traditionally, physicians provided direction for client care activities through *physician orders.* These orders are instructions to be carried out by the nursing staff and ancillary departments such as radiology and respiratory therapy. However, with the advances in nursing practice, such as nurse practitioners, the term *physician orders* might be considered to be outdated. Many institutions are using the new term *client orders.*

Authorized persons such as physicians can write the orders themselves or tell an authorized person (an RN) to write the order as a "verbal order."

Client orders are followed until they are changed. For example, if an order for a regular diet was written, this diet order would be considered current because no other diet order has been given.

Some client orders, such as those that order narcotic medications, have a timeframe for which they are ordered. Federal laws state that narcotic orders must be rewritten every few days. Other situations in which client orders are altered would be client transfers to another unit or after surgical procedures. Many institutions have policies that all pretransfer and preoperative client orders are considered to be discontinued after the transfer or surgery. A new set of orders must be written. This helps to ensure that they will be pertinent to the client's condition.

There is usually a specific format used when writing client orders. Figure 11–1 shows an example.

Must All Client Orders Be Followed?

In the past, nurses were expected to follow physician orders without question. In keeping with the increased responsibility of nurses, however, this has certainly changed. Nurses today are responsible for their own actions and cannot use the outdated excuse, "But the doctor ordered me to do it! I didn't know it was wrong!" An RN or LPN is obligated by each state's nurse practice act to ensure that he or she is providing safe, appropriate nursing care. In fact, many courts are stating that not only are nurses expected to follow standards of practice, they are *required* to do so. You need to know specifically how the nurse practice act in your state guides your practice, because this varies from state to state.

In addition to providing safe, appropriate care, you are obligated to monitor the client care delivered by other practitioners and report any lapses from standards of practice. Nine states (Delaware, Florida, New York, Minnesota, Rhode Island, Massachusetts, Nevada, Texas, and Oregon) have laws requiring nurses to "blow the whistle" on incompetent medical care practitioners (Trudeau, 1994). With ever more public scrutiny being placed on health care providers, this trend is expected to continue.

You will need to know what is within the scope of RN/LPN practice in your

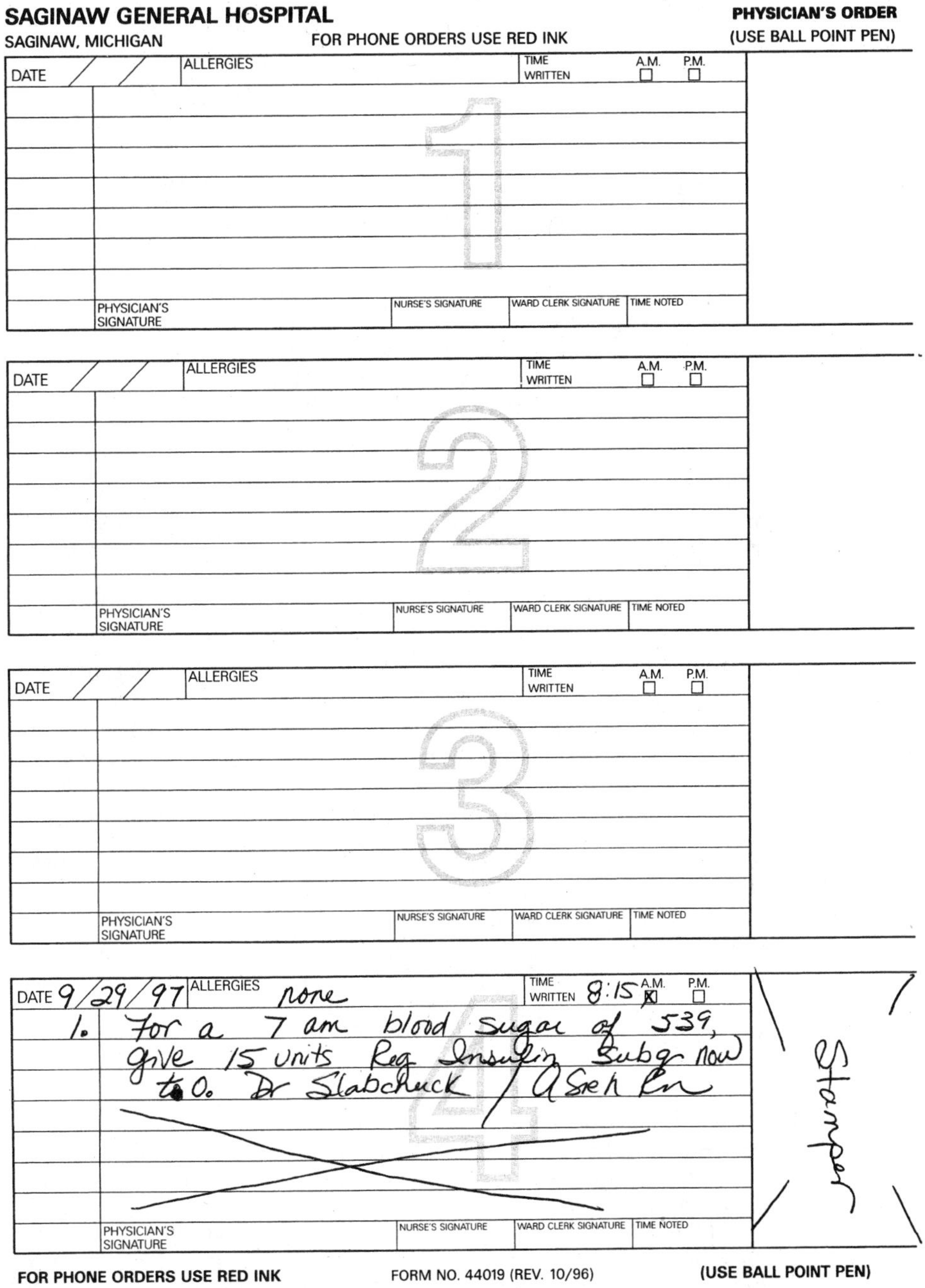

SAGINAW GENERAL HOSPITAL   **PHYSICIAN'S ORDER**

SAGINAW, MICHIGAN   FOR PHONE ORDERS USE RED INK   (USE BALL POINT PEN)

DATE //	ALLERGIES		TIME WRITTEN	A.M. ☐	P.M. ☐	

PHYSICIAN'S SIGNATURE   NURSE'S SIGNATURE   WARD CLERK SIGNATURE   TIME NOTED

DATE //	ALLERGIES		TIME WRITTEN	A.M. ☐	P.M. ☐	

PHYSICIAN'S SIGNATURE   NURSE'S SIGNATURE   WARD CLERK SIGNATURE   TIME NOTED

DATE //	ALLERGIES		TIME WRITTEN	A.M. ☐	P.M. ☐	

PHYSICIAN'S SIGNATURE   NURSE'S SIGNATURE   WARD CLERK SIGNATURE   TIME NOTED

DATE 9/29/97   ALLERGIES *none*   TIME WRITTEN 8:15 A.M. ☒ P.M. ☐

1. *For a 7 am blood sugar of 539, give 15 units Reg Insulin subq now to O. Dr Slabchuck / A Sieh RN*

Stamper

PHYSICIAN'S SIGNATURE   NURSE'S SIGNATURE   WARD CLERK SIGNATURE   TIME NOTED

FOR PHONE ORDERS USE RED INK   FORM NO. 44019 (REV. 10/96)   (USE BALL POINT PEN)

Figure 11–1   An example of a physician order (client order). (Courtesy of Saginaw General Hospital, Saginaw, Michigan.)

state in regard to client orders. Some items to determine, and institutional policy will also guide you, include:

1. Who is allowed to write verbal orders?
2. In all states, medical physicians and osteopathic physicians can write client orders. But how about dentists, medical students, physician assistants, nurse practitioners, respiratory therapists, pharmacists, and dietitians?

When you are looking at a client's order that has just been written, check it carefully for the following:

LEGIBILITY   Can you read it? If it's not legible, you'll have to call the physician to interpret the poor penmanship, so it's a good idea to check the order for legibility before the physician leaves the area. Illegibility of physician handwriting is such a problem that the American Medical Association suggests that physicians print or type client orders to prevent errors in transcription (American Medical Association, 1994).

COMPLETENESS   Did the physician order everything? The client may have asked the physician to write an order for a sleeping medication, and if the physician forgets to write an order for this, you will have to make a phone call to the physician to clear up the matter.

LEGALITIES   Is the order written in an appropriate format? Was the order written by an authorized person? Did that person sign the order?

APPROPRIATENESS   What is the reason the physician ordered the medication, lab tests, health care provider consult, etc.? Is this an appropriate action? Nursing students are frequently surprised to discover that they must be able to determine whether a physician's or nurse practitioner's order is accurate and appropriate before the order can be implemented. If the order is for a medication, is it the correct dosage, route, timing? Is the client allergic to the medication?

DUPLICATION   Is the new client order duplicating another client order? For example, Dr. Andrew Slabchuck ordered a serum blood sugar to be drawn every 6 hours. Later that day, Joshua Brusich, nurse practitioner, ordered a serum blood sugar to be drawn daily. Do these health care providers actually want five blood sugar tests per day or were they perhaps not aware of the other order? If you don't investigate, the client will be charged an unnecessary expense and have to endure the pain of unnecessary blood draws.

Consider This Scenario

Maya Hudson, RN, is providing care for a client in the intensive care unit, hospitalized with respiratory distress. She notices that the client is having severe respiratory difficulty and calls the pulmonology fellow, Dr. Cohen, in to see the client. He comes to see the client and states, "Give 40 mg of Lasix IV now." Ms. Hudson responds, "You're ordering me to give Mrs. Farragut 40 mg of Lasix IV push now. Is that correct? If so, I'll go get the Lasix and the chart so that you can write the order."

The resident tells you that this is accurate and you go get the chart and the medicine. While you are gone, Mrs. Farragut's condition continues to deteriorate. Dr. Cohen begins to insert an oral endotracheal tube so that Mrs. Farragut can be connected to a ventilator for ventilatory assistance. Because the physician is busy in an emergency situation, you give the Lasix *before* writing the verbal order.

However, this should be done only in an emergency. In all other circumstances, the physician should write the order before you perform the intervention.

Client Orders Given Verbally

There are occasions when physicians want to alter the current orders for the client but they aren't physically present at the medical facility. They may call the nursing unit and ask for an RN or a graduate nurse (GN) to write a telephone order.

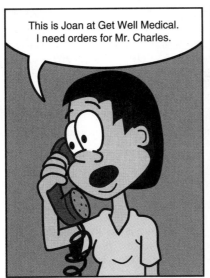

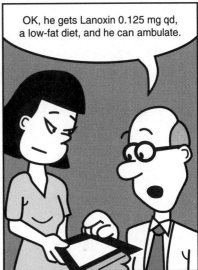

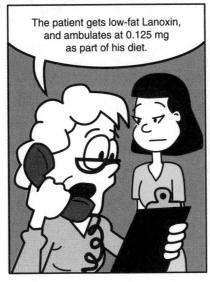

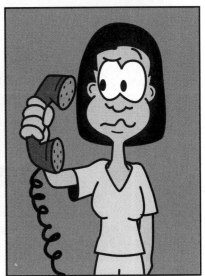

A verbal order would occur in a similar instance, except that the physician is physically in the medical facility and tells an RN to write a client order, rather than writing the order himself or herself.

In most states, RNs and GNs can receive and write a verbal or telephone order for all areas of health care practice. Pharmacists can write verbal orders that relate to medication delivery, dietitians can write orders relating to nutrition therapy, and respiratory therapists can write orders concerning respiratory care. LPNs and nursing students cannot write verbal or telephone client orders. If a physician gives a student or LPN a verbal or telephone order, the physician must be told that only an RN is legally able to receive such orders. The student or LPN can tell the physician that he or she will find an RN to receive the verbal or telephone order.

In some states and institutions, certain orders cannot be given verbally or over the telephone, such as no-code orders, narcotic orders, and orders for client commitment to a mental health unit. There can be wide variances in this from state to state and institution to institution. Before you receive verbal or telephone orders as an RN, check to see if there are any circumstances that cannot be written as this type of order.

In most circumstances, you will want to speak with the physician yourself, instead of communicating through intermediaries such as the office nurse or spouse. Obtaining client orders from someone other than the party directly giving the order might cause miscommunication by the other person and therefore miscommunication by you.

Protecting Yourself When Verbal Orders Are Given

Because a client order obtained verbally lacks the objectivity of a document written by the person giving the order, there are precautions you will want to take to ensure that the order is accurate. In many instances, to avoid the problem, it is best to simply say, "Instead of giving me a verbal order, I'll get the chart for you so that you can write it yourself" (Cohen, 1991). Another way to help ensure accuracy would be to have another RN or GN listen to the verbal order with you and co-sign the client order.

One of the most common times for a verbal order to be given is during an emergency situation. Of course, in this type of situation, where people are rushing about and the anxiety level is high, the potential for communication errors is very high. In an emergency situation, you need to use even greater care to ensure accuracy of communication in regard to verbal orders.

If the physician does give the order in person, the RN or GN must first write it down on the report sheet (it would be better to simply write it on the chart, but usually the chart isn't available or the physician would have written the order). Repeat the order to the person giving the order to ensure that you understood the order correctly. Include the client's name and the ordered information (American Medical Association, 1994; Iyer, 1991).

Once you have obtained experience in clinical settings, you will be able to consider the order in light of what you have seen before and ask yourself if it seems reasonable. Depending on the individual client, you will want to consider specific factors that the physician may have neglected or been unaware of. If the order is indeed appropriate, write it in the client orders as soon as possible, using the correct format.

Consider This Scenario

You are providing care for a diabetic client who has capillary blood sugars ordered four times a day. Her 11 A.M. blood sugar was 511. When you check her orders, you note that you are to call the resident on call for any blood sugar greater than 400. You call the resident, who tells you to give the client 15 units of regular insulin subcutaneously. You write the order in the chart as shown in Figure 11–1. Another nurse is caring for the same client on the following day. Once again, the client's 11 A.M. blood sugar is elevated. The nurse sees the order to call the resident in case the client has an elevated blood sugar. One of the questions the nurse anticipates that the resident will ask is, "How much insulin have they been giving her for this level of blood sugar?" Because you were so thorough in writing the client order, the nurse can find this information easily.

This scenario described important features of telephone orders, including:

- What telephone orders are
- How to take telephone orders
- What is included in the telephone order
- How to provide supporting data in the telephone order

Telephone Orders

Telephone orders can sometimes be more difficult than verbal orders because you aren't able to use body language to confirm the communication. If you (after you become a GN or RN) receive an order over the telephone, ask the physician to speak slowly. Write the orders down on your report sheet as soon as you hear them. You will write them on the client order form after you have read them back to the physician. Read the order back, speaking slowly and clearly. Spell any medications or numbers that sound similar, such as Xanax/Zantac and 16/60. If you have any questions about an order, ask the speaker for clarification. You could say, "Dr. Crudder, I don't understand what you want done with Mrs. Splicer's theophyl-line drip. Are you saying that we should stop it?"

If you are having difficulty understanding a physician over the telephone, you might have another RN listen to the conversation. Of course, you must tell the physician that the other person is also on the line. In some institutions, this method is used for all telephone orders (Carson, 1994).

A fax machine and personal computer equipped with a modem may help ensure accuracy of telephone orders. Instead of giving an RN an order over the telephone, the order could be transmitted via fax or modem to the nursing unit. However, there is concern about the legality of client orders transmitted via electronic mail. Also, it may be difficult to maintain confidentiality with these methods.

What Every Order Should Include

To write a client order correctly, you need to become familiar with the format acceptable in your institution. Client orders are written on a specific form in the chart. Look at your forms. Notice that the form is a multiple carbonless document, attached at either the top or the bottom. Is the form you are using attached at the bottom or the top? If it is attached at the top, start at the bottom to write the first client order on a blank client order form. If it is attached at the bottom, start at the top to write the first client order (see Fig. 11–1).

- Using nonerasable ink, write in the date.
- Start writing the client orders, using a new line for each order.
- Include as much supporting data as possible. In the scenario, the nurse added the client's blood sugar level in addition to the order for insulin.
- If the order is a verbal order, write "v.o." (for verbal order), the physician's or nurse practitioner's name, and then your name.
- If this is a telephone order, write "t.o." or "p.o." (for telephone order), the physician's or nurse practitioner's name, and then your name.
- Cross off any blank lines below your signature. This prevents anything from being added at a later date.
- Place the chart in the correct location for the order to be transcribed.

What Happens After the Order Is Written?

The client order form is usually made of duplicate or triplicate carbonless paper. It is done this way so that the copies can serve as communication devices. The original stays in the chart, and one copy of the order usually goes to the room nurse or primary nurse and one copy goes to the pharmacy (or the appropriate department).

Most institutions have methods to show how soon the order needs to be performed. There could be a special place to put STAT orders, perhaps plastic tabs on the chart to pull out, showing the timeliness of the order.

Transcribing and Noting Orders

After the order is written on the client order form, the information must be distributed to the appropriate people and departments. This activity is called transcribing the order (Table 11–2). Unit secretaries and nurses are able to transcribe orders. After the order is transcribed, the information is checked by an RN (or in some states by an LPN) for accuracy. This activity is called noting the order (Table 11–3).

As an RN, you will need to review the client order against the information placed in the Kardex, medication sheet, computer, etc., by the unit clerk. You will need to consider both the accuracy of the transcription and the accuracy of the order itself. If the order is transcribed incorrectly or if the client order is inappropriate, the client could receive an incorrect medication or treatment. You can see that noting an order is a very serious event and must be absolutely accurate.

Hint: Periodically check all charts for untranscribed client orders. Often, after an order is written, instead of being put in the location for untranscribed orders, it gets put back into the chart rack. This could cause a client order to go unnoticed for several hours, creating an unnecessary delay and possibly endangering the client!

Relationships Between Nurses and Ancillary Departments

Nurses increasingly are becoming managers of the client's health care. They need to ensure that the clients are receiving medical services in a timely, appropriate manner. Because of this, nurses must interact on a continual basis with other health

Table 11–2   TO TRANSCRIBE THE ORDER

Activity	Why
Gather your materials. You will usually need the Kardex and the client's medication sheets.	You must have the necessary materials to complete the task.
Place the client order sheet in front of you. Start with the first client order and place the information in the appropriate place (Kardex, medication sheets, computer reports, etc.).	This is how the appropriate personnel will know the new client orders.
Complete your activities for each order before going on to the next order. When you have completed the activities for one order, place a small check mark next to it.	This will help keep you on track if you are interrupted while working.
When you have completed all the activities for the orders, draw a line through all unused lines.	This will prevent anything from being added at a later date.
There may be an area on the client order form for the person transcribing the orders to sign. If so, sign in the appropriate area.	This allows accountability for the transcription of orders. If you have questions about a transcribed order, you can easily find out who transcribed the order.
When you are finished with the chart, leave the Kardex and medication sheets in the chart.	This will make it easier for the RN to review the orders.
If single orders are carried out before formal (complete) noting of the entire order, write the word "done" next to the order and initial it.	This tells the unit clerk and the nursing staff that this order has already been completed and thus prevents it from being done twice.
After all the client orders are transcribed, show that the orders are ready for the RN to review them. There are several ways to accomplish this. Some charts have plastic pull tabs that say "order to be noted." In other institutions, there is a special rack at the nurse's station to place charts that need to be checked by the RN.	This allows for timely noting of orders by the RN staff.

care providers, such as pharmacists, respiratory therapists, x-ray technologists, and laboratory technologists. For example, if an x-ray is ordered STAT, then the nurse must make sure that it is done immediately. Or, if there are problems with medication delivery, the nurse must discuss this with the pharmacy and obtain the necessary medications.

One of the most common methods of communicating with people in ancillary departments is by telephone. As an RN or LPN, you may be calling people in ancillary departments every day of your nursing career.

Table 11–3 NOTING CLIENT ORDERS

Activity	Why
In many institutions, to ensure accuracy, a verbal order must be noted by a nurse other than the one who wrote it.	This allows a second person to check the order for appropriateness.
If the order has been transcribed correctly and if the client order is appropriate, sign the client order form. Some chart forms have a small box in which to sign when you have finished noting the orders. For other client order forms, the nurse writes the word "Noted" and the date and times and signs the bottom of the order.	This allows accountability for the noting of orders. If there are any questions about an order, you know whom to ask about it.
If the order has been inaccurately transcribed, make the appropriate changes.	This ensures accuracy of the information in the computer, Kardex, medication sheets, etc.
If you believe that the order is inappropriate, you must contact the person who wrote the order to have it clarified.	Until you have this clarification, you must not carry out the order.

Consider This Scenario

Before you can speak with someone within an ancillary department, you'll have to determine exactly what you want, who you will need to talk to, and when you need to have it done. In this scenario, the student nurse and a pharmacy technician try to communicate but it seems that each is speaking a different language.

A student nurse discovered that her client's IV medication was not in the medication refrigerator. She decided to call the pharmacy to find out where the IV medication was. The conversation went something like this:

Pharmacy technologist: "Hello, this is Sharon, pharmacy technician. What can I do for you?"

Carol: "I have a question about an IV medication."

Sharon: "OK. Where are you calling from?" (Meaning "What nursing unit are you on?")

Carol: "I'm in the conference room."

Sharon: "What unit is the conference room on?"

Carol: "3 East."

Sharon: "Which client are we talking about?"

Carol: "Oh, I forgot his name. Just a minute." (She puts the phone on hold and goes to get the chart.) "His name is Mr. Dotty."

Sharon: "Can you tell me his room number?" (Starts speaking slowly, as if talking to a person with a poor command of the English language.)

Carol: "I think he's in 312."

Sharon: "What did you say you need? I've forgotten now."

Carol: "I need to talk about an IV medication."

Sharon: "Which IV?" (Starting to sound irritated.)

Carol: "His aminophylline drip."

Sharon: "Well, what about it?"

Carol: "It's not here."

Sharon: "Well, when is it due?"

Carol: "Due for what?"

Sharon: "Due to be hung!"

Carol: "Oh, that! I'm supposed to be putting it up now."

Sharon: "I'm looking in the computer and I show that it was sent up with the pharmacy runner 20 minutes ago. Has she made it to 3 East yet?"

Carol: "I'll go ask someone." (Puts Sharon on hold.) "Yes, she is here now. Sorry to bother you."

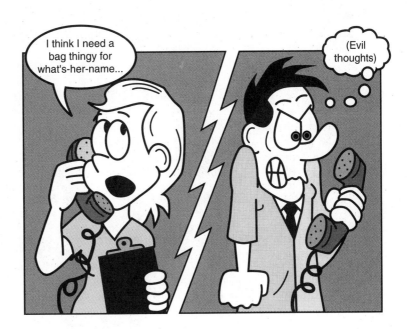

Sharon: "Can I give you some advice? Next time you call us, know what you want before you call. You have wasted a lot of time this way."

What Do You Want or Need?

This is very important to know, because it will help you direct your information search. You'll need to think about what you want so that you can talk to the person able to take care of the problem. In the scenario, Carol needed an IV bag, but didn't articulate what she needed.

To Whom Do You Want to Talk?

Within each department, there are a variety of personnel with differing levels of responsibility. Remember that within each department, there are often a secretary, two or three levels of staff members, and supervisory staff. Each level of personnel is responsible for a different aspect of client care. Refer to Table 11–4 for various personnel responsibilities and when to call them.

When Do You Need It?

Unless it's an emergency situation, you should try to allow as much time as possible for something to be done. Many procedures require a certain amount of time to do, and little can be done to speed this. For example, some IV solutions such as total parenteral nutrition (TPN) have as many as 20 additives. It will take a pharmacist at least 10 minutes to prepare this IV solution. Asking the pharmacist to hurry because you forgot to call earlier won't alter this fact. There's an old saying about how "lack of planning on your part does not constitute an emergency on my part." Carol should have looked for her next IV solution at least an hour before she needed to hang it. This way, if it wasn't available, there would have been time for it to be made.

How Do You Contact Other Departments or Personnel?

It's a good idea to have the client's chart available when you call any department, because there may be information in the chart that you need. Before Carol called the pharmacy, she should have known the client's name and room number and the physician's name. When she called the pharmacy, it would have been helpful to ask for the pharmacy technician assigned to her nursing unit. For other situations, you would ask for the person assigned to the client or someone able to handle this type of problem.

How Should It Be Done? Are There Any Special Instructions?

The nurse is typically the person with the most knowledge of the client's situation. Therefore, if you know any information that will make the job easier, communicate this to the appropriate department. For example, your client also has physical therapy ordered. If you note that your client is exceptionally tired right after meals,

Table 11-4 VARIOUS PERSONNEL RESPONSIBILITIES

Personnel	Job Responsibilities	Educational Requirements	What Is a Typical Reason You Might Call Them?
Laboratory			
Medical technologist	Able to run a variety of laboratory tests on specimens from clients.	Four-year program	Help with interpreting a laboratory result.
Medical technician (certified)	Runs laboratory tests under the direction of the medical technologist.	Two-year program	Is the result available from a laboratory test?
Laboratory assistant	Able to do limited functions within the department.	On-the-job training	Ask whether laboratory results are available yet.
Phlebotomist	Draws blood from the client.	Several-week course or on-the-job training	Notify this person that the client needs blood drawn for a laboratory test.
Nutrition Services			
Dietitian	Assists clients to plan dietary changes, suggests appropriate diet patterns for clients.	Four-year degree	Ask about foods appropriate for a certain diet. Help with determining client nutritional status.
Kitchen worker	Prepares meals, delivers diet trays.	On-the-job training	Substitutions for a client's meal tray; how to obtain a late tray.
Pharmacy			
Pharmacy technician	Prepares oral and IV medications.	Several-month course or on-the-job training	Availability of medication.
Pharmacist	After the pharmacy technician prepares the medication, the pharmacist checks the medication orders for accuracy. Responsible for ensuring that the medication is an appropriate dosage and route.	Five years or more of education	Specific questions about a medication. Compatibility of IV medications.
Discharge Planners			
Nurses or social workers	Specializing in planning the transfer from hospital to home. Usually each discharge planner is responsible for several nursing units.	Nurse—2, 3, or 4 years of education Social worker—4 to 6 years of education	Discharge plans for the client.
Social Workers	Counsels clients, helps them to file financial aid applications, plans client discharge to nursing homes.	Four to 6 years of education	When is the client going to a nursing home?

Table continued on following page

261

Table 11–4 VARIOUS PERSONNEL RESPONSIBILITIES (*Continued*)

Personnel	Job Responsibilities	Educational Requirements	What Is a Typical Reason You Might Call Them?
Respiratory Therapy			
Respiratory therapists (registered)	Able to carry out interventions aimed at improving respiratory function. In most institutions, respiratory therapists maintain and troubleshoot ventilators, although the nursing staff is responsible for the client care.	Two to 4 years of education	Specific suggestions regarding respiratory care of a mechanically ventilated client.
Respiratory technicians (certified)	Can do limited function tasks within the realm of respiratory therapy, such as inhalation treatments.	One-year program	Timing of the client's breathing treatments.
Nurse Specialist	Usually specializes in a specific area, e.g., diabetic management, skin care, ostomy, psychiatric care. Another type of advanced practice nurse is a clinical nurse specialist such as a critical care specialist.	Master of Science in Nursing degree (some do not have this, but have many years of experience in the area)	Specific questions about the caring for the client, e.g., How should we do his ostomy care? What is the best way to do his dressing?
Radiology Technologist	Takes x-rays. Large departments may be divided into specific departments (ultrasound, special procedures, CT).	Two-year program (if specialist, may have several more months of on-the-job training)	What is needed for x-ray prep? When will the test be done?
Physical Therapy			
Physical therapist	Plans and implements a plan of action to enable the client to have maximum use of his or her body.	Four-year program	What is the client's physical therapy treatment plan?
Physical therapy assistant	Implements the plan of action detailed by the physical therapist.	Two-year program	Show me the best way to get the client into a chair.
Occupational Therapy			
Occupational therapist	Assists clients to resume activities of daily living. This could include helping the client learn new ways to dress, feed, and reenter the workforce.	Four-year program	What is the occupational therapy plan of care for the client?
Occupational assistant (certified)	Will provide help to the client as planned by the occupational therapist.	Two-year program	Please show me how the client should put on his shirt.
Environmental Services			
Housekeeping, maintenance	After a client is discharged, the room is cleaned by housekeeping before another person can be admitted to the room. The maintenance person keeps the physical structure of the building in good repair.	On-the-job training	Let me show you the area that needs to be cleaned (or repaired).

give this information to the physical therapy department so that treatments will not be scheduled after meals.

PRACTICAL APPLICATIONS

An x-ray department of a major hospital was having problems with timeliness of the x-rays done in the department. The method for inpatient x-rays was as follows: the unit clerk or nurse entered the client order for an x-ray into the computer. The computer asked for the type of x-ray and whether it should be done in the x-ray department or via a portable x-ray machine. If the client needed to come to the department, the unit clerk or nurse listed how the client should be transported to the department (ambulatory, wheelchair, or stretcher). At the appropriate time, a transporter would bring the indicated transport device to the unit to bring the person to the x-ray department.

The clients were frequently not in the x-ray department until a few minutes after their scheduled times. Most clients were at least 15 minutes late for their x-rays. This was throwing the x-ray schedule off for the rest of the day.

1. What could the nursing staff do to eliminate this problem?
2. Who would need to be included in the decision-making process to eliminate this problem?
3. What would happen if improved communication occurred between the x-ray department and the nursing staff?

(The answers appear at the end of the chapter.)

REFERENCES

American Medical Association. (1994). Report to the board of trustees: Medication errors in hospitals. Resolution 512, I-93.

Burns, L., Andersen, R., & Shortell, S. (1993). Trends in hospital/physician relationships. *Health Affairs, 12*(3), 212–213.

Carson, W. (1994, March). What you should know about physician verbal orders. *The American Nurse,* 30–31.

Cohen M. (1991, June). Why good communication is so important. *Nursing '91,* 18.

Havens, D., & Mills, M. (1992). Staff nurse empowerment: Current status and future projections. *Nursing Administration Quarterly, 16*(3), 58–64.

Iyer, P. (1991, June). Thirteen charting rules to keep you legally safe. *Nursing '91,* 40–44.

MacKay R. (1991). Communication problems between doctors and nurses. *Quality Assurance in Health Care, 3*(1), 11–19.

Makadon, H. (1985). Nurses and physicians: Prospects for collaboration. *Annals of Internal Medicine, 103,* 134–135.

Manisses Communication Group. (1990, Dec 8). Get ready for more nurse-physician conflict. *Brown University Long-Term Care Letter,* 3.

Montgomery, C. (1987, February). Taming a tyrant. *American Journal of Nursing,* 234–238.

Nursing '91 Editorial Staff. (1991, June). The nurse-doctor game. *Nursing '91,* 60–64.

Prescott, P., & Bowen, S. (1985). Physician-nurse relationships. *Annals of Internal Medicine, 103,* 127–133.

Tammelleo, D. (1992, August). Speak up! When silence is negligence. *RN,* 63.

Tammelleo, D. (1993, October). Staying out of trouble on the telephone. *RN,* 63–64.

Tannen, D. (1990). *You just don't understand. Women and men in conversation.* New York: Ballantine Books.

Trudeau, S. (1994, January). The law adds force to your voice. *RN,* 65–68.

Weinfield, R., & Donohue, M. (1989). *Communicating like a manager.* Baltimore: Williams & Wilkins.

ANSWERS TO THE PRACTICAL APPLICATIONS

1. What could the nursing staff do to eliminate this problem?
Communicate more effectively with the x-ray department.

2. Who would need to be included in the decision-making process to eliminate this problem?

The nurses, unit secretary, transport personnel, and x-ray personnel.

3. What would happen if improved communication occurred between the x-ray department and the nursing staff?

The x-rays would be done during their scheduled time. This would decrease wait time and thus increase client satisfaction with the efficiency of the institution.

Discussion

A meeting consisting of the nurses, aides, unit secretary, transport people, and x-ray personnel was held.

It was discovered that the person entering the client order into the computer often stated an inappropriate form of client transport. An average of 41 minutes of transporter time per day was wasted because of an incorrect mode of transport listed in the computer. For example, the computer printout said that Aaron Romicyck could come to the x-ray department in a wheelchair. The x-ray department transporter brought a wheelchair to the nursing unit, but discovered that Mr. Romicyck was comatose and unable to sit in a wheelchair. The transporter had to go back to the x-ray department to take the wheelchair back and bring a stretcher to the nursing unit. It also took longer to place the client onto a stretcher than to get the client into a wheelchair. This made Mr. Romicyck late for his x-ray.

A meeting was held to try to determine solutions to this problem. It was decided that the unit clerks and nurses would continue to show the x-ray transport method in the computer but the unit clerks were to validate modes of transportation with the nursing staff before they put it into the computer. When the client's condition changed, the mode of transport was changed in the computer.

A follow-up study was done to see if the improved communication equated to fewer late x-rays. The late x-ray problem was cut by two thirds.

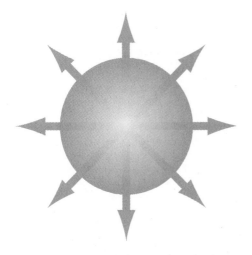

12

With Potential Employers

In this chapter, we will discuss:

- Assessing your needs versus your desires
- Assessing the job market
- Knowing how to interview appropriately
- Knowing what to do after the interview

Probably the most important objective of nursing students, besides passing their nursing courses and boards, is finding a job in the nursing profession after graduation. But, how do you find a nursing job? And even more importantly, how do you find a nursing position that really suits your abilities and your needs?

Well, it helps to determine the specific kind of nursing job you want and to develop a plan to obtain it. Using a plan will considerably improve your chances of obtaining the nursing position you really want. The sooner you begin thinking about this, the more prepared you will be when you finally do graduate and begin job hunting.

In this chapter, we will examine ways to learn what types of nursing jobs are out there and which ones may be right for you. Then we will discuss written communication with potential employers (such as how to write a resume and cover letter) and then move on to verbal communication (such as how to express yourself during the job interview).

Consider This Scenario

In this scenario, a soon-to-graduate student nurse determines where she wants to work after graduation.

Angie Sikarski was in the final semester of her nursing program. Although she had a good grade point average and excellent clinical nursing skills, she was very nervous about searching for a job after graduation. She worried that perhaps the hospitals want nurses younger than she was, or maybe people with more job experience. Although Angie worked as a housecleaning aide for many years before she went to nursing school, she didn't have any experience in the medical field. "How will I ever compete with these younger graduates who have worked as nurse's aides?" she thought.

As graduation drew closer, Angie began to think frequently about a job. Because she felt so overwhelmed by all of the possibilities, she listed her needs and desires, and then drew up a list of what she might find in the ideal nursing job. The box lists what she found.

Angie's Ideal Nursing Job

Needs	Desires
Full-time job	Part-time work until children are out of grade school
Health care benefits paid by employer	
Work any shift	Work day shift
Any nursing unit	Surgical nursing unit
Any type of institution	Hospital
Pay at least $15.00 per hour	Pay as much as possible

Angie thought that her need for a full-time nursing position with health care benefits was the most vital issue. She would like to work the day shift, but she knew that she would need to consider other shifts because she really needed a job. The hospitals in the area were her first choice, and then she would consider the extended care facilities.

Although Angie was overwhelmed by the task of finding a suitable nursing position after graduation, she started her job search in a systematic way: first she assessed her needs versus her desires.

In the next section, we will look at how to decide exactly what you are looking for in your job search.

Assessment

Many people might define the ideal job as one in which they are respected, perform well, and receive appropriate rewards for their labor. But each person's idea of what makes up an excellent job is different. How do you select one position over another?

One way to start is to consider your *needs* versus your *desires,* just as Angie

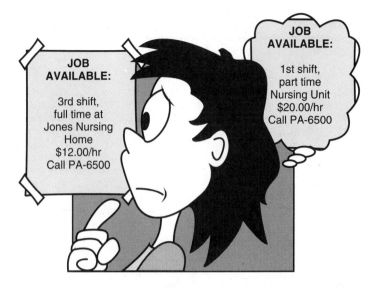

did in the scenario. The *needs* are the things that you (and your family) simply must have to survive. The *desires* are the things you (and your family) would like to have if you were given the choice—items that would be nice to have but you can do without them. Of course, each person's *needs* and *desires* are unique. What is a vital *need* to one person might be a frivolous *desire* to another. Even though you probably could live without meeting your *desires,* it would be more pleasant to have a job include some *desires* along with the things that you simply must have.

What Are Your Needs Versus Your Desires? (Table 12–1)

What type of institution do you want to work for? Hospitals, extended care facilities, industrial locations, and home care agencies are but a few of the places that hire nurses. Traditionally, it was suggested that graduate nurses work in a hospital for a year or two on a medical-surgical nursing unit before taking a position in home care or extended care. Although it is great to gain medical-surgical experience upon graduation, you have to consider your options. You might prefer the arena of home care nursing over that of hospital-based care. If you are unsure of what to do, visit each type of organization and ask questions.

Do you need full-time employment or can you work part time? If you need full-time employment, and no full-time positions are available, consider taking a part-time position anyway. In many institutions, part-time nurses can work additional hours, and if a full-time position becomes available, they are frequently offered the position first. You might also consider working several part-time positions to equal one full-time position. Remember, though, that this can be confusing, and many employers may not want to work around your schedule at another institution.

Do you need health care benefits? Usually this type of benefit is given only to full-time employees. However, many institutions offer health care benefits for part-time employees, perhaps at a reduced rate.

What type of pay do you expect to receive? Although everyone would like to

Table 12–1 FACTORS TO CONSIDER IN SELECTING A NURSING POSITION

Locale
  Region
  Urban, suburban, rural, remote
Type of institution
  Non-profit, for profit, parochial
  Health care sites: major medical center, local hospital, full service or limited service
    hospital, outpatient clinic, extended care facility, hospice, rehabilitation center
  Non-health care sites: non-profit agency (American Red Cross, Diabetes Association,
    Heart Association), industry, elementary/high school, military, home care
  Size (by number of beds, number of services offered, number of clients seen daily)
Type of nursing activity
  Adult, pediatric, geriatric, obstetric
  Medical, surgical (inpatient or ambulatory), post anesthesia care unit (PACU), surgery,
    emergency, intensive care, critical or cardiac care unit (CCU), mental health
  System/disorder specialty (cardiac, orthopedic, cancer, AIDS)
  Inpatient, outpatient
  Administrative: supervision, staff development, patient advocacy/education
Type of employment
  Full time, regular part-time, intermittent (on-call) part time
  Day shift (7 A.M. to 3 P.M.), afternoon shift (3 P.M. to 11 P.M.), night shift (11 P.M. to 7 A.M.)
  Rotating shifts
  Eight-hour shifts, 12-hour shifts
  Weekdays only, weekends only, combination
Other personal variables in your decision
  Do you need health care benefits?
  What pay range are you willing to settle for?
  Do you want to work for an institution that has union representation?
  Will you require child care? Does the institution offer child care?

receive more money, you need to be realistic. Most institutions have pay ranges for their nursing employees, and you will be coming in at a certain level with an expected pay range. Some employers pay more than others, but usually similar institutions within a geographic area pay competitive wages.

Do you want to work in an institution that has union representation? There are advantages and disadvantages to union representation. Some people believe that a union helps to ensure that all employees are treated equally. Other people believe that professionals such as nurses should not be members of unions. This is an issue that you will have to consider.

On what type of nursing unit would you like to work? Adult, child, critical care, medical, surgical, obstetric, or mental health? What was your favorite area of your clinical rotations? Think about working on that type of unit. Some graduates worry that they will be "locked" into whatever unit they begin on. This is far from the truth. Wherever you begin your career as a nurse, you can always use the experiences you gain.

Which nursing shift would you like to work? The ideal work time is different for everyone. Someone who hates to wake up with the shrill cry of an alarm clock might like to work the afternoon or evening shift. The day or midnight shift might work out better for people with children. Some units have rotational shifts, i.e., 3 weeks on day shift and 1 week on an afternoon shift. Would you be able to do

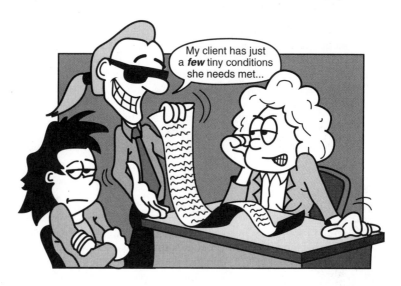

this? Before you answer, consider child care issues, your ability to sleep at different times, and the alterations to your personal schedule.

Would you like to work in a large hospital or a small one? Although large institutions usually have more opportunities for different positions, smaller institutions liken themselves to a "family." For example, if you want to work in a full-service cardiac surgery facility, it is unlikely that this will be found in a small hospital. Which of these types of hospitals has the type of nursing units that interest you?

Should the institution be located in an inner-city, suburban, or rural area? Of course, each type of location has its positive and negative attributes. Inner-city locations will frequently feature a trauma unit, which means you might gain much experience with critically ill individuals. Suburban locations might offer more pleasant surroundings than their inner-city counterparts. Rural locations will offer challenges because of the lack of ready support systems. You might be one of three nurses working on a given shift in a rural location. To help you select a location, remember to factor in driving time and safety issues.

After you have assessed your feelings regarding your future nursing position, it is time to find out what nursing positions are open.

The Job Market

What kinds of jobs are out there? Or perhaps the better question is, are there any jobs out there? The number of nursing positions varies with economy, concerns about health care reform, and the evolution from hospital-based health care to community-based health care. Many students go into nursing with the expectation that they will work in a hospital after graduation. This may not be the case. Many graduates are taking first-time positions in home care, industrial nursing, and extended care facilities.

What Is the Institution Looking for in an Employee?

Many nurse recruiters will tell you that the number one quality that *any* new employee should have is the ability to be flexible. This is especially important because the health care system is in a state of evolution. As the institution evolves, it needs its employees to evolve along with it. An institution will not want to hire you if you have a very limited focus and refuse to learn anything else.

Another important factor to consider is whether you meet the minimum qualifications. For example, a home care agency was looking for a nurse to work with home-based peritoneal dialysis clients. The minimum requirement for the position was 2 years of experience as a dialysis nurse, yet many applicants had never worked with dialysis clients. Therefore, they were not even considered for the position. If you do not meet the minimum requirements, do not apply for the position.

How Can You Find Out Where the Jobs Are?

To begin with, it is important to find out which institutions are currently hiring. It just does not make sense to spend a lot of time courting an employer that isn't currently hiring. If you need to get a job in a reasonably short timeframe, you must concentrate your search on those institutions that have open positions. Of course, if you are very specific about the nursing position you require, consider such an institution although it currently does not have any open positions. Do recognize, though, that while this method may get you the job you desire, you may have to wait to get it.

What Are Some Ways Institutions Communicate Their Job Openings?

One of the most common ways for any employer to indicate job openings is through newspaper advertisements. In fact, in many institutions, job openings *must* be listed in the paper. Get the newspaper for the geographic area and scan the ads, especially in the Sunday paper. The ad will list the job, minimum qualifications, and any specifics about the position.

Another method institutions use to advertise their positions is the job board located within the facility. This is a board that shows available positions within the institution. This board is usually in a conspicuous place, perhaps near the main lobby or cafeteria. Make it a point to locate the job board the next time you are in the institution.

You might hear of job openings via word of mouth. An especially good way to hear of job openings is to talk to the nurse manager during the end of your clinical rotations. Another way is to phone the health care institutions in your area and ask if they have job openings.

Also consider ads in nursing journals. They can be very helpful for an out-of-town job search.

If you are looking for a specialty position in nursing, consider attending the national conventions for the particular interest. For example, if you are looking for a position in an emergency department of a large trauma center, it could be very helpful to attend a conference for trauma nurses. Many nurse recruiters attend these conferences.

You may at times be discouraged, but try to remember that there is a job out there for you, very likely one that suits you perfectly. You will have to go out there and find it.

Plan

Potential Employers

After you have assessed your needs and those of the job market, it is time to take action! By now you should have a list of what you want in a job and what jobs are out there. To help you narrow your job search, visit each possible employer. The goal of this visit is to do a critical analysis and check out the attributes of the employer. This process can be as complex or as simple as you want it to be. Call the nurse recruiter and tell him or her that you would like to visit the institution. The nurse recruiter might offer to accompany you or perhaps will tell you to go by yourself. Bring a notebook to record your observations, and wear comfortable walking shoes.

Walk around the place. Look at the people who are working there. Stop and talk to some of them, especially the nurses. Do the employees feel that it is a good place to work? Stop in an empty client room. Does it look clean and well maintained? Is the institutional security adequate? If you could walk around the institution unnoticed for a length of time, perhaps the security needs improvement. Notice how the nurses and physicians interact. Are their voice levels appropriate or are they speaking in angry voices with each other?

Another method to use to compare institutions would be to go to the office of a large newspaper in the area. Many newspapers keep an index of all their articles. It might be helpful to look in the index to see what has been written about the local hospitals in the past year. Are they having fiscal problems, starting new programs, engaging in important research, hiring, or laying off? Are they having a crime wave in their geographic area? Do they have a history of labor problems?

You could also ask your instructors about possible job sites. They probably are very familiar with the institutions and might have good information for you.

If you have further questions about an institution, consult with its human resources department. Remember, though, that employees probably will not say unfavorable things about their own institution.

After all this research, compare the institutions against your list of needs and desires. How do they measure up? If one is adequate, you might want to apply for a job.

What Is the Actual Process of Applying for a Job?

In many institutions, it goes like this: You fill out an application. A human resources employee looks it over and decides whether you fit the minimum qualifications for any position currently available or available in the future. If you fit the minimum qualifications, you will be contacted via telephone or in writing and asked to come for an interview. The first interview is usually with the nurse recruiter or human resources representative. This interview serves as an initial screening to determine your suitability to the institution. You might have a second interview with the nurse manager or with nursing staff members. This interview is to determine suitability for the specific nursing position. Sometimes this interview involves more than one interviewer.

The human resources department will check on your references and the validity of your nursing license. If the interview, references, and nursing license are acceptable, you might be offered a job. If you accept, you are asked to undergo a physical exam. If the exam results are acceptable, you may be hired.

The Scenario Continues

Ms. Sikarski began to develop her resume. She was told that she needed one, but deep inside she thought that it was a waste of time because the hospital had a job application. It had all the information they would need on it, didn't it? She called GetWell Medical Center and they sent her an application. Just as she was finishing it, her son spilled his breakfast cereal on it. But after she wiped it off it looked OK, so off it went in the mail. After she mailed it, she realized that she had forgotten to include the resume, so she mailed it separately. A few days later, she received a phone call from the nurse recruiter at GetWell Medical Center. They wanted to interview her! A date was set up for the following Thursday.

During the week, Angie tried on her clothes to decide what she would wear to the interview. She wanted to look her best. Finding an interview outfit was not an easy task because she had gained 30 pounds while in nursing school, and none of her nice clothes fit. She tried on her entire wardrobe, and she came up with a pair of slacks and a sweater that did not look too bad. She remembered that she had worn a similar outfit for her interview with the manager of the bookstore where she currently worked. Angie debated wearing makeup to the interview. Although she did not normally wear it, she thought that it might be expected of her and so she put some on.

Because she had never been to GetWell Medical Center for her clinical rotations, she was not really sure where it was. On the way, she missed the freeway exit and got lost. The appointment was for 10:00 a.m., but at 9:55 she was still trying to find a parking place. She had no idea that parking would be so hard to find because there were no parking problems at the hospitals where she had done her clinical rotations. Angie ran through the door of the human resources department at exactly 10:00 a.m. sharp!

She had not quite caught her breath when the nurse recruiter came out to greet her. "Hello, I am Phyllis White, the nurse recruiter for GetWell Medical Center. I take it that you are Angie Sikarski." Angie said that she was.

"Angie, will you come with me, please."

As they walked toward Phyllis's office, Angie said, "The parking here is really bad. Why don't you improve it?" Phyllis said that this was being considered. Angie sat when they came to the office.

"Boy, I am tired! Nursing school is really hard. They make you write all of these care plans, which will never be used anyway. I can't wait until I get out of there!"

"Angie," asked Mrs. White, "can you tell me why you want to work at GetWell?"

"Well, I hear that you pay really well and that you need nurses," replied Angie.

"OK, tell me what positions are you interested in?"

"Oh, I don't care, I need a job so I'll take anything you have that is full-time. And, by the way, I don't want to rotate shifts or work midnights or evening shifts. I have little kids, so I want to work the day shift."

"Angie, we currently don't have any day shift positions available. I'll contact you if a suitable position does become available for you. Thank you for your time." Ms. White stood up and indicated that the interview was over.

As Angie walked down the hall, she was puzzled. "Boy, that sure was a short interview. I feel like I wasted my time."

What went wrong here? Many things! In the next section we will look at how Angie *should* have communicated with her potential employer. We will examine the aspects of:

- Job application forms
- Writing a resume
- Writing a cover letter

Implementation

Job Application Form

There are two basic ways to obtain a job application: call the nurse recruiter and ask for one to be mailed to you or go to the institution and fill one out. No matter how you get the application, ask for two copies in case you make a mistake when filling it out.

At the top of the form, there are usually instructions on how to fill it out. It is vital to do this correctly. Employers are looking for people who know how to follow instructions. Use a blue or black ink pen to fill out the form, and be very neat. Keep the job application clean. If you have poor handwriting, type the form or ask someone else to fill it out for you. (Of course, you must sign it yourself.) Do not fold or staple the application. Because first impressions are important, make sure that everything is spelled correctly. Fill in all appropriate spaces and be sure the information is correct. If a section does not pertain to you, write N/A (not applicable) in the area. Do not leave any areas blank.

If you plan on filling out the application at the institution, take your work history, education history, and names of references with their addresses, telephone numbers, and other pertinent information. Much of this information will be available on your resume, so take a copy of it with you.

Develop a Resume

To begin with, what is a resume? A resume (sometimes called a curriculum vitae) is your introduction to potential employers. It tells the employer who you are, what you have accomplished, and what you would like to do in the future. Because there may be a great number of applicants for nursing positions, your resume must sell you as an excellent job candidate or you may not get the chance to interview with the nurse recruiter for the institution.

You might wonder if you need a resume because many institutions also have a generic job application that is used by all applicants. But remember that you will be applying for a position as a professional nurse. As a professional, you need to also submit a resume besides the job application. Preparing your resume will allow you to organize and analyze your assets and liabilities according to the kind of job you want.

Your resume needs to be written in a concise, logical format. It should be typed and professionally printed on white or light-colored paper. The resume should look conservative. This is not the time to let your personality show through with unusual type styles or paper colors.

The length of the resume should be one page if possible. Many students are tempted to list all the skills they have learned in nursing school, but this is unnecessary because nurse recruiters know the skills taught in nursing school.

It is essential that everything listed on the resume be the truth. Do not make the mistake of stretching the truth to cover up a perceived "hole" in your back-

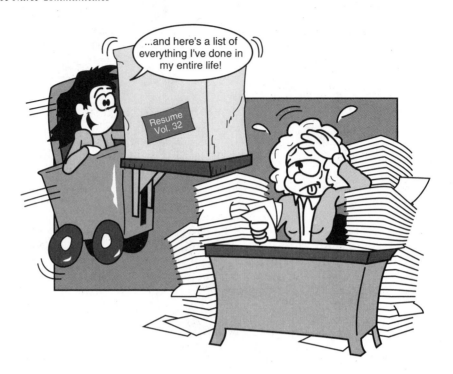

ground. Falsifying information on a job application or resume is grounds for dismissal.

To develop your resume, it is helpful to first collect the information you will need and then consider what type of format to use. Table 12–2 shows the six basic sections of a resume.

There are two basic types of resumes: chronological and functional (see boxes). The chronological resume is arranged by listing the most recent job experience first. This type of resume is useful for a person with a continuous work record. If you have any lapses in employment or your experience is limited, this type of resume may not be the best for you to use.

The functional resume is designed to highlight work experience according to areas of skill. This type of resume is best for persons with varied work backgrounds or accomplishments. It can be very helpful when you are showing how your background experience will contribute toward a job in a different field.

After you have decided which format to use for your resume, write a rough draft of it. Then critique the rough draft. Will it fit onto one page? Does it really give the picture of you that you want it to give?

If you need further help with writing a resume, consider going to the career center at your college or asking an instructor for help. Another source of help would be the college's English or business faculty. They have experience writing resumes.

After you have a resume that you think accurately represents you, have it typed and professionally printed. This can usually be done inexpensively at the student services center within your college. Have several copies of the resume made, because you may need to give them to several people within each institution at

Example of a Chronological Resume

Angela Marie Sikarski
1366 Westgate Drive
Melvindale, Michigan 48665
(808) 385-2296

JOB OBJECTIVE	Entry-level staff nurse position
EDUCATION	LearnMore Community College, 8378 Education Avenue, Melvindale, MI. Associate Degree in Nursing. Expected graduation December 1996. Grade point average 3.4.
WORK EXPERIENCE	LearnMore Community College Bookstore, 8378 Education Avenue, Melvindale, MI. (808) 774-3522. Cashier, 1993–present. Supervisor—Evelyn Walker. Assist customers, run cash register, stock shelves.
	Clean-House Inc., 934 Blenda St., Westlawn, MI. (808) 377-3580. House cleaning personnel, 1978–1993. Supervisor—Helen Malek. Cleaned houses for customers.
ACTIVITIES/SPECIAL SKILLS	Able to work without direct supervision
	Speak conversational Spanish
	Know several word processing programs
REFERENCES	Available upon request

which you are interviewing. (Decide at how many institutions you will interview and multiply this number by three or four.) It is frequently cheaper to have many copies made at once than several batches of a few copies.

Each copy must look professional. Don't make the mistake of using poorly made copies. If the resume looks sloppy, this will reflect upon you.

Write a Cover Letter

A cover letter is a business letter that will accompany your job application and resume (see box). Like your resume, the cover letter must have perfect spelling and grammar. It should look professionally typed, be no more than one page long, and be printed on white or light-colored paper.

Cover letters should be written in a business-letter style. At the top of the page put the date and the name and address of the person to whom the letter is going, usually the nurse recruiter or human resources director. Call the institution and ask for the name of the appropriate person. Make sure you have it spelled correctly.

The first paragraph of the letter should state that you are applying for a position within the institution and give a brief comment on why you are looking for a new nursing position. Examples of this could be, "I am moving to your area" or "I just finished nursing school and am looking for an entry-level position."

The next paragraph or two should detail your qualifications for the position. This might include your educational level and your work experience.

The last paragraph states your plan of action, such as calling the nurse recruiter

Example of a Functional Resume

Angela Marie Sikarski
1366 Westgate Drive
Melvindale, Michigan 48665
(808) 385-2296

JOB OBJECTIVE	Entry-level staff nurse position
ACTIVITIES/SPECIAL SKILLS	SUPERVISION Clean-House Inc. Monitored daily work of a cleaning employee EVALUATION Monthly evaluation of employee RECORD KEEPING Keep inventory of bookstore SKILLS Speak conversational Spanish Know several word processing programs
WORK EXPERIENCE	LearnMore Community College Bookstore, 8378 Education Avenue, Melvindale, MI. (808) 774-3522. Cashier, 1993–present. Supervisor—Evelyn Walker. Assist customers, run cash register, stock shelves. Clean-House Inc., 934 Blenda St., Westlawn, MI. (808) 377-3580. House cleaning personnel, 1978–1993.
EDUCATION	LearnMore Community College, 8378 Education Avenue, Melvindale, MI. Associate Degree in Nursing. Expected graduation December 1996. Grade point average 3.4.
REFERENCES	Available upon request

for an appointment. Your name, address, and telephone number should be at the bottom of the letter.

Preparing for the Interview

After the human resources department has looked over your application and resume and determined that you meet the minimum qualifications for the position, they will contact you for an initial interview.

Because interviewing is a learned skill, you might want to rank the institutions you are considering and interview at your least likely position first. By doing this, you will increase your chances of doing a polished interview at the institution of your choice.

It is really vital to be prepared for the interview. Before the day of the interview, it is important to find out some basic information about the institution. This information will help you to decide if you and the institution will be a "good fit" for each other. The following information can easily be obtained from the secretary in the human resources office.

- Type of institution (nonprofit, for-profit)
- Size of the institution (for hospitals and nursing homes, this would be the number of beds they have)
- Focus of the institution: trauma center, general hospital, etc.
- Number of nursing positions
- Directions and parking locations

The Interview

Because first impressions are so vital, it is very important to dress appropriately for the interview. When you are applying for a position as a professional nurse, you must dress in a professional manner during the interview. The key to appropriate

Table 12–2 WHAT TO INCLUDE IN YOUR RESUME

Heading

Include:
    Full name
    Complete address (include home address if you are a college student)
    Telephone number (home and work)

Job Objective

This should describe the job that you are applying for. An example: "Entry-level staff nurse
    position"

Education/Training

Start with the highest education first, then list the others. Usually you do not need to go
    back further than high school. Include:
    Name and address of the college
    Graduation date
    Degrees
    Grade point average (if better-than-average grades)
    Any education or training related to the job

Work Experience

Start with your most recent job, then list the others. Include full-time and part-time
    employment and volunteer work. Include:
    Names and addresses of employers
    Job title
    Dates of employment
    Supervisor's name
    Duties and responsibilities

Activities/Capabilities

This tells the employer what you bring to the job above your education and work
    experience. Include:
    Personal accomplishments (club awards, computer knowledge, ability to speak a foreign
        language)
    Awards and honors received
    Activities that indicate job-related skills such as organization and leadership

References

State that references are available on request. Use former instructors, employers, or
    someone familiar with your skills. (Make sure that you ask people *before* you include
    their names as references.)

Cover Letter

December 9, 1996

Ms. Phyllis White
Nurse Recruiter
GetWell Medical Center
1189 Health Avenue
Westgate, Michigan 48455

Dear Ms. White,

As you can see from my attached resume, I am nearing completion of my Associate Degree in Nursing curriculum at LearnMore College. I would like to apply for a position as a Graduate Nurse/Registered Nurse within your institution.

I have really enjoyed my nursing education and have been able to maintain a grade point average of 3.4 despite working full time during nursing school. In addition, I have excellent references from prior employers.

I feel that I will be well suited to your institution.

I will be calling you in two weeks for a possible appointment. Thank you for your consideration.

Sincerely,

Angela M. Sikarski
1366 Westgate Drive
Melvindale, Michigan 48665
(808) 385-2296

clothing for a nursing interview is to dress conservatively. The ideal interview outfit for both men and women is a dark-colored suit. However, for men a pair of dark pants and a shirt and tie are acceptable. Women could wear a dress or skirt and blouse that are suitable for an office. Skirt lengths should be to the knee or below.

For both men and women, it is very important to look neat and tidy. To do this, clothes should be pressed before the interview. Make sure that your clothes fit correctly. They should not be too tight or too loose. The styling should be conventional, no bright colors or loud patterns. Women should use no more than a moderate amount of makeup and perfume. It would be better to use too little makeup and perfume than to use too much. Hair should be styled in a business-like fashion.

If you wonder whether your interview outfit is appropriate, ask for help from a person who dresses in a conservative fashion. Try on your outfit for that person and ask his or her opinion. It is important to spend time to develop an appropriate interview outfit. Practice sitting and standing in it to check for ease of movement and how the outfit flows with different postures.

What should you bring to the interview? It would be good to bring two copies

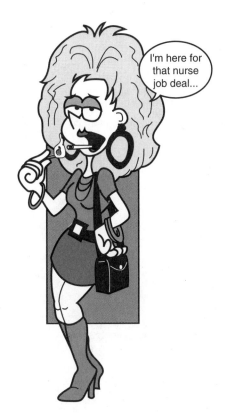

of your nursing license or proof of graduation (copy of the diploma will do) and several letters of reference from prior nursing instructors, nurse managers, or employers. One of the copies is for the interviewer and one is for you. Although the institution will still have to determine the validity of your nursing license or college completion and check your references, bringing these materials with you to the first interview may save weeks of time. Several nurse recruiters said that if they are considering two job applicants with equal backgrounds and one brings these materials, then the more-prepared applicant would have a better chance of being offered the position. Coming to the interview prepared says something about your organizational skills.

These materials should be put into a manila file folder and placed in a briefcase if possible. If you don't have a briefcase, just bring them in a manila folder. Leave large handbags at home.

What should you *not* bring to the interview? The answer: Your children. The interview is a chance for the interviewer to get to know you, not your children. Bringing them gives the impression that you might have problems with child care and may not be a reliable employee.

Plan to arrive about 15 minutes before your interview time. This will give you time to use the restroom and gain your composure before the big moment. While in the restroom, comb your hair and check to see that your clothes look tidy. If you are chewing gum, now is the time to get rid of it. Do not smoke. While you are waiting, take a few deep breaths to help yourself remain calm.

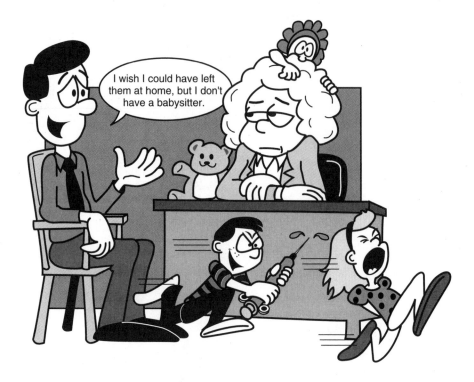

If you cannot arrive early, at least be on time! Coming late for your interview is an absolute turn-off for any nurse recruiter who would then wonder about your ability to be on time for work.

The interview process has several stages. The first stage is simply a "get acquainted" time. The interviewer will come to the waiting area and greet you. Stand up, look them in the eye, and greet them with a friendly smile. Say "hello" and introduce yourself. "Hello, I am Angie Sikarski." Offer your hand for a handshake.

Most likely, the interviewer will ask you to come into his or her office. When in the office, remain standing until asked to sit. The interviewer might ask you if you would like a cup of coffee or soda. It is perfectly fine to accept or decline, as you wish. If you are very nervous, perhaps you should decline the offer. Otherwise, you might spill it!

During the next stage of the interview, the nurse recruiter will ask you some basic questions. Practice active listening before answering anything. If you do not understand or did not hear the question, ask the interviewer to repeat it. Think carefully before answering.

There are some basic questions that your interviewer is likely to ask (Table 12–3). Before the interview, practice answering these questions until you feel comfortable doing so. Remember that all questions should be answered in a positive tone. One of the most common questions a nurse recruiter will ask is: "What type of position are you looking for?" Because many nursing students have "getting a job" as the primary goal, they might answer, "Any position you have open." What the student means is that he or she will accept any job offered, but the nurse recruiter might take this comment to mean the student is desperate for a job. A

Table 12–3   WHAT ARE SOME COMMON QUESTIONS ASKED DURING AN INTERVIEW BY NURSE RECRUITERS?

Question	Good Answer	Poor Answer
Why are you leaving your present job?	I would like to have increased job advancement that is not possible with my current job.	I don't like the people I work with. They are jerks.
What position are you interested in?	I would like to be considered for a surgical nursing unit, but I am open to other areas.	Anything that you have open. I need a job real bad.
What is it about you that will make you successful with us in this position?	I get along well with others and think I will really enjoy being a nurse here.	I don't know of anything.
What is your educational background?	I have an associate's degree in nursing from LearnMore College.	Just an associate's degree.
What types of work experiences have you had?	I've worked at the college bookstore for 3 years and at a cleaning service for 12 years. I have excellent references from both.	As a cashier and as a maid.
Of all the candidates we will interview for this position, tell me why you will stand out in our minds.	I have always been an excellent worker in every job I have had. I know that I will be an excellent nurse, and I would like the opportunity to demonstrate this to you.	I don't know. I can't even think of an answer.

better way of responding would be to discuss your ideal position but to include that you are open to other positions.

Consider the questions in Table 12–3 and read over the sample answers. Try to develop your own set of answers for each question. Practice answering them before a mirror or by asking a friend or other nursing student to be the interviewer.

The third phase of the interview occurs when the interviewer asks you if you have any questions about the job or the institution. Asking intelligent, well–thought-out questions suggests to the interviewer that you have given serious consideration to the job and its requirements. For a list of suggested questions to ask an interviewer, see the box.

Questions to Ask Interviewer

1. What types of positions are currently available?
2. Can you tell me some of the specific skills you would like to see in a person hired into this position?
3. What types of clients are on the nursing unit?
4. What management style is used on the nursing unit?
5. What are the usual hours for the shift?
6. What is the usual staffing ratio for the shift?
7. Can you tell me a little bit about the people with whom I might be working?
8. Does this unit have a higher turnover rate than other units of the institution?
9. May I have a copy of the job description?

Close this segment of the interview by asking whether the interviewer has any further questions of you. Perhaps the interviewer has questions about something you have said. If you don't take this chance to clarify things, the interviewer might walk away with an incorrect impression of you.

The fourth phase of the interview occurs after both you and the interviewer have answered each other's questions. At this time, decisions are made. For the nurse recruiter the question is: Is this person suitable for the position? For you the question is: Would I want to work here?

At the close of the interview, the nurse recruiter will probably tell you what the next step of the process is. You may need to interview with another person. They might need to wait for your references to be supplied, or others might need to be interviewed before the interviewer can decide on the best candidate for the position. Whatever the case, the recruiter will indicate when you will next hear from the institution. If the interviewer does not offer this information, ask for it. Do not call back until after this time has passed.

While you are waiting to hear from them, send a brief thank-you note to the interviewers. This is a nice touch that keeps your name in an interviewer's mind.

Rerun of the Scenario—The CORRECT Way!

In this scenario, the student nurse develops her resume, obtains an interview, and makes a great impression on the interviewer.

Ms. Sikarski began to develop her resume. She knew that she needed one, and was

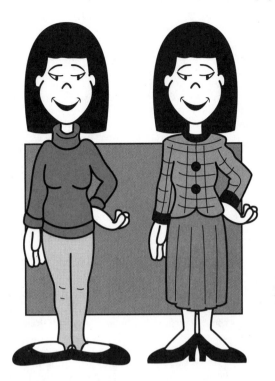

concerned about this because she had never prepared one before. She went to the career center at the college, and they helped her to write the resume. Her friend had a computer with a laser printer and together they were able to print a professional resume. Angie took a copy of the resume to her instructor who critiqued it. Angie made the appropriate changes and printed 10 copies of the corrected resume.

Angie heard that GetWell Medical Center was hiring, so she called and asked them to send her two copies of their application. Just as she was finishing the first one, her son spilled his breakfast cereal on it. She was glad that she had a spare, and she completed it and sent it along with her resume. A few days later, she received a phone call from the nurse recruiter at GetWell Medical Center. They wanted to interview her! A date was set up for the following Thursday.

During the week, Angie tried on her clothes to decide what she would wear to the interview. She wanted to look her best. Finding an interview outfit was not an easy task because she had gained 30 pounds while in nursing school, and none of her nice clothes fit. She tried on her entire wardrobe, and she came up with a pair of slacks and a sweater that did not look too bad. But she knew that this was not appropriate for the interview. She did not know what to do. She did not have the money to buy new clothes, yet she did not have anything suitable to wear. Then it occurred to her that her sister might have something that would be suitable. Together, they found a dress for Angie to wear. It was not new, but Angie made sure that it was clean and pressed. Angie's sister suggested that she wear makeup to the interview. Because she did not normally wear it, Angie decided not to do so. She was afraid that it would not be applied correctly and she might look odd.

Because she had never been to GetWell Medical Center for her clinical rotations, she was not really sure where it was. Two days before the interview, she drove to GetWell Medical Center so she could find it on the big day. On the day of the interview, Angie pulled into the parking lot at 9:30. She could take her time because the interview started at

10:00. When she got to the Human Resources department, she went into the restroom to comb her hair.

At 10:00 the nurse recruiter came out to greet her. "Hello, I am Phyllis White, the nurse recruiter for GetWell Medical Center. I take it that you are Angie Sikarski." Angie stood up and held out her hand. "Hello, I am glad to meet you."

"Angie, will you come with me, please."

As they walked toward Phyllis's office, Angie said, "This is really an attractive building. It is pleasant to have so many flowers outside."

"Oh yes, our gardeners do a fine job with that. Can I get you some coffee?" Angie stood in Phyllis's office until she returned with the coffee. "Angie, you can sit right there if you want." Angie sat down.

"Angie, can you tell me why you want to work at GetWell?"

"Well, I hear that you have a fine reputation as a trauma center and I would like to be a part of that."

"Oh, I see. Tell me, what position are you interested in?"

"Well, I would really like to work in the critical care areas, but I am open to other areas."

"Angie, tell me what your strongest and weakest areas were in nursing school."

"Let me think. The strongest area was in my ability to figure out the important data as opposed to the not-so-important data. The weakest area was in pediatrics. I would really prefer to work with adult clients."

"Angie, I would like you to meet the nurse manager for adult surgical intensive care. Could you come back next Friday at 2 p.m.? By then, I will have had a chance to check on your references."

"Ms. White, I have copies of my college diploma and my references. I know you must have these verified, but I thought they would be helpful to you."

Ms. White said, "Yes, these copies will be helpful. I am impressed and will see you next Friday."

"I'll be here. Is there anything else you would like me to bring?"

"Just yourself. I'll see you then. Thank you for your time."

As Angie walked down the hall, she felt good. The long haul was nearly over. Soon she would have the job she had always wanted. She thought to herself, "I am so glad I learned how to apply for the job!"

Evaluation

The evaluation for this chapter is easy: Were you offered the job that you wanted? Or perhaps several job offers? If you did receive several offers, how should you choose among them? Look at the job offer carefully against your list of needs and desires. Which job best fits into what you see yourself doing in a year or two? You might need to rely on your intuition. Which position gives you the best feelings?

On the other hand, if you don't get a job, you should think about reasons that might have impacted the situation. Although it is very difficult, it might be helpful to call the nurse recruiter and ask for suggestions for improving your interview or resume skills. The key to this is your attitude when calling the nurse recruiter. If you sound angry and defensive, the recruiter probably will not offer you suggestions for improvement. If you are sincere in your desire for self-improvement, then they might provide help.

Remember also that if another person was offered the job instead of you, the other person may be more experienced or may have had more education than you. It doesn't always mean that you did something wrong!

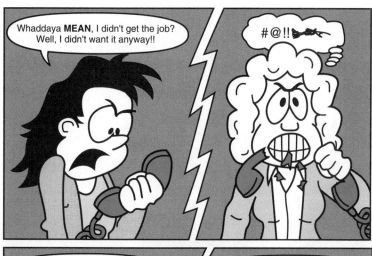

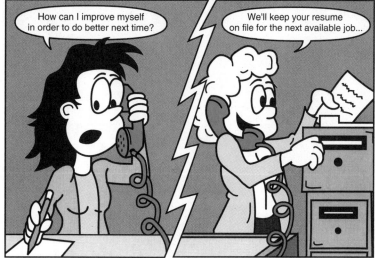

In closing, you can see that nursing school is just the beginning of your adventure in the profession of nursing. Using a planned method for obtaining this position will increase the likelihood of obtaining your dream nursing job. Getting a nursing job that provides you with self-fulfillment and also financial compensation will be worth the efforts that you have made.

PRACTICAL APPLICATIONS

To help narrow your choices in a possible nursing position, fill out this table:

The Ideal Nursing Position	First Choice	Second Choice	Third Choice
Type of institution			
Full- or part-time			
Health care benefits			
Amount of pay			
Union representation			
Type of nursing unit			
Nursing shift			
Large or small hospital			
Inner-city, suburban, or rural			

REFERENCES

Anderson, J. (1992). Tips on resume writing. *Imprint, 39*(1), 30–31.

Cosgray, R., & Hanna, V. (1990). Tips on resume writing. *Imprint, 37*(3), 94–95.

Daniels, C. (1990). *Developing a professional vita or resume.* Garrett Park, MD: Garrett Park Press.

Delta College Career Development and Placement Services. (1992). *Communication! Your key to successful employment.* University Center, MI.

Goodman, J., & Hoppin, J. (1990). *Opening doors: A practical guide for job hunting.* Rochester, MI: Continuum Center, Oakland University.

Fry, R. (1991). *Your first interview.* Hawthorne, NJ: Career Press.

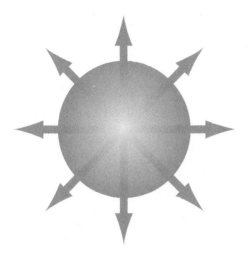

13

Within the Home

In this chapter, we will discuss:

- What home care is
- What does it take to be a home care nurse?
- Differences between home care and the institutional environment
- Common home care communication methods
- Communication difficulties
- Specific environmental issues
- Promoting communication with the client and family members

A major shift is occurring as to the setting/location where we are delivering health care services. In the near future, most of the health care delivered to clients will be provided in their homes and community instead of being delivered in an institutional setting, such as a hospital.

In this chapter, we will look at how communication methods and styles are altered because of the home care setting. To give an understanding of the home care environment, we will discuss common aspects of home care. Then we will consider differences related to home care communication, specific home care communication issues, and methods to promote communication with clients and their family members. Many concepts for communicating in the home care setting are the same as for other settings. For example, treating the client with respect is a universal concept. Reviewing communication concepts in other chapters of the book may be helpful.

What Is Home Care?

There are many definitions of home care, but a general definition is *providing health care assistance to ill clients in their home environment.* Just as in the institutional environment, home care nurses are managers of the client's care. This includes coordinating the care provided by other specialities such as physical therapy, occupational therapy, social work, and speech therapy. The nurse may also be supervising the activities of home health care aides and chore providers. Rehabilitation activities are also supervised.

What Is the Usual Sequence of Events for Home Care?

To begin with, the client must display the need for nursing care. This could occur after hospitalization or simply be the result of the client's chronic condition becoming worse. Clients are also increasingly being referred from physicians' offices.

Besides requiring the services of a nurse, the client must meet the specific requirements of his or her insurance carrier. For example, several requirements must be met for Medicare eligibility. The client must be under the care of a physician and require care that is reasonable and necessary for the medical condition and can be met by intermittent care visits. In addition, the client must be homebound to receive services.

When it is decided that the client will benefit from home nursing care, and the client agrees to such, the physician writes an order for home nursing care. Institutional personnel (usually the discharge planner) contact the home care agency. Once the actual date of client discharge from the hospital is determined, the home care nurse contacts the client to set a time for the first appointment. Usually, during this initial conversation, the home care nurse tells the client that the first visit will last between 1 and 2 hours. During the first visit, the nurse will conduct an extensive history and physical. The plan of care will focus only on priority areas, because many clients have multiple problems. The nurse describes the proposed plan of care to the client and asks the client and family for their ideas. With this information, the nurse, client, and family develop the final plan of care.

At this time, the nurse discusses the responsibilities of the client, family, and nursing staff. The Client Rights and Responsibilities, finances, the number of visits, and the approximate time for the visits are discussed. The client and the nurse are both expected to keep their scheduled appointments. The client is taught how to telephone the nurse at the home care agency, his or her physician, an ambulance, or other emergency services so assistance can be provided if problems develop related to his or her health situation.

Based on the plan of care and the extent of their health insurance coverage, the nurse, along with the physician, determines how often the client will need to receive a nursing visit. During or shortly after the first visit, the client and nurse set up a schedule for subsequent visits. Depending on the client's condition, just a few visits might be required, or the client might need ongoing care. The nursing visit

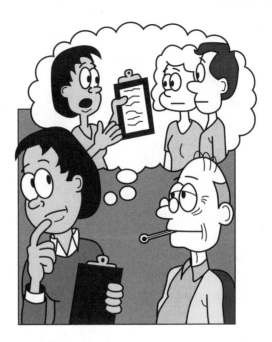

might last only 30 minutes or be around the clock. A "visit" is classified by many agencies as anything lasting less than 2 hours. Anything longer than that is classified as "shift work." The client's case is closed if any of the following occur:

- Client outcomes are met
- The health care team's goals are met
- The client is not showing improvement (this would not be a concern if the client is terminally ill)
- The client no longer wants the care
- The client is unwilling to comply with the care dictated by the nurse or physician
- Financial/insurance coverage is no longer feasible. If the client's finances do not permit continuation of visits, the client, nurse, and physician must develop an alternative plan.

At the end of the visits, the nurse conducts an exit interview, which brings closure to the nurse-client relationship. The nurse might ask that the client fill out an evaluation of the health care provider's performance and mail it back to the home care agency.

What Does It Take to Be a Home Care Nurse?

It takes more than nursing knowledge to be a good home care nurse. Excellent communication skills and confidence in one's own abilities are valued characteristics. Confidence is necessary because the nurse usually works independently out in the field. In the hospital, there are often other health care providers available as resources. By contrast, consultation is accessible in home care, but it must be accomplished in a long-distance fashion. Because of this, home care nurses need

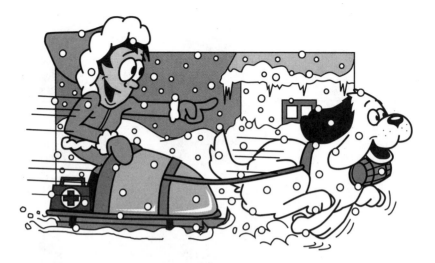

to know the difference between what they know and what they do not know and when to ask for assistance. They also need to know how to obtain the help that is needed.

A home care nurse needs to be able to adapt to varied situations easily. A normal day could include a client visit in an extremely well-to-do home followed by one in a home that is very ill kept. Besides the variety of client situations, the home care nurse also has to contend with the weather. It doesn't matter whether there is a blinding snowstorm or 95° heat, the home care nurse must still visit the client.

Because home care is always conducted at a distance, home care nurses need to be able to describe situations and events over the phone. They also need to be able to communicate accurately without the benefit of seeing the receiver's body language. This can be difficult, especially when talking to a person who has difficulty describing his or her problem accurately. Another problem with telephone communication occurs when speaking to a person who speaks English with an accent. In this situation, environmental cues are lacking that would help to understand what is being said.

Another difference between home care and institutional nursing is the age range of the clients. Although some home care nurses specialize, most see a wide variety of clients, ranging from newborns to the elderly. Most clients, however, are elderly.

Consider This Scenario

This scenario will demonstrate how a nurse provides home care services to a variety of clients.

Meribeth Marek is a home care nurse who works for a home health care agency. At the beginning of her day, she notes that she has six clients to see—a normal day! The first client is an 88-year-old woman who is being evaluated after a serious exacerbation of congestive heart failure. Meribeth parks directly in front of the client's apartment building because it is in a high crime area. She is glad to note that Mrs. Canneli is watching for her through the front window. Although she has never been accosted, Meribeth is always very cautious.

Meribeth does a physical assessment and notes that Mrs. Canneli is much more congested than 2 days ago. Meribeth uses her mobile telephone to call Mrs. Canneli's physician, and she decides to stay with Mrs. Canneli until the physician returns the call. Twenty minutes later, he calls. Meribeth explains the situation and the physician orders an increase in Mrs. Canneli's diuretic medication. Meribeth explains this to Mrs. Canneli. As Meribeth gets ready to leave, she ensures that Mrs. Canneli knows what to do if her breathing gets worse (call Meribeth's home care agency, her physician, or an ambulance). Mrs. Canneli has a home health aide who comes twice a day for personal care. Meribeth also leaves a note telling Mrs. Canneli's home health aide not to give Mrs. Canneli a shower until her breathing gets better. Meribeth tells Mrs. Canneli that she will return tomorrow to assess her breathing and activity levels.

Her next visit is to Mr. Jamison, who is a newly diagnosed diabetic. Although he was supposed to be home for their appointment, he is not. His son tells Meribeth that his dad is at the physician's office. Meribeth makes a note to call Mr. Jamison later to tell him to notify her when he cannot make his appointments.

Her next visit is to Mrs. Peskily, who has a slow-healing venous leg ulcer. Mrs. Peskily needs a dressing change on her leg. Mrs. Peskily's regular home care nurse is on vacation, and Meribeth is providing care during the nurse's absence. Because Meribeth doesn't know where Mrs. Peskily lives, she consults the map provided to her. She is especially grateful that Mrs. Peskily's regular home care nurse took the time to write on the map that Mrs. Peskily has a large dog that must be tied up before the nurse can enter the house. Through the closed door of her home, she tells Meribeth that the dog is tied up and that Meribeth can come in. Meribeth consults the plan of care contained in the traveling chart and the teaching materials that were left in the in-home chart to provide direction for the home care visit. Meribeth does a physical assessment and notes that it is basically unchanged from that noted by her regular nurse. One of Mrs. Peskily's nursing diagnoses is social isolation, and as a nursing intervention, Meribeth spends a few minutes talking to Mrs. Peskily, inquiring how she is managing the care of her leg wound. When she is done with the dressing, Meribeth sits for a while and discusses the weather with Mrs. Peskily, who says, "I'm so glad that you came to see me. Not many people come anymore."

After her visit, Meribeth eats the lunch she brought in a cooler in the car. She brings her lunch because she found that a fast-food lunch adds too many calories to her diet.

After lunch, Meribeth visits a paraplegic man who needs an IV antibiotic. She performs a physical assessment on him and gives the antibiotic. During the IV infusion, she quizzes him on the information she provided yesterday. She is gratified to note that he remembered nearly all of it. This is the shortest visit of the day, as she is there for only about 30 minutes.

The next call is a mother-baby check-up. The local hospital is discharging new mothers 6 hours after a vaginal delivery, and a home care nurse visits them the following day to see how they are doing. This is the part of the job that Meribeth loves the best. She spends a lot of time showing the new mother how to bathe and feed the baby.

Her last visit of the day is to a new diabetic. She helps the woman draw up her insulin and watches as the client injects it. Meribeth offers suggestions on how to improve her technique, saying, "Here, let me show you another way to do that."

After this, she goes back to the office to hand in her paperwork. On a typical day, Meribeth usually spends an hour at the end of the day completing client paperwork. She is on call for the next 16 hours.

Because she is the on-call person for the home care agency, she receives a call from the answering service asking her to call a client, John Tomsik. The phone call to Mr. Tomsik reveals that he is having increased difficulty with breathing. Because of the breathing difficulty and the stroke he had several years ago, he is very difficult to understand over the telephone. With Mr. Tomsik's permission, Meribeth calls his daughter. The daughter tells Meribeth that her father isn't taking his medication properly and agrees to go to his house to check on him.

After a few minutes, Meribeth calls Mr. Tomsik back and asks about the medication. When confronted, he tells Meribeth that he can't remember how to take it. Meribeth asks to speak to his daughter, who tells Meribeth that her father is running a fever of 103° and coughing up large amounts of green sputum. Mr. Tomsik is unable to talk very much because of his extreme shortness of breath. Meribeth suggests that the daughter call for an ambulance or take her father to the emergency department. The daughter agrees to call an ambulance. When this is all completed, Meribeth calls Mr. Tomsik's physician to report on this.

What Is Different About Providing Care in the Home Environment as Compared to the Inpatient Setting?

Probably the most obvious difference is simply the environment. The client is in his or her own setting, as compared with being within the institutional environment. The implications of this environmental change are many.

One of the most important issues is that the nursing staff are guests within the homes of the clients. It is their home, not ours. Therefore, the nurse must act as a guest and respect the client's home even if the nurse comes from a very different background. This isn't always easy, because people have many different types of lifestyles. Many of us believe that our own lifestyle is the preferred one. However, nurses must express acceptance of lifestyles and values different from their own.

When visiting client homes, you will find a variety of differences. Some homes

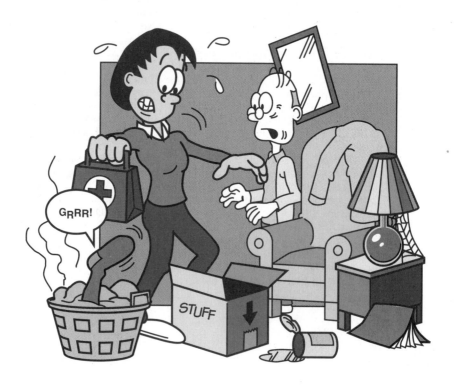

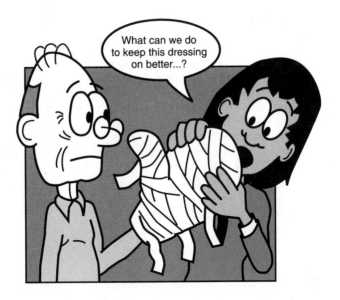

will be very up to date and others might be barely livable. Perhaps the house may be unkempt or dirty, or the size and location of the home may not be what the nurse is used to seeing. No matter what the house looks or smells like, it is the client's home and therefore must be treated respectfully. However, the nurse might need to be very creative in achieving medical asepsis in such situations!

Another issue in home nursing care is related to the sense of who is in control. Although we suggest that clients have an active role in activities regarding their health, in reality the health care staff is in charge of clients while they are in the hospital. There are rules that they expect the clients will follow. For example, most institutions expect clients to wear hospital gowns, although they probably wouldn't choose to do this without that expectation. But when clients are within their own environment, they are on their own turf, and they are the boss.

In the hospital, nurses plan their workload around the activities that need to be done. This type of planning also occurs in home care. The home care nurse has to plan client visits, taking into account the client's physical needs, schedules, preferred visit times, and the client's family needs. Is the client at his or her best in the morning or perhaps after lunch? Is the client an early riser or does the client sleep late? For example, let's look at a client who needs a daily dressing change. The nurse calls the client's house to set a good time to change the dressing. The client might suggest that the nurse come between 1 and 2 P.M. This must fit into the nurse's schedule as opposed to the client altering his or her plans to fit into the nurse's schedule. However, there must be some room for negotiation between the nurse and client.

Another noticeable difference between home care and institutional nursing is that the home care nurse must accomplish much of his or her communication over the telephone. This means that the home care nurse must be able to listen carefully and respond accordingly without the benefit of environmental cues.

In home care, the nurse often resolves many issues via a flurry of phone calls.

For example, a client tells you of a problem. You call his daughter to obtain her insight on this problem and then call the physician. After you receive the call from the physician, you call the client and his daughter. As part of the solution to the client's problem, you might need to call various health care team members, who might not be currently available. If this is the issue, you might need to leave a message or call them at another time. You can see that the telephone is a vital piece of equipment to the nurse! (Safety note: if you are calling a client from your home, use a blocker code, for example ✱67, before dialing the client's telephone number. Otherwise, the client will have your home telephone number if the client has caller ID. It is not wise to let clients have your home telephone number. If they have problems, they need to call the nursing agency, not call you at home.)

Common Communication Methods in Home Care Nursing

Plan of Care

The plan of care (POC) that is developed by the registered nurse, client, and family on the first visit provides the initial direction of the client's care. Subsequent visits may result in modifications and revisions in the POC. The POC also provides direction for other nurses to provide care to the client. Although every attempt is made to have the same nurse visit the same clients, sometimes other nurses make the visits. So you can see how vital it is to keep the POC up to date and accurate! The POC is also used to provide direction for the nurse's aides. The POC will give specific direction as to what they are supposed to do.

Teaching is a major focus of home care. The plan of care spells out what the client needs to be taught and how and when to teach it. After teaching, the nurse assesses the client's retention of information and notes this in the goal assessment area of the plan of care.

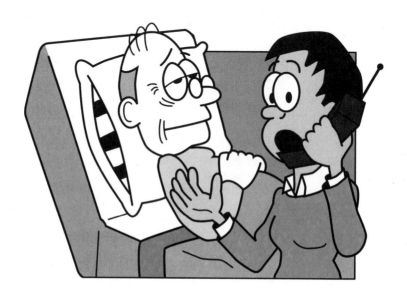

Telephone/Fax

The mobile telephone has changed how communication occurs in home care. Many home care nurses have a cellular phone and beeper. Both are used extensively. Though not all home care nurses have them, many nurses say that they could not do their work without them. Although the nurse could use the stationary telephone at the client's home, having the mobile telephone allows the nurse to leave the client's home before the physician returns the call. The telephone is used to contact other therapists, call physicians, and report back to the home care agency.

If the physician calls you on your cellular phone, take great care to ensure confidentiality. Take the phone to a private place before you converse. If you are talking about another client, do not use names. Even if you think that you are in a private place, it could be possible for others to hear you. Also remember that cellular airways are not considered secure. With the proper equipment, listening in on a cellular conversation is relatively easy, so don't consider it as a method of transmitting confidential information.

In the hospital, client orders are usually written in a very timely fashion. In home care, most client orders are sent through the mail service. Obviously, this can create problems with timeliness. However, if an order needs to be done quickly, the registered nurse can write a verbal order or send a fax transmission. The physician verification of the verbal order is sent by mail or fax. Some health care agencies are issuing portable fax machines to their nurses. This will help to ensure timeliness of physician orders. It can also be used to send lab results back and forth.

Written Messages

Written messages are a common way for home health care personnel to communicate. If you are using this method, determine a location to place all the messages,

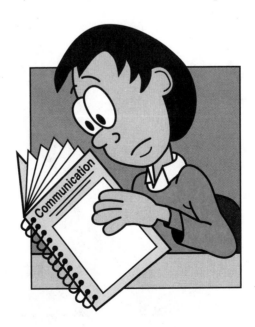

otherwise they might get lost. Consider placing a spiral-bound notebook in a convenient location for messages. Or place the messages within the client's in-home chart.

Information Sheets/Maps

To visit clients, you first have to find their homes. Before the first visit, directions to the client's home are obtained. In some agencies, a map is also developed after the first client visit. A map is a wonderful tool for anybody who has difficulty following verbal or written directions. When drawing a map, provide both main thoroughfares and specific directions. Provide visual cues, such as, "Turn left after the red barn. It is the second house on the right. Tan house, brown roof, lots of flowers in the front."

Many nurses also provide information on the map or direction sheet such as how to get in, whether they have dogs or cats, and whether the animals are friendly and are allowed out. This type of practical data will be helpful when the nurse makes the client visit.

Monthly Case Conferences

Depending on the agency policy, the home care agency schedules weekly or monthly case conferences. Although these conferences are very important, it is very difficult for all the therapists to attend because they are out in the field with clients. Often the therapists write messages or use their mobile phones to call the agency office during the conference time. However, attendance at case conferences is vital because this is a condition for agency participation in the Medicare program. During the case conference, goals are measured, care is discussed, and the care plan is updated as necessary.

Client Care Documentation

One of the more common complaints of any nurse is how much paperwork is required. In home care, the paperwork is even more extensive because of federal

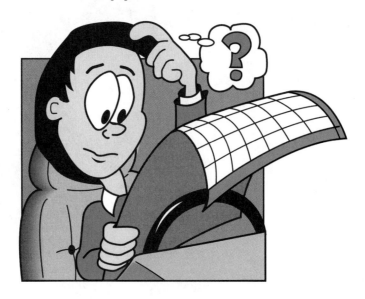

regulations and insurance regulations. Besides the federal and insurance requirements, all agencies have their own documentation methods that must be followed. Regulatory policy also dictates that updates are sent to the referring physician regularly.

Although each home care agency is different, there are similarities in the documentation. For many agencies, the home care client's chart is composed of three sections. The first part is the agency chart, which contains the client orders, nurse's notes, and other ancillary notes.

The next part is called the "traveling chart." This chart contains a summary of the client orders, a medication profile, and teaching records for the client. It also has a map or direction sheet showing how to find the client's home. Be very careful to keep the charts in a secure place in your car. Bring only the traveling chart of the client you are currently visiting into the client's home. Leave the others in the car, and keep the car locked when any records are in it.

The third section of the chart is kept in the client's home. It contains the POC and client education materials. If the client has a home health care aide, the POC would provide direction for his or her actions. The in-home chart also has helpful information that will be useful for the client and his or her family. A major difference between this portion of the chart and an institutional chart is that in the institution, the client and family usually cannot see any portion of the chart until after the hospitalization. In home care, the client and family are *encouraged* to read the portion of the client's chart that is kept in the home.

Because the client and family are encouraged to read the chart, you need to be very cautious about what you write in it. Be extremely careful of using abbreviations, because the family may misinterpret them. For example, the abbreviation "SOB" means "shortness of breath" to health care workers. The family may think it means something else. So you wouldn't use this type of abbreviation.

Calendar

It is not unusual for a client to have a visiting nurse, a home health aide, a home physical therapist, and a home social worker in addition to the previous health care team. Having so many people in the home could easily lead to confusion. To prevent this, make a simple calendar showing who is coming to the home and when they are expected. The key here is coordination of care and planning care so that many people are not in the client's home on the same day and certainly not at the same time!

Communication Difficulties

All the home care nurses interviewed for this chapter agreed on the biggest communication problem in home care. Without question, all related problems inherent to long-distance communication. Walcott-McQuigg and Ervin (1992) reinforced this finding in a study. Instead of talking to a physician or client on a face-to-face basis, much of the communication between the nurse and others has to occur through written notes, fax machine, or telephone calls.

The biggest difficulty when calling a physician is getting through the office staff. This requires a great deal of time spent building positive relationships with the doctor's office staff.

Often telephoning another person involved in the client's case will result in a message left on voice mail or on an answering machine. Although voice mail is useful, it also can result in a phenomenon known as *phone tag*. Phone tag is when successive messages are left on voice mail. This can go back and forth several times before anyone actually talks to another live person. This delay in communication creates problems. You can see that leaving detailed messages on voice mail is vital.

If you find that you often play phone tag with another person, you might suggest that the person call the office and talk to the RN. There is always an RN in the office (at least during business hours). This RN could obtain the information and communicate it to you.

Another communication difficulty related to long-distance communication concerns location. When you have to leave a message to have someone contact you while you are out with clients, where do you want them to call? The client's house, your car phone, your mobile phone, your pager, or the agency office? If you really had this many options, the choice would be simple: have everyone call you on the mobile phone.

However, not everyone has all these electronic conveniences. Student nurses, for example, might not have access to them. If you do not have a mobile phone, car phone, or pager, you will need to figure out an alternate form of communication in the field. Perhaps you could agree to call the agency office from a pay phone every 2 hours. If you are calling a physician from a client's home, you might need to wait until the physician returns the call. (Do tell the office that you are doing this or you might be at the client's house for a long time!)

Specific Environmental Issues

Safety

As a home care nurse, you will be providing care to clients in many geographic areas. No matter how affluent the area, violence against health care workers is a concern for all nurses. Some interventions you can use:

- Plan your visit schedule in advance and have others be aware of your schedule.
- Keep to the schedule.
- Have the clients know your anticipated arrival time. If you will be late, call them.
- Have them watch for you. If you have to make a visit during the night, have them put an outside light on.
- If you have an expensive or frequently stolen type of car, consider borrowing a less obvious car to use for home care visits.
- Wear conservative, nonexpensive clothing. Leave your jewelry and money at home. Just bring enough money to get you through the day. (Do keep your gas tank full!)
- Know where you are going and park in a well-lighted area so that your car remains in full view.
- Walk confidently, but pay attention to others around you. Trust your instincts. If a particular house or group of people appears dangerous to you, do not go near it. Instead, go to a safe place and call the client and your agency to report the problem. (You can see how a car phone would be really useful for a situation like this!)

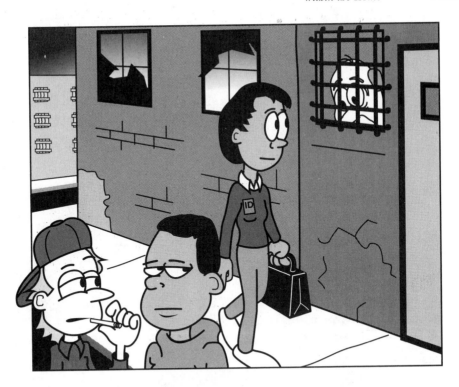

Safety is also an issue for the clients. We all know that we shouldn't allow someone into our house without proper identification. Be sure to wear your appropriate uniform with your identification prominently displayed. Otherwise the client should not let you into his or her home!

Many homebound people leave their doors open when they know that the home care nurse is coming. Even though this is convenient, try to convince them that this is a dangerous practice. Anyone could come through the door! Make sure that you close the door behind you when you leave. Ask if the client wants it locked.

Sensitive Issues

There are many topics that people consider private. For example, many people will not freely discuss their income level or the adequacy of their housing. (Remember, too, that there are people who will volunteer this information without hesitation.) The home care nurse has a broader responsibility and must become business-oriented to some extent and deal with financial and reimbursement issues. Data such as income level, employer, adequacy of housing, and other resources are needed by home care nurses for insurance purposes and to ensure that the client has the resources to obtain needed supplies. You must develop a relationship with the client before you begin to discuss sensitive topics. If possible, ask for this information later in your initial visit or on subsequent visits.

If you need this information, explain why you need it and what you will do with the information. If you will give the information to others, explain who will receive it. Explain what will happen if they do not provide the information. (Often, clients cannot receive services from the home care agency if they do not provide the needed information.)

Accessibility

Because of the very nature of home care, the clients are at a distance from the health care institution. Although being in a familiar environment is helpful to the client, the distance can also create hardships for both the client and nurse.

Depending on the situation, the client may lack close neighbors who could be very helpful to the client. Or the client may have close relationships with neighbors and friends who do not live in close proximity. You will need to teach them to use the telephone as a tool for reaching help. Tell them how to contact you, other health care providers, and emergency aid.

Another issue that relates to distance is the availability of supplies. Remember to call your clients to ensure that they have all needed supplies before you go to see them. Finding specific medical supplies out in the rural areas will be very difficult.

Promoting Communication With Client and Family Members

Assessment

With whom are you communicating? The client, family, or perhaps neighbors? If so, it is often helpful to have them present when you work with the client. This way, you can be a role model and show them how to provide the needed care. (Having the client or family able to assume responsibility for care is one of the most common home health care goals.)

Does the client have animals? Many homebound people have pets for companionship and security. They might consider their dog or cat as a member of the family. Remember the old adage "Love me, love my pet." This is often the case. If so, you will be expected to address the dog or cat in addition to talking to the client and the family. Ask the client for the pet's name and write it down.

What are the client's priorities? Although you are at the client's home to do a dressing change, the client might be so worried about the lack of food in the house that he or she may be unable to concentrate on the instructions for the dressing change. Remember Maslow's hierarchy of needs? If you can't satisfy the more basic needs, the higher level needs will remain unfulfilled. The nurse simply has to work around the client's other priorities.

How do you find out what the client's priorities are? Ask! Just say, "Mr. Frank, what would you like us to do today?" or, "Mr. Frank, what is the most important thing for us to do?"

Clients often have been providing self-care for chronic conditions for a length of time, and they might have novel approaches to their care. It is common for a home care client to say, "I have been taking care of this for years and this is how I do it." Although their suggestions might fall outside the usual practice, consider them anyway. Without actively listening to the client's suggestions, how can you expect the client to listen to your suggestions? Other approaches to this might be: "Tell me how you think this should be," or, "What do you think will work?"

Intervention

Perhaps the most important intervention is a quiet one: simply provide a listening ear. The clients must be homebound to receive Medicare-paid home care services. Because of this, they might lack visitors. Many homebound clients and their families look upon the home care nurse as a cheerful face and a break in the monotony. Many clients report that the home care nurse's visit is the high point of their day.

Although time will not always allow it, if possible, use treatment time to sit and visit with the client, even if it is only for a minute. A lonely client will much appreciate this increased social contact, and many important health care issues will be identified through this type of communication. Remember, also, that you can interact with the client and family while performing care.

Besides spending time with the client, providing emotional support to the caregiver will also be very much appreciated. Although many family members want to provide care for their family member, it is easy for them to feel overwhelmed. Smith, Moushey, Ross, and Gieffer (1993) found that home health care nurses give caregivers a sense of confidence in their own abilities.

Another useful nursing intervention is the inclusion of humor. Although much of health care has a dramatic aspect to it, use of humor can be very beneficial. Try to tune in to those in the environment. Are they making humorous comments? If so, use of humor may be appropriate.

Remember that the goal is to laugh *with* the client and family, not *at* the client and family. Avoid stereotypical jokes or any that are mean-spirited. For more suggestions on the use of humor, see Chapter 2.

Interventions for communicating with pets come easily to some people, yet others are not comfortable around animals. Whatever your comfort level, you will need to be able to do your work in the presence of house pets. Some suggestions:

1. Ask the homeowner if the pet is friendly. (Remember that this does not mean that the pet doesn't bite. It just means that it hasn't bitten anyone yet.)
2. If the client says that it is not friendly, tell the client that it must be locked or tied up before you can come into the home or yard.
3. If the client says that the pet is friendly, approach it slowly. Stand still and let it smell you. Walk slowly into the house.

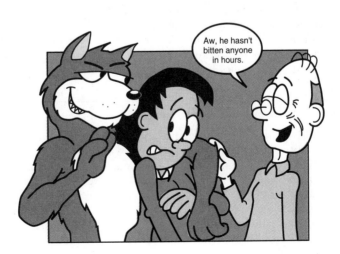

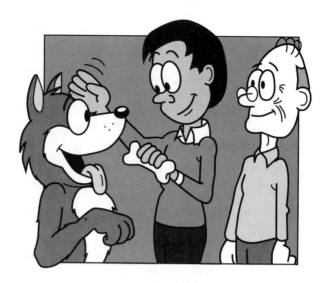

4. Talk calmly to the pet, using its name (if you know it). You could just say, "Hello, Ubby."
5. Ask where the pet lies down. Do not set your things in this area; otherwise the pet may feel that you are in its territory.
6. Before you approach the client, tell both the client and the pet that you are approaching. Many dogs view their job as protection of their owner. If you move toward the owner without warning, it could be perceived by the animal as a threat to its owner. Some animals have to be placed in another area or tied up before they will allow anyone near their owner.
7. Bring small and large dog biscuits and a carton of cat treats in your bag. Ask the pet's owner if you can give one to the pet. If it is acceptable, give the pet a treat. A very astute home care nurse uses this trick and reports that it gives her an instant relationship with the pet owner. (If you start this, you might have to do this every time you visit the client.)

In conclusion, communication in home care has many similarities to communication in any setting. The differences relate to the environment, communication from a distance, and using high technology to talk to others. Although the communication methods may be different, home care is very rewarding. Several studies have shown that the majority of home care nurses are highly satisfied with their work.

PRACTICAL APPLICATIONS

Read the following scenario and consider communication methods to help this family cope with their situation. Answers appear at the end of the chapter.

Frank Biscenni is 86 years young. Because he has been in excellent health, he is able to help provide care for his wife, Muriel, after her stroke. However, recently Mr. Biscenni has been having difficulty with his vision, which his physician diagnosed as resulting from a small stroke. The stroke left him with some speech difficulty and weakness on his left side. It was decided that a home care nurse would visit Mr. Biscenni three times a week to assess his neurological status.

Mr. Biscenni was quite amenable to this plan because he was familiar with the home care nurses who provided care for Muriel. However, because of a scheduling mix-up, a different nurse was assigned to Mr. Biscenni than was assigned to visit Muriel. When she came to visit Mr. Biscenni, she discovered that his speech therapist was working with him, and the physical therapist was in the driveway, waiting for the speech therapist to finish.

Even so, Mr. Biscenni's nurse talked to him. "I'm so sorry I'm late. I couldn't find your house. Did you know that your street sign is missing? I'm going to have to come back in about 2 hours. That way, the physical therapist and speech therapist will be done with you."

"I'm so tired," Mr. Biscenni said, "do you have to come back?"

The speech therapist told the home care nurse that she was the sixth home health care provider to visit the Biscenni household, and it wasn't even 11 A.M. yet! Mr. Biscenni's morning activities of daily living (ADL) aide, Mrs. Biscenni's morning ADL aide, Mrs. Biscenni's speech therapist, Mrs. Biscenni's physical therapy aide, and the social worker had already been there. No wonder Mr. and Mrs. Biscenni were tired!

What communication strategies could be used to help the Biscenni family cope?

REFERENCES

Bernal, H. (1993). A model for delivering culture-relevant care in the community. *Public Health Nursing, 10*(4), 228–232.

Brown, P. (1991). The burden of caring for a husband with Alzheimer's disease. *Home Healthcare Nurse, 9*(3), 33–40.

Cale-Lawrence, J., Peploski, J., & Russell, J. (1995). Training needs of home healthcare nurses. *Home Healthcare Nurse, 13*(2), 53–61.

Carr, P. (1991). A whole different world. *Home Healthcare Nurse, 9*(4), 28–31.

Carter, S., Carroll, M., & Hayes, E. (1994). Environmental safety preparation for community based nursing educational experiences: Measurable indices. *Public Health Nursing, 11*(5), 300–304.

Ceslowitz, S., & Loreti, S. (1991). Easing the transition from hospital nursing to home care: A research study. *Home Healthcare Nurse, 9*(4), 32–39.

dela Cruz, F. (1994). Clinical decision making styles of home healthcare nurses. *Image: Journal of Nursing Scholarship, 26*(3), 222–226.

Horner, S., Amrogne, J., Coleman, M., Hanson, C., Hodnicki, D., Lopez, S., & Talmadge, M. (1994).

Traveling for care: Factors influencing health access for rural dwellers. *Public Health Nursing, 11*(3), 145–149.

Humphrey, C., (1988). The home as a setting for care. Clarifying the boundaries of practice. *Nursing Clinics of North America, 23*(2), 305–339.

Pasquali, E. (1991). Humor: Preventative therapy for family care givers. *Home Healthcare Nurse, 9*(3), 13–16.

Shuster, G. (1992). Job satisfaction among home health care nurses. What they report and what it means. *Home Healthcare Nurse, 10*(4), 33–38.

Smith, C.E., Moushey, L., Ross, J.A., & Gieffer, C. (1993). Responsibilities and reactions of family care givers of patents dependent on total parenteral nutrition at home. *Public Health Nursing, 10*(2), 122–128.

Wagnild, G., & Grupp, K. (1991). Major stressors among elderly home care clients. *Home Healthcare Nurse, 9*(4), 17–21.

Walcott-McQuigg, J., & Ervin, N. (1992). Stressors in the workplace: Community health nurses. *Public Health Nursing, 9*(1), 65–71.

ANSWERS TO THE SMALL GROUP ACTIVITY

What communication strategies can be used to help the Biscenni family cope?

It would be important for someone to assume the job of coordinator of their care. Some factors that need to be coordinated:

- It would be much easier for everyone if the same aide, speech therapist, and physical therapy aide were assigned to provide care for both clients. This would reduce the number of people entering the Biscenni home.

- A calendar needs to be developed so that every health care provider doesn't come at the same time. Because their physical therapy is performed on a three-times-a-week basis, and the speech therapy is twice weekly, it can be arranged so that one therapist comes on Monday-Wednesday-Friday and the other comes on Tuesday-Thursday.
- Because the Biscennis' street sign is missing, a map needs to be drawn that provides visual cues for the nurse. It also needs to note that they own a large dog that shouldn't be let outside (not mentioned in the scenario).

Index

Page numbers in *italics* denote illustrations; page numbers followed by t refer to tables.